T0319535

"This book is packed with clinical wisdom, scholarship, case studies, and detailed neurodevelopment correlates of relational trauma that illustrate the effective use of Chapman's Art Therapy Treatment Intervention. The author makes an irrefutable case for art therapy's place in the treatment of PTSD, acute and chronic trauma, and abuse in infants, children, and adolescents. A must-read and an inspiring contribution."

—George Halasz, MD, Adjunct Senior Lecturer, School of Psychology and Psychiatry, Monash University, Melbourne, Australia

"In this well-researched book, Linda Chapman articulates a neurobiological understanding of trauma and a theoretically grounded model for the treatment of children and adolescents. Chapman uses moving case examples to illustrate how art can bypass left-brain activity and utilize regions of the brain where traumatic memories are stored. She describes how brain processing affects therapy at different stages, providing depth and clarity. Her style of working is informed, intuitive, theoretically grounded, and relational. This book is a long-awaited contribution to the field."

—Gussie Klorer, PhD, ATR-BC, HLM, LCPC, LCSW, Professor Art Therapy Counseling Program, Southern Illinois University Edwardsville; author of *Expressive Therapy with Troubled Children*

Neurobiologically Informed Trauma Therapy With Children and Adolescents

The Norton Series on Interpersonal Neurobiology
Allan N. Schore, PhD, Series Editor
Daniel J. Siegel, MD, Founding Editor

The field of mental health is in a tremendously exciting period of growth and conceptual reorganization. Independent findings from a variety of scientific endeavors are converging in an interdisciplinary view of the mind and mental well-being. An interpersonal neurobiology of human development enables us to understand that the structure and function of the mind and brain are shaped by experiences, especially those involving emotional relationships.

The Norton Series on Interpersonal Neurobiology provides cutting-edge, multidisciplinary views that further our understanding of the complex neurobiology of the human mind. By drawing on a wide range of traditionally independent fields of research—such as neurobiology, genetics, memory, attachment, complex systems, anthropology, and evolutionary psychology—these texts will offer mental health professionals a review and synthesis of scientific findings often inaccessible to clinicians. The books advance our understanding of human experience by finding the unity of knowledge, or consilience, that emerges with the translation of findings from numerous domains of study into a common language and conceptual framework. The series integrates the best of modern science with the healing art of psychotherapy.

A NORTON PROFESSIONAL BOOK

NEUROBIOLOGICALLY INFORMED TRAUMA THERAPY WITH CHILDREN AND ADOLESCENTS

Understanding Mechanisms of Change

LINDA CHAPMAN

Foreword by Allan N. Schore

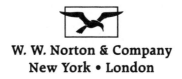

W. W. Norton & Company
New York • London

Note to Readers: Standards of clinical practice and protocol change over time, and no technique or recommendation is guaranteed to be safe or effective in all circumstances. This volume is intended as a general information resource for professionals practicing in the field of psychotherapy and mental health; it is not a substitute for appropriate training, peer review, and/or clinical supervision. Neither the publisher nor the author(s) can guarantee the complete accuracy, efficacy, or appropriateness of any particular recommendation in every respect.

Copyright © 2014 by Linda Chapman

All rights reserved
Printed in the United States of America
First Edition

For information about permission to reproduce selections from this book, write to Permissions, W. W. Norton & Company, Inc., 500 Fifth Avenue, New York, NY 10110

For information about special discounts for bulk purchases, please contact W. W. Norton Special Sales at specialsales@wwnorton.com or 800-233-4830

Manufacturing by LSC Communications Harrisonburg
Production manager: Leeann Graham

Library of Congress Cataloging-in-Publication Data
Chapman, Linda, 1951–
Neurobiologically informed trauma therapy with children
and adolescents : understanding mechanisms of change / Linda Chapman ;
foreword by Allan N. Schore. — First edition.
pages cm — (Norton series on interpersonal neurobiology)
"A Norton Professional Book."
Includes bibliographical references and index.
ISBN 978-0-393-70788-5 (hardcover)
1. Psychic trauma in children—Treatment.
2. Psychic trauma in adolescence—Treatment.
3. Biological psychiatry. 4. Neurobiology. I. Title.
RJ506.P66C43 2014
618.92'89—dc23
2013039706

ISBN: 978-0-393-70788-5

W. W. Norton & Company, Inc., 500 Fifth Avenue, New York, N.Y. 10110
www.wwnorton.com
W. W. Norton & Company Ltd., 15 Carlisle Street, London W1D 3BS

2 3 4 5 6 7 8 9 0

The best discovery the discoverer makes for himself.

Ralph Waldo Emerson

Contents

Acknowledgments

It is an honor to be invited into the lives of children, teens, and families during a time of crisis and stress. I thank all of those who have taught me how individuals experience, perceive, express, and heal from trauma in their lives. A special thanks to the children and families who allowed me to publish their art in this book. Although names are not evident, it is an act of courage, and I am deeply grateful to be able to include the images created in their therapy sessions.

A sincere thank-you is offered to Deborah Malmud, vice president and director of Norton Professional Books and a kind, patient, and talented editor. Her vision for the project and knowledge of the material were instrumental in guiding me with the book.

A heartfelt thank-you is extended to California author and FEMA disaster worker Marcia Sanderson. As my writing coach and first reader, Marcia helped in ways too numerous to mention. In addition to helping with details, Marcia's gifts as a writer and visionary thinker were so very helpful with organizing and completing the manuscript. As a dear and honest friend, Marcia helped keep the focus of my writing, offered abundant support, and helped make the book a better volume with her contributions.

There are so many physicians and mental health professionals who have been instrumental in my clinical training. I am unable to mention every one of them; however, collectively I would like to thank all of my colleagues at the Department of Child Psychiatry, UC San Francisco, and in particular I offer a special thank-you to Lois Herman Friedlander, MFT; Graeme Hanson, MD; and the late Delmont Morrison, PhD.

I greatly appreciate and thank all my colleagues at San Francisco General Hospital who taught me so much about trauma, medicine, and the human condition. In particular, I thank Moses Grossman, MD, Chief of Pediatrics Emeritus, who devoted his life's work to the care and protection of children and families. His recognition of the need for psychological services in pediatric medicine was ahead of its time, and I am honored to have known and learned from Dr. Grossman. I want to thank M. Margaret Knudson, MD, Chief of Pediatric

Surgery at SFGH, for taking me under her guidance with outcome research, along with Herbert Schreier, MD. I thank neurologist Donna Ferriero, MD; pediatrician Kevin Coulter, MD; and supervisors Catherine Kennedy, MD, and Margarita Woodbury, MD. I greatly appreciate the contribution to my learning from social workers Mark Brand, LCSW, and Rose Yee, LCSW. Additionally, I thank the nurses and specialty staff for their important contributions to my knowledge of pediatric medicine and pediatric trauma.

Although it would be impossible to name all those who have contributed to my knowledge of neurobiology and trauma, I thank Allan Schore, PhD; Daniel Siegel, MD; Robert Pynoos, MD; Michael DeBellis, MD; Hans Steiner, MD; and Lenore Terr, MD.

I would like to thank Director Kim Dunster and the Volunteers to San Francisco General Hospital for ongoing financial support.

Thank you to Brad Kammer, MFT, for his affinity for collaboration and sharing his knowledge and skill.

I thank the art therapy community, my students and supervisees, and, in particular, my friend and art therapist colleague Bob Schoenholtz, MS, ATR. I also want to thank Redwood Children's Services in my community, and my colleagues at Arrowhead Ranch.

To those who helped with reviewing chapters of this manuscript, I want to thank San Francisco occupational therapist Sheila Stosick; neuropsychologist Matthew Bowen, PhD; Margaret Rossoff, MFT; and my sister, Marilyn Miller.

Thank you to my immediate and extended family for their support and encouragement, especially my mother Doris Chapman. Last and most important, thank you to my husband, Robert Gates, for his unending support and encouragement.

Foreword

ALLAN N. SCHORE

This groundbreaking book documents the evolution over the last three decades of Linda Chapman's important clinical contributions on the use of art therapy in the treatment of acute and chronic relational trauma in toddlers, children, and adolescents. The structural organization of the volume mirrors the progression from her early work on the Chapman Art Therapy Treatment Intervention (CATTI), a highly effective short-term intervention for acute trauma in hospitalized children, to her more recent creation of a Neurodevelopmental Art Therapy (NDAT), a long-term intervention for the treatment of childhood disorders associated with the enduring negative impact of early yet chronic relational trauma on brain development. Throughout the upcoming chapters Chapman offers a coherent, creative, and ultimately compelling clinical model of child psychotherapy. This integrative model is solidly anchored not only in classical principles of art therapy and child psychotherapy, but also in recent developmental models of modern attachment theory and early relational trauma, ongoing relational trends in psychotherapy, updated neuropsychoanalytic studies of the human unconscious, and, at the core, interpersonal neurobiological studies of right brain affect regulation. As complex as it is, this research-based child intervention comes alive in a very large number of clinical case studies.

The opening chapters offer a valuable overview of child and adolescent PTSD research. Too often models of PTSD in younger clinical populations are based on the effects of trauma on adults, overlooking the important differences in the subjective experience of overwhelming stress in toddlers, children, and adolescents. It is not uncommon for child clinicians to mistakenly frame their interventions as if they were treating the brain of a miniature adult with the cognitive, verbal, and reflective capacities of an adult mind. But here Chapman focuses both on expanding the developing mind's nonverbal capacities for coping with the interpersonal stressors of childhood and on enhancing the neuroplastic maturational processes that are highly active in the still developing brain. Throughout the book, she differentiates the untoward effects of acute and chronic relational trauma on the child's brain/mind/body, moving from "single-hit" to relational trauma treatments.

Beginning in the very first section of the book Chapman integrates relevant theoretical and research data on trauma with astute observations of the overt and more importantly subtle manifestations of trauma in child psychotherapy cases. Toward that end, she provides the reader with numerous (and I would say fascinating) in-depth portraits of both the individual and the universal clinical manifestations of trauma-induced emotional disturbance in childhood, as well as the unique defensive strategies and coping capacities that are available in the very early stages of human development. Using an interdisciplinary perspective she elaborates upon a neurobiologically informed theoretical model of the change mechanisms of art therapy. As an added bonus the early chapters also provide the reader with a clinically relevant "glossary of terms" that inform her intervention, a significant contribution that can be used in any child clinical model.

One of the many unique contributions of this creative volume is its expansion and transformation of art psychotherapy, long known to be an effective intervention for all forms of childhood disorders. Art therapy is theoretically centered in the affect-laden properties of the visual image, an important potential access point into the child's inner world. It should be noted that although all psychotherapies work with internal imagery, an emergent property of the right brain, that imagery can be imprinted by any sensory modality, and by a variety of psychobiological, motivational self states. A fundamental tenet of this volume is that the "concrete image on the paper allows the child to objectify the images, creating distance and allowing her to speak about an external event, rather than an internal one. This objectification of the image eliminates the flooding of disturbing images and sensations" (p. 28). This therapeutic mechanism highlights the unique role of nonverbal psychodynamics in working with traumatized children. It also underlies the clinical principle that effective work with a traumatized child can only take place in a therapeutic alliance that provides a conscious and, indeed, unconscious sense of interpersonal and intrapsychic safety and trust.

Building on the work of major past theoreticians of art psychotherapy, Chapman proposes a four-level hierarchical treatment intervention. Expanding earlier forms of art therapy that were available before "the emotional revolution" and the creation of modern trauma theory, Chapman incorporates information from contemporary neuroscience to model how the processing of bodily-based emotional images in the child's consciousness within a psychobiologically attuned relational context represents a powerful therapeutic mechanism. Indeed she argues that this emergent growth-facilitating relational mechanism activates more complex processing of sensory affective processes from the lower to the higher levels of the child's developing right brain.

As mentioned, the structural organization of the book reflects the progression in Chapman's work from the short-term treatment of acute trauma to the more complex long-term treatment of chronic relational trauma. Over the course of the opening chapters she elaborates a basic four-stage interpersonal neurobiological model. In the early stages of the treatment the focus is on early-forming kinesthetic/sensory activities (bilateral scribbling) that stimulate the lower brain stem structures of the right brain. These visual representations of internal sensations are achieved nonverbally through the body via rhythm and movement. Following this, the brain shifts information processing to the affect/perceptual level—the limbic system—whereby emotions are expressed, released, and subjectively experienced in response to the art media. This subsequently activates cognitive/symbolic information processing at the cerebral cortical level. Lastly the patient's maturational processes allow for the higher prefrontal levels of not only creativity and integration, but also joy and surprise.

This model fits well with my work in regulation theory on the hierarchical processing of bodily-based affective states within the right-lateralized limbic system (Schore, 2003a, 2003b, 2012). A strong argument can be made that this progression occurs not just in art therapy, but also in any child intervention that attempts to deeply enter into and join with the child's bodily-based subjectivity in order to facilitate the progression of developmental processes, including more complex right brain maturation. Thus, Chapman's model rests upon and reflects the known interpersonal neurobiology of the developing social-emotional right brain that stores and is shaped by attachment experiences, including traumatic attachment experiences.

Over the last three decades Chapman's significant leap forward from the treatment of acute to chronic trauma represented a significant advance as she focused increasingly on child cases with a history of relational attachment trauma, an area of intense clinical interest. As the reader will soon note, the NDAT model presented in Chapter 3 now evolves into four stages of treatment: the Self Phase involving brain stem reflexive kinesthetic/sensory visual information processing mechanisms, the creation of safety, and the improvement in engagement; the Problem Phase involving limbic, affect/perceptual emotional processing and the creation of emotional homeostasis; the Transformation Phase associated with higher cerebral abstract cognitive symbolic processing; and ultimately the last phase of treatment, Integration, activating prefrontal abstract creative/integration, and thereby visual information processing associated with improved affect tolerance and new methods for emotional coping. Again, psychotherapeutic changes in the child's affect, cognition, and behavior reflect changes in brain function.

In the later chapters, Chapman describes even more extensively the clinical terrain of each stage of treatment. She again offers numerous clinical examples that create emotionally evocative images in the reader of the right brain-to-right brain bodily-based affective communications within the co-constructed intersubjective field between child patient and therapist. These stage-specific case notes (as well as numerous visual images actually created by child patients) bring alive the theoretical model, reflecting the fine-grain moment-to-moment clinical observations of an expert child psychotherapist gleaned from hundreds of cases of toddler, child, and adolescent psychotherapy.

As in her earlier work on acute trauma work the NDAT model for the treatment of relational trauma is grounded in current neuroscience. In every case Chapman describes the rapid-acting spontaneous right brain dynamics that are transacted within the therapeutic alliance. In my own work I have suggested that the emotional right brain is dominant in all forms of psychotherapy, but this is especially so in child psychotherapy that is centered in the creation and perception of right lateralized visual-emotional self-images. In his masterful volume on brain laterality, *The Master and His Emissary*, the neuropsychiatrist Iain McGilchrist provides an overview of a large body of neurobiological studies which demonstrate that "the link between the right hemisphere and holistic or *Gestalt* perception is one of the most reliable and durable of the generalizations about hemispheric differences. . . . Its holistic processing of visual form is not based on summation of parts" (2009, p. 46). These studies document the visuospatial abilities of the right hemisphere (Young & Ratcliff, 1983), and the differences in right hemispheric global versus left hemispheric local visual information processing (e.g., Evert & Kmen, 2003; Lux et al., 2004; Yoshida et al., 2007).

With direct relevance to the use of art therapy in children McGilchrist observes that "a child comes to understand the world, to learn about it, by seeing the shapes—both literally, the visuospatial shapes, and metaphorically, the structures—that stand forward in its experience, using a form of *Gestalt* perception, rather than by applying rules" (2009, p. 171). It is now established that the child's essential early learning about the social world involves her early developing right brain, which is used to rapidly and holistically recognize and distinguish faces as well as places on an unconscious level. According to McGilchrist, "It is precisely its capacity for holistic processing that enables the right hemisphere to recognize individuals. Individuals are, after all, Gestalt wholes: that face, that voice, that gait, that sheer 'quiddity' of the person or thing, defying analysis into parts" (2009, p. 51).

The intense arousal alterations of relational trauma dysregulate the complex cortical functions of the infant's, child's, and adolescent's right brain (Schore, 2003b, 2009), and shatter its ability to holistically process and integrate intensely negative and thereby traumatic emotional images, breaking them into affectively charged part images. This reflects the well-established principle that intense negative emotion interferes with perceptual processes, of all sensory modalities. Chapman delineates specific deficits in not only visual but also tactile, gross motor, fine motor, auditory, vestibular, and proprioceptive development—valuable information for any child psychotherapist.

There is currently an intense interest in the mechanisms of therapeutic action that enhance the neuroplasticity of right brain limbic structures. Chapman notes that the NDAT model can revisit earlier critical periods of right brain development in order to repair early sensory motor delays and attachment deficits. She specifically underscores the importance of not only interactively regulating the patient's traumatic arousal, but also providing an opportunity for the child to experience sensory motor experiences that were lacking in early development. In this manner the therapeutic alliance can promote a right-lateralized core mind/ body attachment system that was not fully developed in the early relationship with the primary caregiver. Thus, Chapman's focus on the affective power of images in her treatment does more than reduce trauma symptomatology; it also allows for an expansion of previously blocked right brain social-emotional development.

The evolution of Chapman's model into a psychodynamic, attachment-focused treatment of early-forming self pathologies is charted in Chapter 5. Her use of "left eye to left eye communication" that re-creates the physical sense of "being with" the other and serves as "a pathway to an intersubjective space" echoes the focus on intersubjectivity in current psychodynamic treatment models of right brain relational trauma in adults. This commonality is also seen in her description of art therapy's ability to activate limbic structures that express emotional fragments of the self in concrete imagistic form, and that nonverbally and unconsciously communicate dissociated affect (Schore, 2012). As in adults, Chapman writes, "Staying in the right hemisphere long enough for the affect to arise and be tolerated can be done safely with images. The image is a reflection of the self" (p. 113). In this relational process the role of the therapist is to facilitate dialogue that engages the child to then reflect upon and discover the meaning of the symbolic content of the image. Echoing the current relational trend in psychoanalysis and psychotherapy, Chapman observes, "The symbolic and metaphorical content of the image is not found; it is revealed through the interactive process between client, therapist, and image " (p. 114).

In every chapter Chapman offers the reader updated clinically relevant information about attachment and relational trauma side-by-side with numerous case notes in order to more deeply explicate the deeper nonconscious mechanisms of change of her art therapy interventions. In case after case she documents in exquisite detail her sensitive right brain-to-right brain moment-to-moment attunement to the traumatized child's states of mind/brain/body. These careful observations of psychobiological process, more so than any theoretical orientation or verbal content analysis, give us important glimpses into how acute and chronic trauma alter the child's subjective states, and thereby the child's inner world. Numerous clinical vignettes clearly demonstrate the important differences between the impact of trauma on the developing mind and the adult mind, and why art psychotherapy is particularly effective with traumatized children.

The book culminates in three chapters with the effective long-term treatment of a toddler, and then a child, and finally an adolescent. In the first of these .Chapman gives an in-depth description of neurobiologically informed trauma therapy with a three-and-a-half–year-old. The child's early history includes severe relational trauma (abuse and neglect) by substance-abusing parents. In the very first session, the onset of what she calls the Self Stage of treatment, Chapman accesses an empathic "passive observational stance" in order to co-create a relational context that optimizes the expression of affective attachment communications. This relational context also allows for the co-creation of the therapeutic alliance that provides interactive regulation of the child's "physical homeostasis and comfort." Chapman observes,

> I always deferred to her state of physical homeostasis rather than attempt to engage her in play. . . . Any pressure, no matter how subtle, for her to talk or take a preferred course of action would be picked up by her right amygdala that was tracking below the surface. (p. 135)

In her discussions of "dissociation as unconscious communication," Chapman contends that art allows "access to the dissociated affect with subsymbolic, nonverbal information processing from the subcortical right amygdala" (p. 112). Indeed, throughout the following chapters she repeatedly refers to the critical role of the right amygdala in both the child and the clinician in the treatment, as well as the effectiveness of art therapy in tapping into the child's right-lateralized unconscious, the storehouse of early relational trauma.

As the reader may soon deduce, Chapman has worked very closely with me for some time now, and cites a good deal of my studies on the interpersonal neurobiology of attachment, relational trauma, and regulation theory—a model of the development, psychopathogenesis, and treatment of the implicit self. Let me take this opportunity to briefly describe my more recent work in these areas. Over the past two decades I have presented a large body of interdisciplinary data indicating that the right brain is the locus of unconscious functions (Schore, 1994, 2002, 2011, 2012). This conception is echoed in recent neuroscientific writings by Tucker and Moller: "The right hemisphere's specialization for emotional communication through nonverbal channels seems to suggest a domain of the mind that is close to the motivationally charged psychoanalytic unconscious" (2007, p. 91).

In 2003 I offered a neuropsychoanalytic update of Freud's topographic (1900) model of stratified conscious, preconscious, and unconscious systems. More recently I have expanded this conception, suggesting that the right lateralized implicit (unconscious) self represents a nested system, with an outer later-developing orbitofrontal-limbic regulated core, an inner earlier developing cingulate-limbic regulating core, and an earliest evolving amygdala-limbic regulated core that lies deepest within, like nested Russian dolls (Schore, 2013). These three levels of organization of the right brain represent three levels of the system unconscious: the preconscious, the unconscious, and the deep unconscious. The unconscious systems of the hierarchical three-tiered cortical-subcortical limbic core thus reflect the early developmental history of the self.

In this ongoing work I continue to apply the perspective of developmental neuropsychoanalysis, the study of the development of the unconscious mind, to clinical models of the treatment of infants, children, adolescents, and adults (Schore, 1994, 2003a, 2011, 2012). This integration of developmental psycho-analysis and developmental neuroscience explores the experience-dependent maturation of unconscious right brain-to-right brain intersubjective, implicit affect-regulating mechanisms, offering a psychoneurobiological model of the development of the right brain, the "biological substrate of the human UCS." Although in my early work I described cortical-subcortical limbic circuits, more recently I have increasingly focused on the early development of the subcortical areas of the right brain. This perspective shifts from higher preconscious and unconscious systems to the core of the "deep unconscious" and the unique essential functions of the right amygdala. The brain matures in a caudal to rostral direction, with subcortical areas maturing before cortical areas. Similarly the core of the unconscious develops before the higher levels. The early critical period of right amygdalar reciprocal connectivity with brainstem arousal and hypothalamic neuroendocrine systems parallels the relationally induced primor-dial organization of the "deep unconscious."

Indeed, neuroscience now demonstrates that throughout all later stages of development "the right amygdala may subserve a high-speed detection role for unconscious stimuli" (Costafreda et al., 2008, p. 66), and for processing "uncon-scious emotional learning" (Morris, Ohman, & Dolan, 1998). This includes the unconscious processes encoded in internal working models of attachment, a central focus of psychotherapy (Schore, 1994). Indeed current neurobiological research shows that human attachment security is mediated by the early matur-ing amygdala (Lemche et al., 2006). Other studies document that the right amygdala, a limbic structure located in the right temporal pole, is centrally involved in emotional autobiographical memory (Calabrese et al., 1996), and in the storage of perception-emotion linkage and the reactivation of relevant per-sonal information when emotion is aroused (Olson et al., 2007). Interestingly, right (and not left) amygdala activation occurs during the processing and identi-fication of ambiguous, emotionally laden visual images in the Rorschach inkblot test, an instrument that assesses the mechanism whereby intense unconscious emotion interferes with perceptual processes as well as the individual's capacity to integrate fragmental visual features into a whole elaborated response (Asari et al., 2010). Chapman's work taps directly into this right lateralized unconscious subcortical system.

The essential adaptive functions of the amygdala, now described by neurosci-ence, are relevant to all clinical models, including Chapman's:

> Traditionally, the amygdala has gotten a lot of "bad" press. Popular wisdom has portrayed the human amygdala as the center of an ancient animal id that drives us to rapid impulsive action before our more reasoned judgments can kick in. For a long time, it was considered to be a fear center or threat detector that is instrumen-

tal in allocating processing resources to potentially harmful events . . . . More recent studies in humans suggest that it is responsive to positive and arousing rather than to strictly negative events, as well as to ambiguous events . . . . The connectivity of the amygdala places it at the center of the brain, a physical hub linking numerous distant regions, and it is positioned to allow emotions to influence how the rest of the brain works, from the first stages of stimulus encoding to regulating social behavior. (Todd & Anderson, 2009, p. 1217)

Mirroring the current relational, intersubjective trend in psychodynamic models, these authors further describe "the amygdala's role in regulating interpersonal distance. People automatically regulate the distance between themselves and others on the basis of feelings of personal comfort" and refer to "invisible social force fields that regulate close physical proximity, suggesting that the amygdala is crucial for the sense of interpersonal space . . . [and that] the amygdala should be more active at close interpersonal distances" (Todd & Anderson, 2009, p. 1217). These data fit well with my model of right brain-to-right brain unconscious communication and regulation across a co-created intersubjective field (Schore, 2012). They also support Chapman's assertion that "[t]herapy with young children is a moment-to-moment, intimate corrective experience that takes place in an intersubjective space where . . . both are active participants" (p. 146).

Neuroscientists are now characterizing the amygdala as "a hub of a network" that "via its multitudinous connections with cortical and subcortical areas forges the integration of emotion, perception, cognition and behavior and might contribute to a sense of unitary self" (Markowitsch and Staniloiu, 2011, p. 728). With direct implications for treatments of all early-forming relational trauma, Vrticka and colleagues conclude that the amygdala encodes patterns of both negative and positive social images, and that "this encoding pattern is not influenced by cognitive or behavioral emotion regulation mechanisms, and displays a hemispheric lateralization with more pronounced effects on the right side" (2013). This clearly implies that neither child cognitive-behavioral techniques nor mentalization can directly impact or alter the deep core of the human unconscious.

On the other hand, relationally driven changes in the right brain unconscious are a central focus of Chapman's neurobiologically informed art therapy, wherein "the organism unconsciously responds to the experiences that promote the developmental trajectory" (p. 155). Concordant with my own work on the right orbitofrontal regulation of right amygdala emotional states, Chapman notes, "Once the affect is validated, welcomed, and felt as shared experience, information processing moves to the higher structures and cognition" (p. 146), thereby acting as "an effective tool to facilitate the maturation of the underdeveloped right hemisphere of the brain" (p. 179).

In the upcoming chapters the reader will encounter numerous descriptions of childhood trauma, dissociative defenses, and rupture and repair. In this age of cultural over-emphasis on child psychopharmacology and devaluation of child psychotherapy, it is refreshing to read the clinical insights of an expert child psychotherapist working with difficult clinical cases. A gifted, creative, and intuitive psychotherapist, Chapman describes the subjective and intersubjective forces that are activated in working with childhood trauma, both in her patients and in herself. In numerous clinical vignettes and extended case histories she describes her rich clinical experiences of translating an interpersonal neurobiological theoretical model into an effective and pragmatic treatment intervention for childhood trauma. The reader will enter into the minds of both the patient and therapist as they jointly encounter the child's traumatized subjectivity and dissociative defenses against overwhelming affect. Perhaps most revealing of her relational transformation of art therapy, Chapman's skillful negotiation of rupture and repair in reenactments of affect-dysregulating relational trauma offers deep insight into how this master child clinician's skill co-creates an interpersonal context that promotes emotional growth and indeed more complex maturation of the emotional right brain.

Readers with an art therapy or more general psychotherapeutic practice are in for a fascinating intellectual and emotional journey into a highly effective treatment model for traumatized infants, children, and adolescents. In fact, I would argue that Chapman's clinical model, which sits atop an interpersonal neurobiological research foundation, describes the mechanism of action of all forms of child psychotherapy that attempt to facilitate right brain growth and development, and thereby emotional well-being.

REFERENCES

Asari, T., Konishi, S., Jimura, K., Chikazoe, J., Nakamura, N., & Miyashita, Y. Amygdalar modulation of frontotemporal connectivity during the inkblot test. *Psychiatry Research*, *182*, 103–110.

Costafreda, S. G., Brammer, M. J., David, A. S., & Fu, C. H. Y. (2008). Predictors of amygdala activation during the processing of emotional stimuli: A meta-analysis of 385 PET and fMRI studies. *Brain Research Reviews*, *58*, 57–70.

Evert, D. L., & Kmen, M. (2003). Hemispheric asymmetries for global and local processing as a function of stimulus exposure duration. *Brain and Cognition*, *51*, 115–142.

Lemche, E., Giampietro, V. P., Surguladze, S. A., Amaro, E. J., Andrew, C. M., Williams, S. C. R.,...& Phillips, M. L. (2006). Human attachment security is mediated by the amygdala: Evidence from combined fMRI and psychophysiological measures. *Human Brain Mapping*, *27*, 623–635.

Lux, S., Marshall, J.C., Ritz, A. Weiss. P. H., Pietrzyk, U., Shah, N. J.,...& Fink, G. R. A. (2004). Functional magnetic imaging study of local/global processing with stimulus presentation in the peripheral visual hemifields. *Neuroscience*, *124*, 113–120.

Markowitsch, H. J., & Stanilou, A. (2011). Amygdala in action: Relaying biological and social significance to autobiographical memory. *Neuropsychologia*, *49*, 718–733.

McGilchrist, I. (2009). *The master and his emissary: The divided brain and the making of the western world*. New Haven, CT: Yale University Press.

Morris, J. S., Ohman, A., & Dolan, R. J. (1998). Conscious and unconscious emotional learning in the human amygdala. *Nature, 393,* 467–470.

Schore, A. N. (1994). *Affect regulation and the origin of the self.* Mahwah, NJ: Erlbaum.

Schore, A. N. (2002). The right brain as the neurobiological substratum of Freud's dynamic unconscious. In D. Scharff (Ed.), *The psychoanalytic century: Freud's legacy for the future* (pp. 61–88). New York, NY: Other Press.

Schore, A. N. (2003a). *Affect regulation and the repair of the self.* New York, NY: Norton.

Schore, A. N. (2003b). *Affect dysregulation and disorders of the self.* New York, NY: Norton.

Schore, A. N. (2009). Relational trauma and the developing right brain. An interface of psychoanalytic self psychology and neuroscience. *Annals of the New York Academy of Sciences, 1159,* 189–203.

Schore, A. N. (2011). The right brain implicit self lies at the core of psychoanalysis. *Psychoanalytic Dialogues, 21,* 75–100.

Schore, A. N. (2012). *The science of the art of psychotherapy.* New York, NY: Norton.

Todd, R. M., & Anderson, A. K. (2009). Six degrees of separation: The amygdala regulates social behavior and perception. *Nature Neuroscience, 12,* 1217–1218.

Tucker, D. M., & Moller, L. (2007). The metamorphosis: Individuation of the adolescent brain. In D. Romer & E. F. Walker (Eds.), *Adolescent psychopathology and the developing brain: Integrating brain and prevention science* (pp. 85–102). Oxford, UK: Oxford University Press.

Vrticka, P., Sander, D., & Vuilleumier. (2013). Lateralized interactive social content and valence processing within the human amygdala. *Frontiers in Human Neuroscience,* doi: 10.3389/fnhum.2012.00358

Yoshida, T., Yoshino, A., Takahashi, Y., & Nomura, S. (2007). Comparison of hemispheric asymmetry in global and local information processing and interference in divided and selective attention using spatial frequency filters. *Experimental Brain Research, 181,* 519–529.

Introduction

It was a singular event that caught my attention and captured my interest in child abuse, violence, and posttraumatic stress disorder (PTSD). In 1976 a group of school children were kidnapped and buried in a boxcar in Chowchilla, California. I began to wonder about the psychological impact of such a horrific experience. How would it affect the children over time? I followed the work of child psychiatrist Lenore Terr of the University of California, San Francisco, who, after the children's escape, assessed and documented the reactions of the child victims (Terr, 1979, 1981, 1983, 1990). Hers is a unique and comprehensive study of the immediate and long-term effects of child trauma. There was scant literature and research on childhood trauma and PTSD prior to that time.

This book is about the practical application of neurobiology for work with traumatized children and teens in the clinical setting. The evolution of this book has spanned over 30 years of continuing education and my clinical practice. The material in the book is based on the model of treatment I developed, Neuro-developmental Art Therapy (Chapman, 2002). The treatment model is based in neurobiology and the advances gained through research in the fields of psychiatry and trauma combined with my skills, knowledge, and experience as an art therapist and play therapist. I am fortunate to have worked as an art therapist in outpatient practice, inpatient child psychiatry, inpatient pediatric medicine, and trauma.

BACKGROUND AND SIGNIFICANCE

The statistics published by the Children's Defense Fund in 2012 are stunning. Every day in America 5 children are killed by abuse or neglect; 5 children or teens commit suicide; 8 children or teens are killed by firearms; 32 children or teens die from accidents; 80 babies die before their first birthday; 186 children are arrested for violent offenses; 368 children are arrested for drug offenses; 2,058 children are confirmed as abused or neglected; 3,312 high school students drop out; and 4,133 children are arrested (Children's Defense Fund, 2012).

Adolescents are tragically underserved. They have the highest rate of homicides in the United States. Approximately 6,900 teens commit suicide annually, and 1.8 million youths enter the juvenile justice system each year. Between 1992 and 2006, 116 students were killed in school violence, and in 2008 more than 656,000 youths ages 10–24 were treated in emergency departments for injuries sustained from violence (Centers for Disease Control, 2011).

The current crisis in the mental health of American children is staggering, with over 15 million American children and adolescents affected by a mental or behavioral health problem (Centers for Disease Control, 2006). Unfortunately, less than 25 percent of affected children and youth receive any treatment (Burns et al.,1995).

The trauma that results from these violent acts has created a crisis that must be addressed if we are to counter the crippling impact on the mental health of these young people. This is my primary motivation for writing this book.

As a mental health provider to children and teens, I am concerned about the lack of resources for the development of psychological assessments and the pre-scribing of medication before less-invasive treatments are utilized to control symptoms. I am concerned about the number of young children who are asked to learn academic skills that are beyond their developmental level, their information-processing capacity, and their cognitive ability. I am concerned about the number of children who are exposed to domestic violence, video game violence, film violence, television violence, and the transgressions of those who bully them in their schools and communities. I am concerned about the severity of the cases that cause therapists to feel inadequate when traditional methods of therapy prove ineffective for their clients.

I began my clinical training at University of California San Francisco (UCSF) in the Department of Child Psychiatry. I was trained by and worked with child psychiatrists, social workers, psychiatric nurses, occupational therapists, creative arts therapists, and other mental health professionals. All contributed assessment data over a period of weeks or months as we worked together to formulate and implement consistent treatment goals.

In early 1988 I co-created and directed an art therapy program at San Francisco General Hospital (SFGH) to offer inpatient psychological services to the 1,200 annual pediatric patients. Then, too, there was an epidemic of gang violence. Physicians were observing stress symptoms and readmissions with repeated injuries. Working in this acute medical setting afforded me the unique opportunity to learn about trauma from impact to symptom reduction. I was again fortunate to be able to learn from and work with exquisitely skilled physi-cians, child psychiatrists, nurses, psychiatric nurses, social workers, occupational and rehabilitation specialists, and the specialty services: surgery, neurology, orthopedics, child life, and critical care providers.

In the 1980s, there was no child psychiatry or child psychology literature about treatment for acute injuries. My goal was to learn the child's perception of an event. I offered children and teens structured art materials: paper, pencils, colored pencils, and markers. I asked children and teens to draw a series of images associated with their acute event. From my patients, I learned how children and teens perceive, recall, and express traumatic images. The children were able to tell their story in narrative form by referring to the images in their drawings. Their stories included many misperceptions, rescue and revenge fantasies, and signs of shame, blame, and guilt. Hence, I tailored the intervention to address a variety of issues. Giving children the opportunity to draw and tell their own stories resulted in a dramatic reduction in observable symptoms, including those of withdrawal, anxiety, fear, and hypervigilance.

At the same time, my interest in neurobiology and psychotherapy was growing. I was formulating a protocol for an acute trauma treatment intervention based on how children and teens experience traumatic events, their reactions and responses, and how they integrated the experience. There were times when I was puzzled by a particular reaction during an intervention session. Neurologist Donna Ferriero was often able to offer a neurological definition or description for my observations of idiosyncratic symptoms of childhood and adolescent trauma. Fascinated with this new information, I eagerly sought out and attended conferences that offered neuroscience presentations.

In 1992, I heard Daniel Siegel speak at the American Academy of Child and Adolescent Psychiatry Conference. His presentation examined the science of the development of the human brain and mind and the impact of trauma on brain development and subsequent functioning. Drawing on this information, I began to look for correlations to the dramatic changes in children and teens I was seeing in the drawing intervention sessions I conducted. At the same time, Bruce Perry was writing about the neurobiology of violence. His descriptions of the neural process, symptoms, and associated behavior further added to my understanding of what was occurring in the clinical setting in which I worked. With this knowledge, and my clinical experience with children and teens, I continued to refine my drawing intervention approach.

Others were working concurrently and influenced and contributed to the material for this book. Robert Pynoos and his colleagues at University of California at Los Angeles were publishing papers and conducting research on childhood PTSD, acute PTSD, and violence. Michael DeBellis was doing groundbreaking neurobiological research on the effects of violence and child abuse on neurodevelopment. Lenore Terr was a major source for knowledge and clinical techniques for treating childhood PTSD.

Another early influence on the development of my treatment model was a day-long training with Joseph Chilton Pearce and his introduction to the work of Paul McLean. Dr. Pearce beautifully explained the relationship between brain development, information processing, and traumatic stress. This, too, enhanced my understanding of what was occurring in the clinical setting and validated my approach to the treatment of PTSD.

Finally, and most significantly, have been my years of study with Allan Schore. Since 2007 I have attended his ongoing study group. Dr. Schore has shared his gifted understanding of the physiology of the brain, the relational aspects of neu-

rological body/mind development, the effects of trauma and abuse on development, and regulation theory. His lectures and guidance have afforded me a
deeper understanding of my role as a therapist and of how to participate in the
therapeutic dyad.

I offer these visionary pioneers a great deal of gratitude. They were all
approachable and generous with their time and knowledge as they answered my
many questions. Each of these individuals contributed greatly to my current
knowledge of neurobiology, trauma, abuse, and violence. Each offered material
that helped me scientifically articulate the rationale for my intervention that was
demonstrating remarkable results in the hospital setting. The intervention protocol is described in Chapter 2.

A NEURO-DEVELOPMENTAL MODEL
OF ART THERAPY TREATMENT

The Neuro-developmental Model of Art Therapy (NDAT) (Chapman, 2002)
grew out of the acute intervention protocol I created while assisting pediatric
trauma patients and served as the beginning of a treatment protocol for art therapy outcome research. As I continued to define and refine the model, I expanded
it to include interpersonal neurobiology and attachment theory. Interested in
conceptualized treatment protocols for art therapy outcome research, I extended
the model to treat relational trauma and child abuse in long-term therapy.

Art therapy practice is congruent with the neurobiology of trauma. It is common knowledge that the body-based sequelae of trauma are stored in the right
hemisphere of the brain, (Siegel, 1999; van der Kolk, 1994). Art therapy, along
with the other right-brain–activating creative arts therapies (music, dance/move-
ment, drama, poetry therapy), along with play therapy and sand tray therapy,
utilize the brain's integrative capacity (Jones, 1994). Activation of the right hemisphere offers access to the stored physical and emotional traumatic memories,
internal sensations, feelings, and thoughts that can then be expressed in visual
form. In my clinical experience, I have witnessed that kinesthetic and sensory
experiences activate the right hemisphere of the brain, followed by the limbic
system, cognitive, and prefrontal structures (Chapman, 2002). It is this concept
that is the basis for the NDAT approach to treatment of trauma in children and
teens, the focus of this book.

PTSD TREATMENT

Two decades of PTSD research fostered the creation of many approaches to
child and adolescent PTSD treatment. Randomized and randomized-controlled
treatment trials demonstrated success in reducing PTSD symptoms for children
3 to 5 years old and their parents (Lieberman, Van Horn, & Ippen, 2005). School-
based treatment protocols were examined (Berger, Pat-Horenczk, & Gelkopf,
2007; Kataoka et al., 2003; Stein et al., 2003) and treatment for sexual abuse

were studied (Cohen, Berliner, & Mannarino, 2000; Deblinger, Steer, & Lippmann, 1996; Trowell et al., 2002). There were investigations with inpatient adolescents with chronic PTSD (Lyshak-Stelzer et al., 2007) and with children and teens who experienced disasters, (Goenjian et al., 1997). Eye-Movement Desensitization and Reprocessing (EMDR) treatment (Chemtob, Nakashima, & Carlson, 2002; Greenwald, 1999), and treating PTSD with hospitalized children (deVries et al., 1999; Chapman et al., 2001) were also investigated.

The infusion of new, highly refined scientific knowledge of how the brain functions was interfaced with the practice of therapy and resulted in new treatment models that are neurobiologically and developmentally informed. Effective PTSD treatment of complex, relational trauma is now focused on the right hemisphere, the primacy of affect, the importance of relationships at critical times in development, and ways to dynamically apply these concepts in psychotherapy. In the opening pages of his 2012 book, *The Science of the Art of Psychotherapy*, Allan Schore writes of a paradigm shift occurring across all sciences, from conscious, explicit left-brain discourse to the unconscious, nonverbal, body-based expression of the right hemisphere:

> This paradigm shift from behavior, to cognition, to bodily based emotion has acted as an integrating force for forging stronger connections between the disciplines of psychology, social neuroscience, and psychiatry, all of which are now focusing on affective phenomena. (Schore, 2012, p. 4)

The concept of technique has not been abandoned (Bromberg, 2011), but the focus is now on the "affective, nonverbal, body based processes of the right brain" (p. 6). Examples of early models of mind/body therapy for PTSD included somatic therapy (Levine & Kline, 2007), sensory motor (Ogden, Minton, & Pain, 2006), and EMDR (Greenwald, 1999).

This book has theoretical and practical information for the beginner and the seasoned clinician. The first chapter includes a review of the past and current literature on PTSD. Chapter 2 is devoted to Chapman Art Therapy Treatment Intervention (CATTI) (Chapman, 2001), the intervention developed in the medical setting for reducing observable, acute PTSD symptoms in hospitalized children. Beginning with a theoretical overview, the intervention is described in detail, along with case examples. The outcome data from a randomized controlled investigation of the efficacy of the intervention are found in the Appendix.

The neuro-developmental model of treatment is introduced and described in detail in Chapter 3, which describes the four phases of treatment along with specific examples of the interventions utilized in a particular stage of treatment.

Chapter 4 is about the practical ways to help therapists, mothers, and caregivers aid the development of infants, children, and teens with sensory processing and sensory integration difficulties. The chapter is not meant to take the place of a formal evaluation by an occupational therapist; rather, it is meant to aid development and help therapists determine the possible need for a formal evaluation.

The right hemisphere is the main topic of Chapters 5 and 6. Chapter 5 is primarily case material to illustrate ways to implicitly re-create attachment and other early developmental experiences in the clinical setting. Unusual yet effective tools are offered. Chapter 6 is also mainly case material presented to illustrate ways to integrate interpersonal neurobiology and art therapy in the clinical setting. The chapter provides techniques showing how to stay in the right-hemisphere information-processing mode using mutual co-regulation between an attuned therapist and the client within an intersubjective space (Schore, 2012). There is also commentary on left-hemisphere language in therapy.

The last three chapters of the book are case studies, one chapter each, illustrating intervention at work with a toddler, a school-age child, and an adolescent. The case material in each chapter is very detailed to illustrate the nuances that affect the therapeutic dyad.

The focus of attention in psychoanalytic treatment is on the right-hemisphere-to-right-hemisphere transactions that occur in the therapeutic dyad. The focus of this book is to offer knowledge and case material that forge a connection between art therapy and the application of interpersonal neurobiology in the clinical setting. Because of my background in medical and psychological PTSD treatment, my attempt is to offer knowledge and skills that contribute to the larger understanding of how to treat those who are suffering and to prevent future acts of abuse and violence.

Neurobiologically Informed Trauma Therapy With Children and Adolescents

PART I

CHILDHOOD TRAUMA: A NEURODEVELOPMENTAL APPROACH

The chapters in Part I are devoted to acknowledging previous research, and to exploring how the early and current research has been incorporated into a model of PTSD treatment that is consistent with development, neurobiology, and information processing.

Chapter 1 begins with an overview of the evolution of PTSD research, citing numerous researchers and clinicians who have contributed to the current body of knowledge on child and adolescent PTSD. The chapter also describes the numerous reactions, responses, and symptoms children and teens exhibit from both short-term and long-term exposure to violence, abuse, and trauma.

Chapter 2 focuses on a drawing treatment intervention that is designed to treat acute traumatic episodes and effective in reducing PTSD symptoms in children and teens who have experienced acute traumatic events. The chapter delves into the theoretical basis for the intervention, as well as revelatory case examples and illustrative data from an outcome study that investigated the efficacy of the intervention.

Chapter 3 describes an art therapy treatment model for long-term exposure to child abuse and violence that was developed as an extension of the intervention illustrated in Chapter 2. Readers are introduced to many art therapy and play therapy interventions, including the Neurodevelopmental Art Therapy (NDAT) treatment model that effectively treats those who have experienced persistent exposure to child abuse, violence, and trauma.

CHAPTER 1

Acute and Chronic Exposure:
Children's Reactions and Responses

Advances in research and imaging technology over the past two decades have afforded us a comprehensive understanding of the mechanism of stress and its effects on the body, mind, and human development. The biological and clinical sciences have contributed to a tremendous body of research that defines, describes, and quantifies the effects of childhood stress. This chapter begins with an overview of the evolution of child and adolescent posttraumatic stress disorder (PTSD) literature and research. It offers a description of the physical, psychological, and cognitive reactions and responses experienced by children and adolescents with both acute and long-term exposure to trauma, violence, and abuse. Case notes illustrate the ways children from across the developmental spectrum exhibit symptoms in response to acute and repeated exposure to stress and demonstrate the effects of that stress on the brain, body, mind, and behavior.

Witnessing children, adolescents, and families in the early stages of dealing with acute trauma in a large, urban Level I trauma center has greatly informed my clinical work with all clients. Offering psychological services in the immediate aftermath of corporal injuries, violence, and abuse has enabled me to learn directly from infants, toddlers, children, teens, and their families about how they perceive, express, and integrate traumatic experiences.

The human organism is designed for survival, and with most acute trauma the individual returns to homeostasis rapidly. Repeated exposure to violence, trauma, and abuse, however, creates intense suffering. The lifetime negative effects of repeated exposure to violence, abuse, and neglect are often misunderstood, minimized, and misdiagnosed. In addition to managing symptoms, knowing what the child experiences and the effects of violence and abuse on the individual, and on society, informs the development of appropriate treatment strategies for healing.

CHILD AND ADOLESCENT PTSD RESEARCH

Early researchers in child and adolescent PTSD conducted studies with children and adolescents who experienced trauma: terror (Terr, 1979, 1990), witnessing of violence (Nader et al., 1990; Pynoos & Eth, 1984, 1986; Pynoos & Nader, 1988; Pynoos et al., 1987), war-related trauma (Nader et al., 1993; Wisenberg et al., 1993; Ziv, Krugalski, & Shulman, 1974), school-based disasters (Gillis, 1993; Klingman, 1987), technology disasters (Yule, 1993), natural disasters (Figley, 1985; Frederick, 1985; Pynoos et al., 1993; Shelby & Tredinnick, 1995). Additionally, researchers examined the relationship between acute injuries and PTSD in hospitalized children (Chapman et al., 2001; Daviss et al., 2000; deVries et al., 1999).

Other pioneers in child PTSD investigated the effects of child abuse, neglect and violence in specific ways. Neurobiological studies investigated the stress response at the cellular level and the effects of stress on the brain. Studies determined the presence and quantity of catecholamines (DeBellis, Baum, et al., 1999; DeBellis, Keshavan, et al., 1999; DeBellis, Lefter, et al., 1994; Perry, 1994; Rogeness, Javors, & Pliszka, 1992) and cortisol in maltreated children (Carrion et al., 2002; Cicchetti & Rogosch, 2001; DeBellis, Baum, et al., 1999; DeBellis, Keshavan, et al., 1999; Hart, Gunnar, & Cicchetti, 1995). Hippocampal volume was the topic of several studies (Bremner et al., 1997; Carrion, Weemes, & Reiss, 2007; DeBellis, Baum, et al., 1999; DeBellis, Keshavan, et al., 1999; DeBellis, Lefter, et al., 1994). Others focused on brain structure, including intracranial volume (ICV) (Carrion et al., 2001; DeBellis, Keshavan, et al., 1999), cerebral volumes (DeBellis et al., 1994), prefrontal right and left amygdala volume, and the size of the corpus callosum (DeBellis, Keshavan, et al., 1999).

Developmental psychologists investigated behavior, emotion, and cognition, including the relationship between rates of exposure and the development of PTSD (Breslau et al., 1998; Nader et al., 1990; Pynoos et al., 1993; Shaw et al., 1995), risk factors (McLeer et al., 1992; Pynoos & Nader, 1989; Wolfe, 1994) and resiliency (Cicchetti & Rogosch, 2001). Others investigated the effects of stress associated with the lack of an attachment with a primary caregiver (Allen & Hauser, 1996; Bokhorst et al., 2003; Carlson et al., 1989; Cicchetti & Barnett, 1991; Lyons-Ruth, 1996; Lyons-Ruth & Jacobvitz, 1999; Main, Kaplan, & Cassidy, 1985; Schore, 2003a; Spangler & Grossman, 1999; van IJzendoorn, Schuengel, & Bakermans-Kraneburg, 1999; Weinfield, Whaley, & Egeland, 2004). Still others investigated gender differences (Bokszczanin, 2007; Green et al., 1991; Springer & Padgett, 2000) and, especially important, how chronological age and the stage of development at the time of exposure affect the onset of PTSD (Eth & Pynoos, 1985; Grych et al., 2000; Pynoos & Nader, 1988; Saigh & Bremner, 1999; Scheeringa et al., 1995). Peer relationships in maltreated children were also examined (Mueller & Silverman, 1989; Howes & Espinosa, 1985).

Several early PTSD researchers developed formal assessment tools to quantify symptoms for diagnostics and outcome research. There are several reliable and valid assessment scales by which child and adolescent PTSD can be formally measured. Among them, and the most widely used, is the UCLA Posttraumatic Stress Disorder Reaction Index (Pynoos et al., 1987; Steinberg et al., 2004) This index was designed for children and adolescents and is used in evaluation and research; it has also been deemed appropriate for disaster and emergency use (Balaban, 2006). The Diagnostic Interview for Children and Adolescents– Revised (DICA-R) (Reich & Welner, 1988) consists of a semi-structured interview that relies on parent/child/adolescent interviews for the diagnosis of PTSD. John Briere's Trauma Symptom Checklist for Young Children (TSCYC) (2001) and the Child Behavior Checklist (CBCL) (Achenbach & Rescorla, 2000) are modifications to assess PTSD in children (Levendosky et al., 2002).

ACUTE TRAUMA AND CHRONIC TRAUMA

In 1991 an important distinction was made between acute and long-term exposure in the child and adolescent PTSD literature. Child psychiatrist Lenore Terr (1991) described *acute* traumatic experiences as Type I events and *chronic* exposure as Type II. The revisions for the American Psychiatric Association's 1994 *Diagnostic & Statistical Manual,* fourth edition *(DSM-IV)* included a diagnostic category for acute stress disorder. Acute trauma, described as a one-time event in a normal life (Terr, 1991), is often of short duration, is severe, and may be accompanied by injuries or loss. PTSD symptoms are common, yet very few children who experience acute traumatic episodes develop PTSD, because symptoms of acute trauma typically abate in one month or less. However, many children have observable symptoms and adverse reactions, warranting assessment and referral for treatment (deVries et al., 1999). Some children initially appear free of symptoms, then have a delayed reaction. Acute traumas may also include significant life changes such as scars or disfigurement, having to live with medical devices, repeated medical and surgical procedures, or loss of limbs or function of the limbs.

Acute traumatic episodes typically result from three general categories: medical trauma, natural disasters, and human-made disasters. Examples of medical trauma include motor vehicle and pedestrian accidents; falls; sports injuries; mild to moderate burns; gunshot, stab, or assault wounds; and hospitalization. A natural disaster may be a fire, hurricane, flood, tornado, earthquake, storm, landslide, tsunami, avalanche, or volcanic episode. Human-made disasters include acts of terrorism, chemical spills, plane crashes, mass shootings, nuclear reactor incidents, disease outbreak, and explosions.

Mass casualty experts are mobilized for most natural and human-made disasters; however medical and other acute traumas typically do not receive due attention. Some children and teens have severe behavior problems as a result of earlier unresolved medical trauma. Research demonstrates that children and teens have PTSD symptoms following even minor medical trauma and that parents tend to underrate their child's symptoms (Schreier et al., 2005). I find remarkable the number of children referred for treatment for behavior problems resulting from unresolved earlier acute traumatic events. One may not see a child or teen in therapy until long after the acute reaction to acute trauma; however, such early body-based states often influence behavior and functioning long after the initial observable symptoms have lessened or abated.

Chronic exposure to trauma is defined as repeated, anticipated events with persistent exposure (Terr, 1991). Neglect, war, repeated child abuse, repeated exposure to violence, multiple transitions and losses, and poverty are descriptive of chronic trauma. Neglect, by far the most common form of abuse (Hildyard & Wolfe, 2002; Levy et al., 1995), is described as failure to provide adequate food, clothing, shelter, and medical and dental care. Neglecting to provide the child with a secure attachment with a primary caretaker creates adverse effects specifically on the "self-organization of the developing brain that occurs in the context of a relationship with another self, another brain" (Schore, 1996, p. 60). It is well established that disruptions to the infant's attachment relationship with a primary caregiver influence the child's neuroplasticity and future psychopathology (Schore, 2012). Inherent in the attachment experience is the development of the sensory and motor systems, fundamental building blocks for emotional and behavior regulation and for learning. Over time, these repetitive sensory-motor experiences increase in complexity. If the sensory systems are not developed adequately, behavior, emotional regulation, and learning are affected.

PHYSICAL STRESS RESPONSES AND REACTIONS

At the onset of an acute traumatic episode, the neurochemical dysregulating stress response shuts down 80%–90% of the brain's function. This is a reflexive activation of the fear response, which is mediated by the autonomic nervous system (ANS) and hypothalamic-pituitary-adrenal (HPA) axis to control the body's state of arousal. The HPA axis consists of two systems: the sympathetic component, which develops during the first year of life, and the parasympathetic, which develops during the second year of life.

The acute stress response creates a state of hyperarousal, with an accelerated heart rate and blood pressure, increased respiration, and eyes wide open in a state of alertness. The stress hormone corticotrophin releasing factor (CRF) is released from the hypothalamus, which in turn stimulates the release of corticotrophin from the pituitary for physiological homeostasis. This causes the adrenal glands to secrete cortisol. By contrast, the parasympathetic response is inhibiting and energy conserving, creating a state of hypoarousal: heart rate decreases, blood pressure drops, and respiration slows.

Pain is inhibited by the release of endogenous opioids (van der Kolk et al., 1989). Perceptual, association, and memory circuits are altered. Right-hemisphere traumatic memories are implicit (Mancia, 2006; van der Kolk, McFarlane, & Weisaeth, 1996) — perceptually and nonverbally organized as sensory memories and memory fragments of the event, or somatic memory (Achterberg & Lawlis, 1980; Ogden, Minton, & Pain, 2006; Schiffer, Teicher, & Papanicolaou, 1995; Terr, 1995; van der Kolk & van der Hart, 1991).

Bessel van der Kolk hypothesized the effects of emotional arousal on declarative memory. The sensory system sends a traumatic experience to the thalamus, an area of the brain that serves as a relay station for incoming sensory information. The amygdala sends the information to the hippocampus for categorizing and cognitive appraisal (van der Kolk et al., 1996). Because of the possible volume loss in the hippocampus during an extreme stress response, hippocampal functioning is inhibited, "leaving the memories to be stored as affective states or in sensory-motor modalities, as somatic sensations and visual images" (p. 294). As a result, there is no neural access to the frontal neocortex for integration and planning. The ability to transfer the material to permanent, explicit memory is compromised.

PSYCHOLOGICAL STRESS RESPONSE AND REACTIONS

There are several models describing the psychological reactions to traumatic experience. I prefer the four-stage model developed by Jane Lee (1970): impact, retreat, acknowledgment, and reconstruction. Based on my clinical experience, her model accurately describes the psychological reactions and stages experienced, from the first awareness of the event through rehabilitation. This model has been applied to art therapy treatment in the medical setting with burn patients (Appleton, 2001). Some psychological reactions to an acute traumatic episode are mislabeled as bizarre or psychopathology by those unfamiliar with particular aspects of a traumatic stress response. Understanding the psychological reactions and ramifications of acute and chronic trauma is essential to the formulation of effective treatment strategies.

The first stage of Lee's model is *impact,* a depersonalized state during the initial encounter with the event. This state may occur at the scene, during transport to medical care, or in the hospital setting. It may also occur in visual flashbacks or other sensory modes years after the event, as in cases of early abuse and neglect. During this stage of awareness, anxiety is high and sensation and emotion are indistinguishable. Children may comment they did not know whether the experience was real or whether they were dreaming. Behavior is often passive or poorly controlled. Dissociation is common.

> CASE NOTE: An 8-year-old girl appeared frozen in a state of shock following the stabbing of many family members. I was summoned to the Emergency Department by the medical staff treating her for numerous stab wounds. The child was immobile, her gaze fixed. I arrived with a small teddybear, knelt down beside her, and repeated, "It is over. No more. It is over. No more." She brought her focus to my face, her eyes wide with fear. I repeated, "It is over. No more" as I held the teddybear within her reach. She accepted the soft bear and held it close. She made and main-

tained eye contact with me. I explained that she was in the hospital and the doctors needed to look at her body and put Band-Aids on her sores and give her some special medicine to help her feel better, and that she would not die. Her eyes remained on mine as I stayed with her. I explained the function of the various monitors and the role of the doctors and nurses and what was occurring. She gradually relaxed and became more aware of herself and her environment.

The second stage is **retreat,** a defensive phenomenon that results in the activation of defense mechanisms in an effort to achieve psychological homeostasis. Among the unconscious defenses employed are repression, suppression, denial, wishful or magical thinking, and fantasy avoidance.

> CASE NOTE: A mother, driving while intoxicated, was involved in a motor vehicle crash that resulted in her young daughter becoming a quadriplegic from injuries sustained in the crash. One morning the mother arrived in the ICU and stood over her child's bed announcing she had purchased a brand new scooter on the way to the hospital and that the scooter would belong to the child when she went home. I immediately recognized the mother's use of magical thinking in an attempt to return to the pre-morbid state. Some hospital staff wondered if the mother was impaired or psychotic. I was able to validate the mother's wish that her daughter would be riding the scooter and gently reminded her of the reality of her daughter's condition.

The psyche is not always able to tolerate the powerful emotions that arise. A psychological retreat or dissociative strategy is common.

> CASE NOTE: A 17-year-old male suffered severe burns on his arms, hands, and torso resulting from injuries sustained in an explosion. Despite being connected to numerous monitors and unable to move, the patient proclaimed he was getting up and leaving the hospital because he did not need any help. I gently validated his wanting to get up and leave and that he would do so one day, but now the doctors had to be sure he did not get an infection and to ensure his burns were healing.

Psychological retreat should also be a consideration when children disclose abuse and then retract the statement. Rather than a retraction, a psychological retreat is a normal part of the psychological stages of integrating traumatic experiences. Allowing space for the child to acknowledge the event may take time. Physicians, nurses, and first responders are likely to see the appearance of a psychological retreat when these normal defenses activate to deny or minimize the experience.

The third stage in Lee's model is ***acknowledgment,*** a mourning period. It occurs when the person experiences the grief and loss associated with the event. This can be the loss of body image, of a sense of body integrity, or of function. Feelings of helplessness and hopelessness result in episodes of existential cycling as an attempt is made to redefine the self.

> **CASE NOTE:** The burned teen described in the previous note made a psychological shift from retreat to acknowledgment when he asked to sit by an open window. When he then asked to have the window opened further and was told it was open as far as it would go, he said in an angry tone, "Damn." When I gently questioned him about his comment, he expressed his desire to jump from the hospital window and commit suicide. Expressing his hopelessness, he looked at his injuries and said, "Look at me. Who will love me now?"

This is the existential cycling that occurs in an attempt to redefine the self.

Lee defines the last stage as ***reconstruction,*** a new beginning with new approaches to living, letting go of the old self-concept and accepting the new self-concept. Mastery is the focus here, and there is a shift toward independence and coping with the new situation. The client becomes future oriented.

> **CASE NOTE:** During therapy, the teen with burn injuries made the shift to reconstruction when he requested that the plastic surgeons fix the contractures of his hands so he could paint, play chess, and do other things that the contractures currently impeded. He was no longer coping via suicidal ideation. He was accepting his newly formed self-concept and was investing in improving his outcome and looking forward.

Lee's model applies to long-term exposure as well. Many adults abused as children are in the retreat stage for many years, some for a lifetime. Adults who do enter therapy commonly experience intrusive images, memory fragments, or other sensory experiences that trouble them.

SYMPTOMS AND REACTIONS WITH ACUTE TRAUMA

The inclusion of acute stress disorder (ASD) in DSM-IV generated attention and prompted research into the symptom presentation and treatment of those who experience acute trauma. However, with no differentiated diagnostic criteria for children and adolescents as opposed to adults, the criteria failed to consider the stages of human development. The *DSM-V* (American Psychiatric Association, 2013) has included a new developmental subtype of PTSD called posttraumatic stress disorder in preschool children. Rather than reiterate the symptoms it describes—reexperiencing, avoidance, negative cognitions and mood, and arousal symptom clusters—the remainder of this chapter describes the observable, developmentally consistent expression of PTSD symptoms in children and teens.

From my observation of acutely injured youth, symptom presentation is often idiosyncratic and severe. Young people may not exhibit symptoms from all three of the identified symptom clusters described in the diagnostic criteria for PTSD in the *DSM-V*, but children and teens do exhibit symptomatic behavior that is consistent with their stage of development.

In infants, acute PTSD symptoms are generally observed as increased needy and clingy behaviors. Other times, however, infants appear withdrawn and avoidant. They exhibit an exaggerated startle response, are irritable, and cry often. Although most parents attempt to ameliorate the effects of traumatic hospitalization and injury exposure with infants, some acute trauma results in their separation from caregivers, painful medical procedures, medication side effects, and an alien environment if hospitalized. Infants express motorically, seeking relief from tension and stress. Loud screams, crying episodes, and repetitious movements with the body or body parts are common.

> CASE NOTE: A 2-year-old girl witnessed the murder of her family members. During her hospitalization, she was withdrawn and mute. When introduced to toys, she would play actively, but following the play times, she sat in her highchair and said, "Mama" repeatedly while rapidly flapping her lower arms and hands. When she requested food, juice, or said "Mama," she would rapidly flap her arms and hands.

Consistent with development, the child was expressing emotions motorically. Young children have neither the cognitive skills nor the vocabulary for verbal expression.

Toddler and preschool-age children experiencing acute trauma exhibit fear and anxiety that is expressed through their body. They may cower in a protective posture, exhibit gaze aversion, or resist comfort. Toddlers and preschoolers are consistently vying for control of their situation, which they demonstrate by refusing to ambulate, eat, or talk.

> CASE NOTE: A 3-year-old girl was hospitalized and placed in a body cast following a car crash. The cast left her immobile with the exception of her arms and head. She was oppositional and refused to cooperate when the nurse attempted to take her vital signs or feed her. To give the child an opportunity for control, I placed a cart with toys and art supplies just out of reach from her crib. I asked her to let me know what she wanted. She proceeded to demand each item on the cart. When I handed her the requested item, she immediately returned it and demanded another. The nurse was able to take her vital signs while the child was distracted, busily ordering me around. When the nurse was finished and offered the child some juice, she drank it.

What toddlers are controlling often does not matter as long as they perceive that they are in control.

> CASE NOTE: A 3-year-old boy was hospitalized after a serious illness that required surgery. Post operatively, the child was hysterical, combative, and uncooperative and refused his mother's attempts to provide comfort. During one screaming episode, he attempted to pull the IV out, complaining of pain in his hand. The nursing staff ascertained there was nothing wrong with the IV. I asked the child what would be the one thing that would help fix the hurt. He said tearfully, "A Band-Aid." I placed a Band-Aid over the plastic cover of the IV. "It doesn't hurt now," he said.

Young children exhibit increased or excessive fear of strangers, increased or excessive separation anxiety, and increased or excessive stranger anxiety. They are often highly irritable and oppositional. They can exhibit cognitive confusion and regressed developmental skills: thumb sucking, baby talk, or bed wetting. They have intrusive images, often precipitated by external reminders, but also self-generated. Some children experience sleep disturbance and nightmares following acute trauma. During this period, young children engage in repetitive posttraumatic play or art, although young children's drawings are motor driven and not representational.

> CASE NOTE: A 3-year-old boy had witnessed his 10-year-old brother become injured in a tractor accident on a farm. The 10-year-old recovered, but the 3-year-old had witnessed a great deal of blood at the scene and subsequently talked constantly about blood. Any pouring of, or the sight of, moving liquids was a traumatic reminder (Pynoos, Steinberg, & Goenjian, 1996) and imagined by the child to be blood. His comments about blood were continuous and illustrated his use of fantasy and magical thinking as a way of coping.

Developmentally, the child was attempting to master his anxiety by repetitiously replaying and retelling the disturbing aspect of the event (blood). A 3-year-old is not capable of reasoning his way out of fear. He manages intrusive images with fantasy.

School-age children primarily exhibit anxiety, fear, shame (Lansky, 1991), and guilt following acute traumatic episodes. Behaviorally, this is observable in averting their gaze, appearing withdrawn, and refusing to participate in normal activities. Shame and guilt are common and often elicit fear and depression. Of the hundreds of children I have treated for acute injuries in the hospital setting, rare is the child or teen who did not believe he or she was at fault for the incident—even when this was obviously not so. Children have trauma-specific fears (Terr, 1991), idiosyncratic and unique to each child.

Acutely stressed school-age children may also exhibit regressed developmental skills. They may seek earlier levels of adult attention and support, exhibit a fear of the dark, and display increased separation anxiety. They report having intrusive images, memories, and memory fragments of the event (Pynoos, Steinberg, & Goenjian, 1996). Reminders brought on by a sound, sight, smell, toy, dream, or body sensation can cause the child to experience fear physically. Some children report that the bodily sensations make them feel as if the event were happening again.

> CASE NOTE: A 9-year-old boy was hospitalized following second- and third-degree burns on his hands and torso sustained while fleeing his burning home. He had nightmares during which he would yell "Fire!" and would attempt to bat away flames from his torso.

School-age children who have experienced acute trauma have high anxiety about body integrity. They exhibit fear of dying, of losing body parts, and of losing body functions. Frequently this concern is revealed metaphorically in their art, stories, or play, but rarely literally.

> CASE NOTE: A 6-year-old girl was hospitalized with severe injuries to her legs after she was hit by a car. Following her surgery, she drew a picture of her grandparents. When I asked if she would like to say anything about the image, she replied, "They died." I asked if she was worried about dying, and she tearfully stated that she thought she would die because her grandparents had died in a hospital.

One might expect a 6-year-old girl to make the cognitive distinction between herself and her grandparents, yet in her neurochemically dysregulated state, it was apparent that she was fearful and worried about survival.

School-age children also exhibit anger. Often it is directed at the perceived perpetrator of the event. For example, toddler and preschool pedestrians hit by a car perceive that it was the car that hit them, while school-age children indicate it was the driver. Anger directed at the driver is often expressed verbally in a loud or angry voice or motorically, by pounding a table or throwing objects.

> CASE NOTE: A 7-year-old girl was hospitalized after being hit by a car. She had watched the driver leave the scene of the incident without offering assistance. She became mute and withdrawn. She kept the sheet over her head while in bed, occasionally coming out from under the sheet to eat or ambulate. She refused all offers to play, engage with art making, or watch television. When she emerged from this state of retreat, she said that she was afraid and ashamed of being hit and that she did not want to look at anything because all she kept seeing in her mind was the car driving away.

Moving from the retreat stage of psychological experience in response to her trauma, the shift to acknowledgment was evident when she expressed her feelings of fear and shame associated with the event. She attempted to ward off the intrusive images by covering her eyes, her problem-solving attempt to cope.

> CASE NOTE: A 10-year-old boy was hospitalized after being hit by a car and sustaining a broken leg. The driver of the car left the scene of the accident. The young boy was furious with the driver and told anyone who approached him, "The guy who hit me is a dumb, bad, stupid person and I hate him."

Children may also have a grief reaction. Sometimes the loss experienced is related to the body, such as loss of function or a change in appearance, or it may be the loss of a bike or personal possession, a surprise to many parents. Or, the loss may be associated with the inability to participate in normal activities such as school or sports. Sometimes the loss is of a friend or family member, and despite being an acute event, it becomes something more than an acute trauma in terms of treatment.

Acutely injured adolescents exhibit many of the same symptoms as school-age children. Additionally, they have a foreshortened view of the future that is different from that of a depressed teen. With violently injured teens, for example, the foreshortened sense of the future is often predicated on their experience of being hurt or having seen their peer group or family members shot, stabbed or killed. They do not expect to live long.

> CASE NOTE: A 17-year-old male was hospitalized following a gunshot wound. When asked about his future, he replied, "I probably won't live long. Everybody on my block dies before 20. There were eleven kids on my block and now there are four. I know I am going to die, so I don't care about the future."

In his view, there was no concept of growing to adulthood, so making a commitment to education or a relationship was pointless. What may have been mistaken for denial or attitude problems was actually a developmentally typical psychological reaction to an acute traumatic event.

Teens often exhibit revenge fantasies, especially when they have been the victim of violence, particularly gang violence. They utilize action-oriented coping mechanisms: they are going to *do something* in response to trauma. They have not yet developed the higher structures of the brain that enable concepts of judgment, right and wrong, and consequences. They are strictly reacting in response to the perceived injustice they have experienced.

> CASE NOTE: A 15-year-old was hospitalized following a gunshot wound to the abdomen. He was a member of a gang. He bragged he could handle

"being shot." He pointed to several fellow gang members in the hospital hallway and stated, "See all those guys? Tonight they are going to get base-ball bats and go after those guys who shot me. Tonight you will see lots of beat-up people at this hospital because they are not going to shoot me with-out getting it back."

Revenge seeking is a common symptom of acute violent episodes. The imma-ture prefrontal cortex development in adolescents is problematic. They lack judgment and cannot comprehend the consequences associated with the action-oriented coping mechanisms that prompt them to retaliate proactively. There-fore, it is critical to understand what acutely injured youth experience so that effective strategies for prevention and treatment can be designed.

SYMPTOM PRESENTATION FOR REPEATED EXPOSURE

The actual symptoms of PTSD resulting from persistent exposure to abuse, neglect, and violence are numerous, though they are only narrowly defined in the *DSM-V*. Taking into consideration the normal stages of human develop-ment, the following description of symptoms and reactions is from my clinical observation and treatment experience.

It is widely accepted that genetics and experience shape the human brain and mind (Cozolino, 2002). Early experiences between infant and caregiver are essential for the development of the early maturation of the self system (Schore, 2003a, 2003b).

Abused and neglected children have core-identity problems. When the infant is exposed to negligent caregiving, or is exposed to violence or abuse, neural development suffers—in particular, the development of the right brain. Right-brain development is associated with the development of the mind/body/self (Schore, 2012). What Schore describes as massive misattunement with caregiv-ers causes hypometabolic dissociative encoding failures (Allen, Hauser, & Borman-Spurrell, 1999) "in the autobiographical memory of the developing self" (Schore, 2012, p. 272). The attachment that develops with an attuned or misattuned care-giver eventually establishes either a stable or an unstable core self (Bromberg, 2006). Abused children and teens have an altered, distorted sense of self that includes self-blame, shame, and often guilt (Ford & Kidd, 1998). Many of the severely abused children and teens I have seen in therapy have little to no sense of self that they are able to describe in art or verbally.

Abused and neglected children often have self-regulation difficulties with body, affect, and behavior. The underdeveloped sensory and motor systems are unable to process incoming sensory information, organize the incoming infor-mation, or control expression. When infants and toddlers are neglected and mal-treated, development of the brain and mind is disrupted. The young child is completely dependent on caregiving and the environment in order to attach with a primary caregiver to complete brain development, and to realize optimal development of the sensory-motor systems. Without the mother as a template for regulation, the infant becomes increasingly stressed. Defensive functioning rapidly shifts the brain from interactive regulatory to autoregulatory modes (Schore, 2003a, 2003b). This is seen in infants with self-stimulating behaviors such as repetitive body movements or sounds. Infants become anxious and cry often, are hypervigilant and clingy, and exhibit an exaggerated startle response. Some infants become withdrawn and avoidant, as seen in gaze aversion, restricted affect, regressed developmental skills, or a lack of response to stimulation from people or toys.

Toddlers and preschool-age children may appear highly anxious and needy or withdrawn and sad. They are highly distressed at reminders of the event, such as seeing someone who has a feature of a perpetrator like a beard or eyeglasses. Victims of sexual abuse may engage in sexual behavior or sexualized play and may have fears or phobias, sleep problems (Hewitt, 1999), or regressed developmental skills. Toddlers and preschoolers may be aggressive toward others, toward themselves, or in play. Young children exhibit behaviors that suggest intrusive images and dissociation. They often replay the event or reenact the abuse or violence in literal or symbolic ways.

> CASE NOTE: A 3-year-old girl with a history of neglect and violence in the home was pretending to feed and care for a doll during play therapy. While the doll was sitting at a small table in a chair, the child suddenly placed her hands around the doll's neck, squeezed her hands tight and yelled, "I said shut up bitch."

As children age, the symptoms are similar but advance developmentally, reflecting the child's broader emotional and cognitive functioning. Abused children and teens have overwhelming feelings that are confusing and produce anxiety and fear. A negative self-concept can result because they feel vulnerable, disempowered, and helpless. This is revealed in self-deprecating comments such as announcing, "I'm stupid." Abused children are highly anxious and exhibit a higher incidence of sleep disorder, eating disorder, panic disorder, substance abuse, suicidal preoccupation and somatic complaints (Putnam, 2003). They also may develop obsessive-compulsive rituals and disorders.

> CASE NOTE: A 13-year-old girl was in the United States after having run away from her home in another country. She ran away with a friend, but the friend soon abandoned her on the streets for a boyfriend. The young girl checked herself into the hospital with severe abdominal pain, which she stated had been occurring for a long time. After a medical workup with no findings, she was invited to explore her pain nonverbally in an art therapy session. The art elicited her story. She tearfully disclosed a long history of severe physical and sexual abuse by family members. She had run away to escape. After the art therapy session, she reported to her physician that she was pain-free.

Allowing the girl a nonverbal means of expression elicited the information from the right hemisphere. This method enabled her to create the images she was then capable of putting into words. I doubt this young girl had the verbal skills or vocabulary to talk about the many years of abuse that had compromised her brain development and brain functioning. She had developed a somatic response. The pain was real, although caused by emotions. She was free of the pain after the 45-minute art therapy session.

Children with histories of abuse, neglect, and violence have learning difficulties. When a child is chronically stressed, cortisol is chronically elevated. High levels of cortisol are damaging to brain cells and may affect hippocampal functioning associated with memory and learning. Persistent exposure to stress requires the child to remain hyperalert, anxious, and vigilant. The right amygdala is constantly scanning for danger (Schore, 2003a, 2003b). Information *not* associated with danger is dismissed. The focus of the child is on the facial expression, tone of voice, or movements of others. Because of the dependence on the right hemisphere for information processing and staying alert to danger, the left hemisphere begins to atrophy, or turn off. Therefore, if the cortex is not active, it will not store information (Perry, 1997). DeBellis and colleagues (2000) determined that abused children have a smaller inner cranium volume (ICV) than nonabused children. The severity and duration of the abuse correlates with smaller ICV: the harsher the abuse, the smaller the brain; the longer the abuse, the smaller the brain. The corpus callosum—the band of tissue that connects the hemispheres of the brain—is smaller in abused children than in nonabused children. The child cannot access the higher structures of the brain for thinking, planning, judgment, consequences, wisdom, compassion, or empathy.

Children and teens frequently present with sensory-motor delays resulting from a lack of maternal input at critical times in development. These delays can greatly contribute to a child's learning problems. The child may be highly sensitive to tastes, sounds, smells, or touch, dislike certain fabrics, or refuse to wear particular clothing. The child may be clumsy, have difficulty sitting upright, or appear to have balance problems. These deficits can cause him or her to appear hyperactive, manic, or depressed or to have attention and focus difficulties. Abused children cognitively underachieve in the elementary school years (Erickson & Egeland, 2002; Veltman & Browne, 2001).

Abused and neglected children have social problems and peer relationship problems (Rogosch, Cicchetti, & Aber, 1995) and exhibit aggression. With limited or no ability to regulate emotions or behavior, these children are often socially withdrawn, are depressed, or have anger control problems (Runyan et al., 2004). They have difficulty attending to social cues and are often aggressive in speech and behavior. Pain and fear reduce serotonin levels, promoting aggression (Lewis, 1998).

In addition to the epidemic of children requiring mental health services, America is also faced with an epidemic of violent youth (Garbarino, 1993).

Approximately 1.4 million youth enter the juvenile justice system each year (Office of Juvenile Justice and Delinquency Prevention, 2013). The prevalence of PTSD in incarcerated youth ranges from 24% (Burton et al., 1994) to 48.9% (Cauffman et al., 1998). In a population of sociopathic juvenile offenders on death row, Mallett (2003) found 60% were victims of abuse and neglect, 74% experienced family dysfunction, and 43% had a diagnosed psychiatric disorder. The neural structures required for memory, learning, wisdom, judgment, compassion, and empathy are not accessible because the cerebral cortex is the last part of the brain to develop and correlates with cognitive functioning (Sowell et al., 2001).

Any deviation in normal developmental milestones is possible, as the neural damage of abuse, neglect, and violence affects each child individually. Collectively, there appears to be a pattern of struggles common among a population of abused and traumatized children and teens. In addition to regulation problems, they appear anxious and guarded, have a defensive behavioral pattern, often have school and learning problems, have a persistent fear response, exhibit behavioral impulsivity, and have conduct problems described as being inattentive, overactive, hypersensitive, hypervigilant, disruptive, aggressive, oppositional, or antisocial (Perry et al., 1995; Pynoos & Nader, 1990; Pynoos et al., 1993).

Along with the pattern of symptoms, there is often a pattern of referrals for therapy that make transparent the etiology of the problems. Symptom presentation alone is not satisfactory information for developing treatment goals. Knowing the child's attachment history and history of previous trauma will help in developing an appropriate diagnosis and treatment plan.

> CASE NOTE: A 14-year-old boy with a history of severe neglect and physical abuse was arrested for hitting a peer whom he said was following him. The boy had been removed from his biological mother and father at age 2 after being found alone on a school playground, malnourished and with multiple bruises. His parents were addicted to methamphetamines. During the intervening years, he had been placed in fourteen foster homes. He had been removed from four of those homes because he was physically abused during his placement. His school performance was poor. He had been barred from several classes because of his highly aggressive and defiant behavior.

This is so very typical of the many cases presented in supervision or clinical practice. It is doubtful that this child had the opportunity to develop a secure attachment with his drug-addicted mother, causing a cascade of stress, deprivation, impaired brain and sensory development, and brain damage from a sustained high level of cortisol. A defensive behavioral pattern is to be expected from a child with such a terrifying and abusive history. This child had most likely been in a state of terror most of his life. His neural pathways developed very differently from those of a child who has been nurtured, comforted, protected, and loved. When children are deprived of a secure relationship with a primary caregiver or are persistently exposed to child abuse, neglect, and violence, the ensuing repetitive stress results in an altered neurochemical homeostasis. Bruce Perry (1995) describes this as "states becoming traits." The child's adaptation to stress makes it increasingly difficult for him or her to attain a state of homeostasis.

Ultimately and unfortunately, these children are likely to have increased adult psychopathology (Caron and Rutter, 2006) and are more prone to become abusive parents of their own offspring (Widom, 1989).

Vincent Felitti confirmed these negative outcomes in his research. He analyzed and documented the consequences of what he refers to as *adverse childhood effects* (ACE) in the home of a child. Later adult behavior is highly affected. Studies of persons from homes in which negative effects such as child abuse, substance abuse, or parental mental illness existed have revealed some alarming statistics. For example, a person with three or more ACEs in the home is 550% more likely to abuse alcohol, 900% more likely to engage in intravenous drug abuse, and 1200% more likely to attempt suicide (Felitti et al., 2010).

It is imperative that we continue to look carefully at the negative ramifications of child abuse in order to develop appropriate prevention and treatment strategies. We must also strive to increase public awareness of the effects of child abuse and violence on children and teens. It must become general knowledge that the negative effects of child abuse are staggering and have lifelong negative consequences for the victims, and by extension, for society.

CHAPTER 2

Treating Acute Traumatic Episodes:
A Brief Intervention for Integration

Although specifically trained mental health professionals respond to natural and manmade disasters, treatment for acute trauma is often overlooked (deVries et al., 1999). The intervention described in this chapter, developed in 1988, was in response to the identified need for a brief method of treating hospitalized children and teens with observable PTSD symptoms following acute trauma—in particular, those who were victims of urban community violence.

Early investigators identified urban trauma as a recurrent disease (Koop & Lundberg, 1992). In adults admitted for violent injuries within a six-month period, there was a 44 percent recidivism rate (Sims et al., 1989). Another study found a rate of 45 percent of recurrent, intentional injuries in a population ages 16 to 45 (Goins, Thompson, & Simpkins, 1992). The term "revolving door" was used to describe the phenomenon of those repeatedly admitted for a violent injury within a short period of time (Cooper et al., 2000). In a study of youth under age 25, of the 16 percent with a prior injury, 94 percent had been reinjured during the prior 5 years, and of those, 44 percent had sustained a gunshot wound (Tellez et al., 1995). Fortunately, many researchers were writing about the issue of youth and community violence (Bell, 1992; Bell & Jenkins, 1993; Garbarino et al., 1992; Osofsky, 1999; Chiland & Young, 1994; Pynoos & Nader, 1988, 1989; Pynoos et al., 1987). However, literature was scant about acute traumatic injuries in the population of violent youth.

The Chapman Art Therapy Treatment Intervention (CATTI) is designed to help children remember, express, and integrate acute traumatic episodes. It evolved from my clinical experience with injured youth in the hospital setting. For two decades, CATTI has been utilized successfully with pediatric patients by clinicians in the United States and Europe. Although originally created for hospitalized children and teens, the intervention has been adapted for other types of acute trauma.

HISTORY OF THE INTERVENTION

In 1987, music therapist Lois Friedlander and I received an offer to create and direct a pediatric therapy program at a large urban community hospital where 1,200 multicultural pediatric patients were being admitted each year. The patients ranged in age from infancy to 18. Seventy percent of the children and teens presenting for treatment at the pediatric service were trauma patients, admitted for gunshot wounds, stab wounds, other acts of violence, severe child abuse, unintentional injuries, motor vehicle crashes and pedestrian accidents, falls, and burns. The other 30 percent of the patients were admitted for acute and chronic childhood illnesses such as asthma, diabetes, sickle cell disease, and neglect.

Physicians recognized the need for early psychological intervention. Many of the children and teens exhibited a strong, defensive behavioral pattern, a grief reaction, and observable symptoms of PTSD. It was hoped that early intervention could reduce the PTSD symptoms and assist the children and teens with the development of adaptive coping mechanisms, thereby increasing compliance with their treatment plan and rehabilitation therapies. It was felt that early intervention would not only mitigate disruptions in normal development but also reduce the "revolving door" readmission and be a step toward prevention. Without in-patient trauma resolution therapy, it was unlikely these patients would receive follow-up therapy. There were few affordable alternatives, and of those, most had long wait lists.

The identified goal of reducing PTSD symptoms in the patients before they left the hospital presented unique challenges. Short-term therapy was not the norm, and many of the patients had short hospital admissions. Many of the young patients were experiencing the neurochemical dysregulation of a stress response, concurrent with the stress of hospitalization, physical injuries, technical devices, pain, and effects of medication.

Once Ms. Friedlander and I began the program, the children received psychological intervention from the time of admission until they left the hospital. The treatment included individual trauma resolution art therapy and/or play therapy, group art therapy, group play therapy, and milieu activity therapy. A graduate intern training program was initiated to recruit students. These interns provided patient services in exchange for training and supervision in medical art therapy and medical play therapy.

Child Life and psychiatry literature was useful for child development, medical play, and issues related to hospitalization and illness; however, no literature or guidance was available for the assessment and treatment of PTSD symptoms in pediatric trauma patients. No treatment protocols for short-term trauma resolution therapy existed, with the exception of *Witness to Violence: The Child Interview* (Pynoos & Eth, 1986), a drawing intervention utilizing an interview designed to treat children who witness violence.

Many of the children and teens exhibited avoidance symptoms. They refused to talk, eat, or ambulate. I began by offering children trauma resolution therapy at their bedside using structured art media such as colored pencils and markers and paper. As I anticipated, they readily, willingly, and easily portrayed their experience in visual form. When I encouraged patients to put a narrative with their drawings, they were able to verbally express their version of the traumatic experience by referring to their images. Learning from the children and teens how they perceived and expressed their traumatic experiences, I gradually shaped a protocol that contained troubling intrusive images, yet facilitated a coherent narrative of the event. The use of CATTI resulted in an immediate reduction in observable PTSD symptoms.

Surgeons, physicians, nurses, and mental health and rehabilitation therapists saw not only a reduction of observable PTSD symptoms but also increased compliance with care plans. It was determined that the intervention warranted documentation of its efficacy. An investigation of the actual incidence of PTSD symptoms in the patient population and an outcome study of the efficacy of CATTI in reducing PTSD symptoms was conducted by University of California San Francisco Injury Center for Research and Prevention and the Children's Hospital and Research Center in Oakland, California. The study was funded by a U.S. Centers for Disease Control Injury Prevention Grant (see the Appendix).

BRAIN ORGANIZATION

The brain consists of a hierarchy of three primary systems: the brainstem, the limbic system, and the cerebral cortex. The brainstem contains vital centers for survival, including cardiopulmonary functions, primary visual and auditory orientation, fundamental pathways for motor function, and neurochemical production centers.

The limbic system is primarily responsible for emotional experience and has a fundamental role in the formation of memories. The system includes the amygdala, hippocampus, thalamus, hypothalamus, and anterior cingulate and has an intimate connection with the pituitary gland. The amygdala is involved in interpreting emotional tone and instincts for fight/flight and approach/avoid. The hippocampus is the primary memory gateway and essential to the consolidation of implicit memory to explicit memory and learning. The thalamus is the brain's complex sensory relay center, and the hypothalamus is crucial for autonomic/endocrine functions that determine overall physiological homeostasis.

The cerebral cortex is made up of its right and left hemispheres, which are bridged by the corpus callosum. The cortex processes the vast range of higher cortical functions composing consciousness as attention, perception, reasoning, and complex memory and learning. The more elaborated and adaptive functional neuroanatomy underpinning these abilities has the capacity, or *neuroplasticity*, to reprogram in response to psychotherapy (Schore, 1999). The prefrontal cortex is the more anterior aspect of the cerebrum and subserves the most complex integration of mental functions, both intellectual and emotional.

Of particular relevance to the CATTI, the frontal lobes of the brain control impulses such as aggression. This part of the brain does not reach maturity until the late second or early third decade of life: "The evidence now is strong that the brain does not cease to mature until the early 20s in those relevant parts that govern impulsivity, judgment, planning for the future, foresight of consequences, and other characteristics that make people morally culpable" (Gur, 2002, p. 2).

INFORMATION PROCESSING AND TRAUMA

It is well established that traumatic sequelae are stored in the implicit memory of the right hemisphere (Achterberg & Lawlis, 1980; Schiffer et al., 1995; Siegel, 2001; Terr, 1995; van der Kolk, 1987; van der Kolk & Van der Hart, 1991). In trauma situations, the brain is primarily processing information visually (Terr, 1991; Tower, 1983), and thus the most common recall of traumatic imagery is in visual form (Cohn, 1993; Terr, 1991).

Proposed by Kagin and Lusebrink in 1978 (Hinz, 2009), the expressive therapies continuum (ETC), (Hinz, 2009; Lusebrink, 1990, 2004) is a conceptual model illustrating the increasing abstraction of image formation, visual information processing, and expression through art media. Based on the work of Bruner (1964) and Horowitz (1970), the ETC consists of four levels that delineate the formulation of images and how images facilitate an increasing complexity of expression from lower to higher structures of the brain. The four levels are

> Creative
>
> Symbolic/cognitive
>
> Affect/perceptual
>
> Kinesthetic/sensory

Adapting the visual information-processing aspect of the ETC for expression in PTSD treatment is consistent with a mind/body approach to treatment. *Kinesthetic/sensory* activities stimulate the lower structures of the right hemisphere, the somatic aspects of memory that activate the formulation of imagery and an awareness of internal sensations. Right-hemisphere visual representation of internal sensations is achieved through the body via rhythm and movement—nonverbal methods of expression.

In my clinical experience, following kinesthetic activity, the brain instinctively shifts information processing to the *affect/perceptual* level of processing. Emotions are expressed and released through the art media and, importantly, the person becomes aware of affect. Incoming stimuli, such as intrusive images, sensations, or memories, become better organized.

Cognitive/symbolic information processing emphasizes the intuitive aspects of concept formation. It involves cognition and allows for the generalization of concrete experience based on previous experiences. This level of information processing involves language, logic, analytical thought, and problem solving.

Lusebrink (1990) proposed that the *creative* level of information processing is a synthesis of all the levels through activation of the self-actualizing forces within an individual and yields creative expression leading to joy. In a trauma model, and in my experience, the creative level corresponds with integration and is evidenced by symptom reduction. Thus, activation of information in a manner that is consistent with brain development, and with information processing and cognition, increases the potential for integration and symptom reduction.

DESCRIPTION OF CHAPMAN ART THERAPY TREATMENT INTERVENTION

The four components of CATTI are described in detail in this chapter. Briefly, the intervention begins with a kinesthetic scribble, followed by the child drawing a sequential depiction of the event and a discussion about each drawing that extends to the child's perceptions of how he will adjust when he is released from the hospital. The child is then engaged in retelling the story while referring to his images. It is appropriate for the therapist to ask for clarification, to normalize physical and emotional reactions, and to respond to questions during this step. This results in immediate, observable symptom reduction of acute stress symptoms.

As can be seen in Table 2.1, the CATTI method is consistent with the flow of information processing from the lower to the higher structures.

CATTI is consistent with the neurochemical dysregulation of a stress response, the storage and retrieval of traumatic memories, and the psychological stages of the emotional reactions to trauma (Lee, 1970). This approach is designed for crisis-intervention trauma-resolution therapy in cases of mild to moderate acute traumatic experiences. Its main goal is to facilitate activation of the right hemisphere to create a nonverbal narrative of the patient's experience through drawings that can be translated into a verbal narrative of the event. CATTI serves as a

Table 2.1 Neurodevelopmental Art Therapy: CATTI

Neural Activity	Cognition	Visual Information Processing	Psychological Reactions	CATTI
Prefrontal	Abstract	Creative/integration	Reconstruction	Symptom reduction
Cerebrum	Abstract	Cognitive/symbolic	Acknowledgment	Retelling with images
Limbic	Emotional	Affect/perceptual	Retreat	Visual drawn narrative
Brain stem	Reflexive	Kinesthetic/sensory	Impact	Scribble

vehicle for expression and containment of the traumatic imagery, accessed in a way consistent with image formation and how such memories are brought to language (Bruner, 1964; Horowitz, 1970; Lusebrink, 1990) and explicit memory.

A specific linguistic manner and order is essential when requesting the drawn images. The structure of the drawing directive helps children contain, organize, and sequence traumatic memories. The right-hemisphere imagery may also elicit the child or teen's own unique trauma-specific fear (Terr, 1991). Retelling the story with the images enables the child or teen to discuss the event in greater detail. Normalizing his responses during this process relieves anxiety, worry, guilt, and shame. Specific issues are addressed in the retelling: misperceptions, shame, blame, guilt, fear, worry, rescue and revenge fantasies, coping, the patient's treatment plan, a follow-up treatment plan, traumatic reminders, and reintegration strategies for returning home or to school. CATTI addresses prognosis and assists the patient with devising adaptive coping mechanisms, preparing for rehabilitation therapies, learning about traumatic reminders (Pynoos, Steinberg, & Goenjian, 1996), and planning for possible future therapy (Pynoos, Steinberg, & Piacentini, 1999).

Before Beginning CATTI

CATTI is designed for use by master or higher-level clinicians, social workers, and psychologists who have a working knowledge of and experience with facilitating trauma-resolution therapy. Although specific art therapy training is not required to utilize the intervention, having some experience using drawings in therapy is helpful.

When facilitating CATTI in the medical setting, it is important to know as much as possible about what occurred during and following the patient's acute injury. It is essential to be cognizant of the extent of the child's or teen's injuries, past and future treatment plans, and prognosis, including specifics regarding a change in the use of, or function of, limbs or other body parts.

Some situations contraindicate the use of CATTI, including chronic injury, injuries requiring complicated medical treatment such as burns, child abuse, traumatic brain injury, and incident-based events that resulted in the death of another person. Additional exclusionary criteria include not having a complete understanding of the event, the treatment regimen, and the prognosis for recovery. There may be medical limitations that prevent the child from participating. There may be times when the child or teen is not well enough to participate willingly and comfortably. It is also important to check with the nursing staff before facilitating the intervention to find out whether doing so would interfere with the care plan or other treatment procedures.

Establishing Safety

In a hospital environment, there is limited opportunity for rapport-building sessions or the time required to develop a sense of trust. With acute trauma treatment, however, it is imperative to develop a sense of physical and psychological safety. To promote a feeling of physical safety, I reassure children that they can stop the intervention at any time if they become tired, if they have pain, or if their arm is tired of drawing. I also tell them they can ask to see their nurse, doctor, or parent at any time. I let children know I am aware of their injury and that I will be careful not to move fast or touch them.

To assure the child or teen of her psychological safety, I reassure her that she can draw any way she wishes, that she can use symbols or X's for people, and that the quality of drawing is not important. I also explain that she can ask for help with any drawing, can refuse to draw any picture requested, and can stop the session at any time. Giving the child full control over the intervention is effective. It is extremely rare for a child or teen to refuse to draw or to stop the intervention, even when stressed.

It is not necessarily detrimental to stop the intervention. However, the child will have a heightened awareness of the event and it is recommended that the therapist bring the narrative to a place of closure.

Facilitating CATTI

The CATTI intervention requires simple, structured media. It is designed to be completed in one session of approximately 50–70 minutes. The following art materials are required: several sheets of 11- by 18-inch drawing paper, a spectrum of eight markers, a #2 pencil with an eraser, and a box of tissues (tears are common).

Following introductions and initial rapport building, I ask the patient to participate in CATTI. I describe it as making a story with drawings about their experience and about being in the hospital. Before beginning, I ask if they have any physical pain or drawing limitations, such as blurred vision from medication. If not, I arrange the drawing materials on a smooth surface usually at the bedside, or in the playroom, in a one-to-one session. CATTI should not be facilitated in a group setting.

Scribble Drawing

The child is offered the markers and pencil and is asked, "Would you please pick one of these?" He is told, "The first picture is a warm-up. I will say 'Go,' and I would like you to scribble like this [therapist demonstrates gross motor movement] until I say stop." The child scribbles on the paper for 15–30 seconds—less if he appears fatigued or chooses to stop—and is then instructed, "Please stop."

The child's ability to pick a color and scribble is a no-fail, no-risk method to engage the child in the drawing process. This nonthreatening kinesthetic experience offers some initial rapport building with a safe, enjoyable experience with the media. It involves a minimum of effort and allows assessment of the child's physical ability to participate in the art therapy intervention. The sensory and kinesthetic experience activates the right hemisphere of the brain, where traumatic memories are stored (Schiffer et al., 1995). The kinesthetic scribble stimulates the awareness of internal sensations, stimulates the formulation of internal images, and releases defensive and anxious energy through body movement and rhythm (Lusebrink, 1990). This may be reflected in physical reactions such as smiles, loud sighs, or an increase in motor movement.

When the scribble drawing is completed, the child or teen is asked, "Did you like to scribble?" or "Do you remember drawing like this when you were little?" This questioning stimulates the recall of sensations and formulates images. It is this subcortical, bilateral activity that activates visual, kinesthetic, and sensory neural pathways. I turn the scribble page face down, indicating that it is the first in a stack of drawings.

Event Drawing

Following the scribble, a second paper is readied. The child is asked, "Would you please draw a picture of what happened, why you had to come to the hospital?" The request is in the form of a question to allow the child to refuse. Also, the question is asked in two parts to allow the child access to the imagery, which may be traumatic, followed by an immediate awareness that he is in the hospital and that the event is in the past. Based on my clinical experience, this eliminates psychobiological reactions that are activated in the form of body sensations and reexperiencing phenomena such as a flood of images of blood, bones, or other injured body parts.

After the child has drawn the event and indicates he is finished, I turn the paper face down and place it on top of the scribble drawing. If the child or teen elects to begin talking about the drawing, I use active listening to convey understanding and validate his reactions as normal responses to what he has experienced. However, most children do not talk about the drawings at this time.

Helper Drawing

I offer a new sheet of paper and ask the child, "Please draw what happened next, who came along to help." Note that the child is not asked *if* she will draw the helper but rather is instructed to do so. This subtle change is designed to facilitate completion of the coherent narrative. It is important for the child to acknowledge that she has received help and that the event is in the past.

What Happened Next Drawing

After the child has drawn the helper drawing, it is turned face down on the earlier drawings, a new sheet of paper is presented, and the patient is told, "Please draw what happened next." This open-ended directive is designed to elicit the child's unique perceptions. Often what surfaces is the patient's trauma-specific fear (Terr, 1991). At this time, children typically draw an image that relates to their own unique perceptions of, or issues relating to, the event, their transport to the hospital, hospitalization, treatment, and prognosis. Some children do not recall details but only remember coming to the hospital and waking up in bed. If this is the case, and the child desires additional information, the therapist offers to draw (not tell) the child what has occurred.

Most children want to know what occurred during the time they were unaware. The therapist may draw general information, such as transport to the hospital, the visit to the emergency department, getting x-rays or a CT scan, surgery, and the recovery room. I generally draw squares on a paper, void of details, to indicate each room, with the goal of completing the missing parts of the narrative. Filling in these gaps helps the child complete his narrative. I take care to avoid giving any specific information about what occurred in those locations, such as suturing, pinning bones, or removing bullets. The child or teen's physician or nurse should be called on if the patient has specific questions about medical issues.

When the child stops asking questions, it is an indication that he has as much information as he can handle. Children need time to integrate that information before they seek additional details.

I do not correct misperceptions at this time unless the child has a psychobiological or other negative reaction, such as panic, anxiety, or fear. If a strong reaction does occur, correcting the misperception will offer new information that can minimize or contain the reaction.

> CASE NOTE: A 17-year-old male was admitted to the hospital following a gunshot wound to the abdomen. While engaged in CATTI, he was drawing his transport to the hospital and going to surgery. He panicked and began yelling, "Those doctors stole my gold! They stole my gold necklaces and I am going to have to get them for that."
>
> I responded, "Hold it. Not true. Your gold necklaces were removed before you went to surgery. They were placed in a sealed envelope with your name and kept with hospital security staff. Before you leave the hospital, you can pick up your personal belongings."
>
> The youth said, "Oh. I thought they stole my gold." He calmed down and we continued with the intervention.

I continue to offer new sheets of drawing paper and request, "Please draw what happened next" until the child or teen brings the images to the present, which is typically a drawing of him in bed waiting to go home.

Most children draw five or six pictures. Children with severe injuries that require extensive treatment regimens sometimes draw images depicting various aspects of their treatment. Others recall earlier memories during the retelling portion of the intervention and add those images. Occasionally, children will add drawings to their narrative after completing CATTI that reflect additional stages of their hospitalization. This is helpful to those who use their CATTI drawings to educate others about their experience.

CASE NOTE: A 7-year-old girl was hospitalized following a car crash resulting in extensive injuries to her leg that required her to go to a rehab facility after her acute hospitalization. Following her successful participation in CATTI, she continued to draw images depicting different aspects of her surgeries and treatment. As she prepared for transfer to the rehab facility she said, "I am glad I have my story in pictures so I don't have to tell everybody at the new hospital over and over about it. I can just have them look at my drawings."

Leaving and Coping Drawing

Once the child has completed a drawing depicting her in the present, she is offered a final sheet of paper and told, "Please draw what it will be like when the doctor lets you go home." This offers an opportunity to learn about the child's imagined course after leaving the hospital and being at home with injuries or pain: how she will cope, and how she sees herself reintegrating into daily living activities.

Retelling

When all the drawings are complete, I say that I would like the child to tell me the story that goes with the drawings. I show her the scribble and describe it as a warm-up activity. I then place the event drawing in front of her and ask, "Would you please tell me this part of the story?" Care must be taken not to ask the child to talk about anything but the image. For example, asking the child or teen, "Can you tell me about the accident?" may cause her to have visual images of the scene of the event, rather than focus on the drawn image. Also, it is not easy to respond with verbal cognition at this time, as the image is from the nonverbal right hemisphere. The concrete image on the paper allows the child to objectify the images, creating distance and allowing her to speak about an external event, rather than an internal one. This objectification of the image eliminates the flooding of disturbing images and sensations.

Careful attention is paid to what the child talks about, what she avoids mentioning, the terminology she uses to describe the event and the perpetrator, and her thoughts, feelings, and perceptions about the event. All questioning is focused on the image, with careful monitoring of the child's physical and psychological reactions to the dialogue associated with each image.

Typically, children will exhibit an affective response such as sadness, anger, or frustration as they describe the image of the event. The affective response is consistent with limbic system processing that occurs following kinesthetic activity. Affect precedes cognition (Chapman, 2001; Jung, 1916; Shelby & Tredinnick, 1995). The affective response is normalized by letting the child or teen know that his response is like that of others who have gone through what he has experienced. Allow for many silent pauses as the child identifies body sensations, expresses feelings, grieves, or formulates a response. For example, a response to a child crying while describing being hit by a vehicle might be, "When kids are hit by a car they have sad feelings and it is okay to cry. Bodies are designed to let those feelings out."

During the drawing of the event or the verbal narrative process, it is common for patients to report psychobiological reactions: smells, sounds, tastes, physical sensations, or pain. They may demonstrate autonomic nervous system responses: wide eyes, shallow breathing, and sweaty palms. Comments helpful to the child at this time include, "Your body is remembering right now when you tell me this, and it is normal," which facilitates affect regulation. If the child is experiencing pain, simple pain-reduction techniques using imagery are offered: "Take a deep breath and blow the pain away." The discomfort usually abates rapidly, as it is a response to the material being recalled. Many children and teens have reported they are relieved to learn that their body is "remembering." The physical sensations or unusual responses can be confusing and sometimes terrifying. Patients have said, "It made me afraid to talk about it," and, "I thought I was going crazy."

If there is a perpetrator in the image—a person, a car, an animal for instance— the patient is asked if there is anything he would like to say to the perpetrator. Be careful to use the exact language of the child when describing the perpetrator. The verbalizations associated with this aspect of the image often elicit anger, sadness, rescue fantasies, or revenge fantasies, as will be seen in case examples.

Shame, blame, and guilt may be represented by changes in behavior, included in the drawings, or expressed during the patient's verbalizations (Feiring, Taska, & Chen, 2002; Lansky, 1991). It is important to reassure patients that they have not done anything bad to cause the event to occur. For example, when a child hit by a car relates that she ran into the street, her perception that she is not supposed to run into the street should be validated. But when the therapist points out that the law states that people who drive cars are supposed to drive slowly enough to be able to stop when children are present, children show relief with loud sighs, smiles, or verbal comments. Some indicate it was "their biggest worry." When their misperceptions are corrected, children are relieved of their feelings of shame, blame, and guilt.

Shame and guilt, functions of the frontal cortex, are often expressed during the retelling portion of the intervention because the higher structures of the brain have become engaged. When told by an adolescent, "I feel guilty because I was shooting at people too," the therapist can address the issue indirectly by stating simply, "Tell me more." As the therapist repeats "Tell me more," the adolescent can move from a defensive retreat to acknowledgment of his role, and then on to a discussion of the future and how he will avoid danger.

More commonly, though, adolescents blame someone else for their violent injuries. A teen cannot be told he is not at fault if he is a perpetrator. The therapist can shift the focus of the discussion to their living or school environment, or past insults, or abuse that has influenced their choices and their methods of behaving, protecting, and coping.

Rescue fantasies are commonly expressed in the belief that if the child had done something differently, he could have avoided the traumatic event altogether or stopped a perpetrator. Reality testing is helpful to alleviate shame, guilt, and remorse for not having been able to protect or rescue oneself or others. I may ask, in response to a child's wish that he could have taken a gun from a perpetrator of violence, "Do you think a boy your size could take a gun away from a big, tall person who is mad and mean and scary?"

Revenge fantasies are also common (Pynoos & Eth, 1984). The younger child often expresses extreme revenge fantasies that abate once the underlying emotions are validated and reality testing is utilized. The patient may require help to discriminate between what is possible or feasible, right and wrong. The adolescent's revenge fantasies are more serious. Teens have action-oriented coping mechanisms and, often, the means to carry out their revenge fantasies. Adolescents are encouraged to talk about their fantasies when the therapist uses the phrase "Tell me more." This is repeated until they stop, or until the higher, prefrontal structures of the brain are engaged and they begin to discuss possible outcomes of their proposed revenge.

During the intervention, many adolescents realize they should not carry out revenge fantasies because of the perceived negative consequences—that is, the fear of retaliation or the wrong kids being killed. They may display feelings of remorse. This demonstrates the neurologically informed premise on which CATTI is based. The higher frontal function has been activated, resulting in a systematic assessment of the traumatic material in a manner consistent with the brain's integrative capacity and how images are translated to cognition. It allows the child to psychologically progress through the power of the imagery (right brain) and language (left brain) to create a coherent narrative that transforms his neurochemistry, promoting a higher form of consciousness about the event. This is reflected in the child's ability to translate the experience into language (Siegel, 1994) and to move to the higher structures of the brain that have the neuroplasticity to change as a result of psychotherapy (Schore, 1999). Combining images with language accesses the prefrontal functions of compassion, wisdom, and judgment. This is evidenced in the child's verbalizations about the event and alterations in behavior. Of course, if an adolescent reveals a plan to harm another, reporting laws apply. In my clinical experience of addressing revenge fantasies hundreds of times while using CATTI, I have never once had to report potential harm to self or others.

Note that the child and therapist review and retell the entire story together. It is important to make accurate references to details, events, and people in the child's story and to allow time for the patient to intervene with additional details or verbalizations about the images, event, self, or others. The child may want to draw additional images, as he is desensitized to the trauma and can often remember and comprehend the depth and breadth of his experience in greater detail.

Closure

Finally, the therapist offers information about traumatic reminders (Pynoos, Steinberg, & Goenjian, 1996). The child is educated about sights, smells, sounds, and experiences that may recall the feelings or physical sensations she has or may have had about the event.

The child or teen is assisted in devising developmentally appropriate coping mechanisms. The school-age child hit by a car will express a specific fear associated with the event, such as of crossing the street again. Utilizing problem-focused coping skills, the child will solve the problem by creating a plan of how to overcome the fear. The child may devise a strategy in which she has control over who walks with her one day, then the next.

The adolescent, with action-oriented coping mechanisms, readily responds to action-oriented therapy techniques to literally act out various possible situations that may occur. For example, the therapist and the teen may role-play saying no to peer pressure to participate in behaviors that may result in additional injuries and hospitalization. Most important, it depathologizes the adolescent and replaces the perceived pathology with information that aids in formulating an understanding of feelings, thoughts, and ideas instead of defending the teen's normal omnipotent and narcissistic stance. The importance of future, possibly sporadic, therapy is presented, along with information for future contacts for evaluation and treatment.

CASE EXAMPLES

The following three case examples will illustrate the facilitation of CATTI. The first case demonstrates the use of the intervention with a very young child, the second case features a school-age child, and the third case focuses on an adolescent. CATTI has been used successfully with individuals across the developmental spectrum. I have used the intervention with children as young as 2 and with adults as old as a woman in her 80s.

Intervention with a Toddler

CASE NOTE: M. is a 3-year-old girl who sustained numerous skin and scalp lacerations following a mauling by a Japanese Akita dog. She required surgery and hundreds of stitches on her numerous wounds. In the hospital, M. was irritable, had severe sleep disturbances, exhibited gaze aversion, and was withdrawn. When medically able, M. was brought to the playroom. She started exploring the toys in a chaotic manner. I sat at a small table and began to make random marks on a sheet of drawing paper, developmentally matching her skill level. She ran to the table and began making random marks on a paper. After several of these drawings, her motor activity and body posture changed. She hunched over the table with her nose inches away from the paper. Her teeth were clenched and bared. She drew a large orange spot with great intensity. When she stopped and looked at me, I commented, "I see you are making a big orange one." She replied, "That's the dog. "

I asked M. if she would like to make a picture about the dog and what had happened to her. She nodded affirmatively. I placed a sheet of 11- by 18-inch drawing paper in front of her and she proceeded to make large, yellow strokes back and forth across the paper as she tearfully related the story of the dog mauling and her terror. She sobbed, "I wanted my mommy." I responded, "That is what happens when girls get bit by a dog. They cry and they want their mommy." After a few moments, she stopped crying. I asked, "Can you draw what happened next, who came along to help?" She drew more yellow lines back and forth across the paper as she described the ambulance and the firetruck, her transport to the hospital, and the doctors. After a long pause, she said, "That dog has to move." M.'s mother told me earlier that the dog had been shot by the owner. I replied, "We must ask mommy about the dog moving." Together we went to M.'s hospital room and asked M.'s mother to return with us to the playroom. The child said to her mother, "The dog has to move." The mother informed her daughter that the dog had already moved and would never be returning. M. stood up, folded her arms, and said, "I got my story and now I will play toys." I asked her if we could tell the story one more time and she agreed. As I showed her the yellow image consisting of lines drawn, she calmly related her story.

After a 40-minute session, M. was symptom-free, talking, eating, and playing with her mother and other children. She did not exhibit any further symptoms of avoidance or sleep disturbance.

Consistent with her level of development, M.'s verbalizations were about people, places, and things, not feelings, thoughts, and ideas (Hewitt, 1999). Since her cognition was concrete, my comments about her drawing were also concrete, "I see you are making a big orange one." My motivation to make this statement was in response to her body: face close to the paper, tension in her muscles, bared teeth, and intense scribbling in one spot. Her drawings were motor driven, so I did not expect her to create images of the dog or ambulance.

The kinesthetic experience of scribbling activated the right hemisphere where images are stored. She immediately had a visual image of the dog, as illustrated when she created the intense orange spot on the paper and identified it as the dog. Her brain shifted the process to the limbic structures as evidenced in the outpouring of emotion as she drew the yellow lines on the paper and tearfully described the attack. My normalizing comments kept her in the present time. I assured her that her responses were normal. Her shift to cognition was evident in her announcement that the dog must move. To a 3-year-old child, if the dog moved, she would not have to worry about being bitten again, an adaptive coping mechanism. There was evidence of cognition when she used this experience to generalize about her future safety and avoiding another such encounter.

Through the activation of the traumatic story in a manner that is consistent with neurological development and information processing (Bruner, 1964; Horowitz, 1970; Lusebrink, 1990), M. had created a coherent narrative about the event that allowed her to integrate the experience, as evidenced in the complete reduction of symptoms and her return to her usual behavior and activity level. Psychologically, the event is in the past.

Intervention with a School-Age Child

CASE NOTE: 10-year-old T. was admitted following a compound fracture of his femur after being hit by a car while he was a pedestrian. He stepped off the curb when the light changed; the driver ran a red light, hit the child, and drove away from the scene. In the hospital, T. was withdrawn, exhibited gaze aversion, and would not talk. His affect was sad, but he willingly participated in CATTI. He began with a scribble, then drew the event with a firetruck, ambulance, and several people in the image. The helper image contained an ambulance, several people, and a man holding his leg. The next image was a drawing of him going to surgery with his mother at his side. The next image was of him in bed waiting to go home. His last drawing of what it would be like when he got home consisted of him sitting in a wheelchair in front of a TV.

When I showed T. the image of the event and asked him to please tell me this part of the story, he immediately burst into tears and stated, "I was on the corner and this lady just drove over me and hit me. She drove away and left me in the street." As he cried, I quietly told him it was normal to be sad, as that is what happens when someone hits you with a car and drives away. I waited quietly as he grieved. When he stopped, I reassured him it was normal to feel sad when drawing and talking about the accident. After he was comfortable, I asked him if he saw the lady in the car, and he said yes, she was from another country. I asked if he could place her in the picture, and he drew her as the driver of the car. I asked if there was anything he wanted to say to her, and he said, "Yes. Why were you driving so fast and why did you drive away?" I asked him if he knew the answer to his question, and he stated, "She didn't like me." I reality-tested by asking if he knew the lady and that she didn't like him. He replied quietly, "No. Why do you think she hit me and drove away?" I replied, "Maybe she was afraid of the police, maybe she was drinking alcohol or doing drugs, but the most important thing is that it is not your fault and you did not do anything bad to cause it to happen." T. smiled broadly and said enthusiastically, "Oh, thank you. Thank you."

I then pointed to the image of him lying in the street and asked, "Do you remember what you were thinking or feeling when you were lying here?" He replied, "I wanted my mom." I reassured him, "When boys are in pain and afraid, they want their moms. I am sorry you had to wait until you got to the hospital to see your mom, but I am glad she was there." I asked if there was anything else he wanted to say to the lady, and he said, "Yes, you are a dumb, bad, stupid lady and I hate you!" I replied, "You are feeling mad at the lady who hit you. That is what boys feel when they get hit by someone. The lady might not be a bad lady, but the lady did do a bad thing. She drove away after hitting you with her car and that is a bad thing."

After a few moments, I showed T. the image of the helper and asked him to tell this part of the story. He described the scene and the people in the image. When I asked if he remembered what he was thinking or feeling while pointing to the depiction of him in the image, he said, "I was scared and in pain and afraid of dying." I reassured him, "It is normal to feel scared, and afraid of dying. I am glad the helpers came and brought you to the hospital where the doctors are. They helped you with your pain and are now helping your leg get better." After a long pause, T. asked, "Do other kids worry about having their leg, you know, cut off?" I replied, "Yes, other boys with a broken leg have been worried about losing their leg. Are you worried about that?" T. replied, tearfully, "Yes, my granny had her leg cut off and then she died." I responded, "You are worried about your broken leg because your granny lost her leg and died. Your leg is broken, and the doctor has set it inside the cast and the bone is knitting back together. You are not going to have your leg cut off and you are not going to die. Were you worried you might die?" T. tearfully replied, "Yes, I thought I might die." I replied, "It is normal to cry and it is normal to worry you might die. Your leg is broken, and the doctor has set it inside the cast and the bone is knitting back together. You are not going to have your leg cut off and you are not going to die." T. sighed loudly. His shoulders dropped and he stopped crying. After a pause, I asked if there was anything else to say about this part of the story and he did not have any other comments.

After a few moments, I showed him the next image of the story of him in bed waiting to go home. I asked him to tell this part of the story and he said, "I woke up after surgery and then my family came and I was glad to see them and my brother. Then my doctor came and told me I would be able to go to someplace to walk on crutches and then go home." I replied, "You were happy to see your family, and the doctor told you about learning to walk on crutches and about going home."

I pointed to the boy in the bed in the image and asked, "Do you know what you think or feel when you wait to learn crutches and to go home?" T. replied, "I worry about going to school. I worry I will get hit again because I will not be able to run with a cast." I replied, "You are worried about school, and getting hit again, and that is normal and what other kids worry about, too. You are right, you cannot run with a cast, and that is why you will have help and have extra time to get from place to place so you will not have to run. Your mom and your aunt plan to help you get to and from school, and you will have extra help and time at school with a cast." T. let out a loud "Whew!" upon learning this information. I then added, "And when you are on the street near where you got hit, it is normal for your body to remember and you might feel scared, worried, and not want to cross the street. Your mom will help you get used to doing that over time. Each day it will get a bit easier." T. said loudly, "Whew!" I asked if he had anything else to add to this part of the story or any other questions, and he did not.

After a moment, I showed him the last picture of himself, in a wheel-chair in front of the TV. I asked T. to tell me this part of the story and he said, "I am home watching my TV, and since I can't walk, everyone will have to do things for me, like get me something to eat." I asked if he knew what he would be thinking or feeling when he was home and pointed to his image of himself in the drawing. T. said, "I will be bored, but everyone will be around to get things for me so I won't be too much bored." I replied, "You think you will be a little bit bored but everyone will be there to wait on you and keep you company." T. said, "Yes," to which I replied, "Well, T., that usually happens for about one day, and then everyone will get busy with what they do and might not have as much time to help you be enter-tained as you may think. Perhaps we can come up with some things you can do when you are alone. And, when you learn to walk with crutches, you will be able to walk so you won't need everyone to wait on you past the first day or so." T. said, "Yeah, you are right that I will be walking and then my leg will get better and I will be just like my dad, who had a broken leg and now you can't see his blood or his bone and he can walk." I agreed, "Yes, you will be able to do most things for yourself and your leg will be better just like your Dad's leg." I asked if he had anything else he wanted to say, and he did not. As the nurse entered the room, T. told her, "I got hit by a car and it is not my fault and my leg will get better and I will be able to walk."

In this case note, many important misperceptions and fears arose in the retell-ing of the story. We moved from kinesthetically activating the right hemisphere and facilitated a nonverbal narrative that can be put into words. Note the fear of loss of body parts and fear of dying. Normalizing the patient's responses creates a space for him to ask other questions. Note that I corrected T's misperception that the lady was a bad lady. I pointed out that it was the lady's behavior that was bad, not the lady. I did not want him to think of people from other countries as bad people who run over children and leave them lying in the street. It is the behav-ior that is bad, not the person. I did not change my language from "bad" when describing the behavior of the lady, because it is important to use the language of the child to validate his intense affect. I also corrected his misperception about going to school alone and helped with anticipatory anxiety and the development of adaptive coping mechanisms.

Intervention with an Adolescent

CASE NOTE: L. is a 14-year-old boy hospitalized after sustaining a gunshot wound to the abdomen, a result of community violence. He was withdrawn and mute, and he refused to cooperate with law enforcement professionals investigating the case. I invited him to participate in creating a story about his injury and hospitalization with the usual preparation and offered him full control over the experience. He agreed and made a scribble drawing. He then drew an image of the event, depicting himself lying on the street next to a car. He added several human figures, one holding a gun on the other side of the sidewalk, and a trajectory of bullets going from the gun into his body.

The drawing of the helper contained an image of himself lying on a gurney being put in an ambulance. The next image was of him lying on his hospital bed watching television with a visitor. The last image consisted of him standing upright on the left side of the page and two human figures on the right side of the page.

Invited to comment on the image of the event, he stated, "I was standing on the corner minding my own business and these guys came around and started shooting at me and my friends. I got shot, and I tried to run away but I couldn't and I had to lie down by the car." I responded, "You were on the corner minding your own business when someone started shooting, and you were shot and tried to run but had to lie down by the car." He said, "Yes, and my friends stayed there with me after those guys ran away." I said, "Your friends were there. It is normal to want your friends with you when you are hurt, and I am glad your friends stayed with you." I pointed to the image of him by the car and asked L. if he remembered what he was thinking or feeling when he was lying next to the car. He replied, "Yes, I was in pain and I was afraid of dying." I said, "It is normal to feel pain and be afraid of dying when you are shot and lying in the street. I am glad you are not going to die." L. said, "Me too." He did not have anything else to say about that image. I showed him the image of the helper and asked him to tell this part of the story. He began, "I was lying in the street and then the cops came and the ambulance came and they took me to the hospital in an ambulance." I said, "So someone called for help and the ambulance came and brought you to the hospital. I am glad you were brought to the hospital right away." Pointing to the person on the gurney, I asked if he remembered what he was thinking or feeling when he was lying on the gurney. L. said, "I was in pain, and I was scared of dying." L. began to get tears in his eyes. I quietly said, "It is okay to let that out. Your body is responding to the emotions inside that want to get out." He cried briefly then stopped. I said, "I just want you to know that it is completely normal for you to be in pain and scared and afraid of dying when you are being put in ambulance after being shot. That is how most teens feel when they get shot." He sighed loudly and his shoulders dropped.

He did not have anything else to say about that image, so I showed him the next drawing in the series. He said, "This is me in the hospital. I've never been in the hospital before. I don't know when I will go home." I replied, "You have never been in the hospital and this image is you waiting to go home when you are better." L. said, "Yeah." I then asked if he knew what he thought or felt while lying in bed waiting to go home and he replied, "Yeah, I think about getting out of here and going home and I think about my friends and how we have to get those guys who shot me. They shot me and my friends." I said, "That is how teens feel when they get shot. They want to get even, so it is a completely normal feeling to have after being shot. Tell me more." L. replied, "Yeah, that is right because if you shoot at me and my friends, we are going to shoot at you back." I said, "Tell me more." L. said, "That is why kids get shot is because we all have to get even." I said, "Tell me more." L. said, "Well then if we shoot those kids then . . . wait . . . then those kids will shoot us . . . wait . . . when will it ever stop?" I said, "You feel like you want to shoot those guys but then you realize they will shoot more kids like you." L. replied, "Yes, then it will never stop. Wait a minute." L. got up, opened the door, and said to his visiting peers lined up in the hallway, "You guys don't go out tonight to try to shoot those guys who did this to me and I will tell you why in a bit. Just wait and don't go and shoot anybody." L. returned to the table and said, "If we keep shooting more kids, then more kids will keep getting shot and then more kids will die like I almost died." I said, "You don't want to shoot more kids because it will never stop and more kids will die." L. said, "Yes, that is how I see it." I asked if there was anything else he wanted to say about that image, and he did not.

I showed him the last drawing, and he pointed to the single figure and said, "That is me at home and these are my friends asking me to go out but I am not going because I don't want to get shot again." I said, pointing to the image, "Your friends want you to go out with them, but you don't want to go out because you don't want to get shot again." L. replied, "Yeah, I don't want to go through this again man, because, I don't want to be in pain again." I said, "You don't want to go because you want to be safe from getting shot and having to go through pain again." L. said, "Yeah." I said, "Let's try it out. Stand up, and I will too, and I am going to pretend to be your friend asking you to come out, and you try to tell me no, that you are afraid of getting shot again." We engaged in a role-play and he began meekly saying no and I kept pushing him by saying, "Oh, so you are afraid of those guys now?" and "Oh, so now you want to stay in and hide instead of fight?" After a few moments, he became more forceful and after several minutes, he was loudly saying, "I am not going to go out and maybe get shot! You don't know what it is like to have that pain, and a chest tube, and I don't care. I am not going to be like this again!" I quietly respond, "That sounds like you mean no."

I talk with teens about how practice will make it easier when they face their friends. I ask if they have any questions. I let them know I will be back to check in later and thank them for sharing their very important story with me, and I tell them that I am glad they are safe and alive.

Here is an example of the incredible ability to reach the higher structures of the brain through imagery and with bottom-to-top processing of information. The youth was able to access the prefrontal cortex and judgment, consequences, and wisdom. It was this aspect of CATTI that qualified the intervention for funding for research into the prevention of violence.

More than one teen has returned to the hospital to get staples removed and has tracked me down in the hospital to tell me, "I am glad we practiced that thing about going out with friends." Having the experience of saying no rather than just thinking about it allows for a faster and stronger response when faced by their friends. Their cognitive responses are now connected to their body-based emotions.

CATTI OUTCOME DATA

The CATTI was investigated in a randomized, controlled trial at University of California–San Francisco Injury Center and the Children's Hospital & Research Center in Oakland, California. The children were pretested for PTSD symptoms and posttested one month, three months, and six months after the intervention. The control group received normal and usual hospital care that included Child Life and art therapy services. Although the symptoms were reduced in all three PTSD symptom clusters described in the *DSM-IV*, there was a significant reduction only in avoidance symptoms from baseline to one month after treatment.

Three supporting and interesting facts were derived from the correlational data. The first was that 89 percent of the children completed the narrative of their experience, indicating that children are willing and able to depict their stories immediately after an acute traumatic event. In the second finding, anxiety was observed in 94 percent of the subjects. After CATTI, 83 percent experienced a decrease in anxiety. Third, 67 percent of the subjects had a misperception that was corrected during CATTI, and it correlated with the presence of an ANS response. This may indicate that a misperception may contribute to a child's stress following an acute event. This finding is indicative of the importance of offering children a nonverbal way to express *their* perception of an event (see the Appendix).

Dr. Lenore Terr (1991) is accurate in her conclusion that children do have a trauma specific fear. In my clinical experience, misperceptions are often associated with that fear, or they arise in the nonverbal images created for their narrative of the event.

As with all investigations, replication of this study is needed. There were many problems with it, including significant errors in the randomization, lack of a determined effect size, and a small sample size. The intervention was designed to reduce observable PTSD symptoms in the acute care setting. Re-testing study participants for PTSD symptoms at future monthly intervals presents challenges, as it is difficult to control for the exposure to other traumatic events that may have occurred, and the attrition rate for retesting is often high.

GLOSSARY OF TERMS

This section identifies words and phrases used when applying the Chapman Art Therapy Treatment Intervention model. It is divided into four parts: medical considerations, physical responses, emotional responses, and cognitive considerations. Examples of ways to respond are suggested.

Medical Considerations

Always check with medical providers prior to the facilitation of any intervention to be certain your treatment does not conflict or interfere with the medical treatment plan. Some aspects of the CATTI may be contraindicated medically. For example, if a child has a chest tube, do not use "deep breath" as an intervention without approval. Or, if the child is NPO (no food or liquids), do not offer juice or water to abate recalled taste sensations.

Deep breath   Breathe slowly, inhaling through the nose, and exhaling through the mouth. I refer to this as a "signal breath" for use when necessary. Do no more than three breaths without a rest.

Pain reduction techniques   Art media and image techniques are utilized to reduce pain. Examples of pain reduction techniques are, in the typical order used:

1. Ask the child to take a deep breath and blow the pain away (usually works) and repeat, slowly, up to three times.
2. Have the child draw the pain, then illustrate how he can make the pain go away (child must alter image).
3. Ask the child what would make the pain go away, and do what he suggests.
4. Request a pain evaluation from the medical staff.

Reassure the child and normalize his response   Nearly all of a therapist's responses during CATTI are intended to merely remind the child or teen that his reactions are normal and typical of anyone who has experienced a similar traumatic event. Avoid eliciting additional information about other traumatic experiences or asking if he has experienced such a response previously.

Reframing with imagery   Reframing is a method of using art media and imagery to stop flooding of intrusive imagery. If a child is flooded with a vision of blood and bone as a result of viewing a compound fracture, I would use art media to quickly draw the bone in place inside a cast and tell the child or teen that this is her bone now. This will immediately stop the flooding, as the reframing is in the visual mode. It is difficult to stop the flooding by switching from visual to verbal reframing of the image.

Physical Responses

Sighs   Most sighs are associated with relaxation, the release of tension and relief from anxiety. Many children sigh after misperceptions are corrected about their body integrity and upon learning that they are not at fault for the incident.

> *Suggested response:* "I noticed you let out a big breath; do you have a feeling or thought that goes with that big breath?" If the child states she is relieved to know the event was not her fault, restate your comment: "You are relieved to know the accident was not your fault" or "You are relieved to know there is nothing you could have done to prevent the accident."

If the child has no feeling or thought associated with the sigh, do not suggest how she *might feel*.

Intrusive images   Flooding of imagery is not typical, as the imagery is contained graphically on paper and externalized, but sometimes a child may have a flashbulb memory (Terr, 1995).

> *Suggested response:* "Sometimes our memories come in pictures or sounds. When you have had a traumatic experience, it is normal to have pictures or thoughts come into your mind when you don't expect them."

Smells   Although rare, some children report olfactory recollections.

> *Suggested response:* "You smell the same smells you smelled at the accident. Your body is remembering the smell and that happens when you have been in an accident."

Asking the child to take a deep breath and blow the smell away usually stops the olfactory sensation. If not, ask the child what would make the smell go away.

Tastes   It is rare for children to have taste sensations; however, sometimes they do recall the taste of blood.

> *Suggested response:* "Your body is remembering the same taste you tasted at the accident, and that sometimes happens after an accident."

Asking the child to take a deep breath and blow the taste away usually stops the taste sensation. If not, ask the child what would make the taste go away.

Tears   Nearly every session utilizing CATTI results in some form of grief reaction prompting tears. Tears usually arise when the child describes the event (drawing #2) but may occur at any time during the intervention.

Suggested response: Reassure the child that his response is normal. "It is okay to cry; that is what happens to boys when they get hit by a car. Your mind and your body are not separate, and they both remember as we talk about it. Your body is designed to release those tense and sad feelings by crying. Just let it out, because your body is doing what it needs to do to make you feel better."

Psychobiological reaction   When describing imagery pertaining to the body, many children will reexperience the injury or physical pain associated with the event. For example, when describing being hit by a car, many children will grab their leg and cry out in pain.

Suggested response: "Feeling [describe sensation in the words of the patient] in your body is normal, as your body is remembering when you draw or talk about what happened. It is completely normal. To get rid of the pain, take a deep breath, hold it for a few seconds, and blow the pain out when you let the air out your mouth."

This typically stops the pain episode. If this fails, I draw the broken bone or other area of the body in a repaired state and explain how the body is healing just as in the drawn image.

Increase in pain   Some children will experience actual pain during a psychobiological reaction or during the recalling or retelling of the event.

Suggested response: Reassure the child that her body is remembering and that it is normal for her body to remember the pain. Asking the child to take a deep breath and blow the pain away will usually stop the pain episode. If not, try pain-reduction techniques using imagery described in the case portion of this book. If those methods are not effective, seek a pain evaluation by the medical staff to determine whether it is associated with the injury. Recalled pain will abate rapidly when brought to consciousness.

Decrease in pain   Following pain-reduction techniques, children often announce their surprise at the immediate reduction in pain.

Suggested response: Reassure the child that the body is learning what parts of the trauma occurred in the past recalled by the pictures, words, or sounds: "I know it seems surprising that your pain went away, but it is normal when we talk about your injury for your body to remember along with your thoughts. As your body and thoughts learn it is not happening again, those sensations and thoughts will both go away."

Autonomic nervous system activation   ANS responses—sweaty palms, shallow breathing, wide eyes—are typical both during the creation of the event (drawing #2) and the retelling of the event. ANS responses often precede psycho-biological reactions. They may also occur during intrusive image episodes. Children often report feelings as though the event is happening again.

    Suggested response: "Your body is remembering and responding to drawing and talking about the accident. Take a deep breath, and blow that feeling out of your body. The accident is not happening now; your body is remembering, and that is normal for boys who get hit by a car. Take another deep breath and blow the fear away."

Pseudo-bulbar affect   This term describes laughing and crying at the same time. This may occur during a discussion of an image or during the retelling of the event. Following an explanation of the phenomena, children and teens have remarked, "I'm glad you told me, because sometimes I think there is something wrong with my brain." Or, "Every time I try to talk about it and cry, this happens, and that is why I can't talk about it because I get scared."

    Suggested response: "I see you are laughing and crying. That is because the chemicals in your brain are not just on one side. When they get mixed up after a scary event, you can laugh and cry at the same time. It happens some-times when kids are talking about what happened, and though it may seem very odd/weird/strange [use child's description if possible], it is normal when you talk about something scary that happened to you. It will go away, usually after we draw and talk about the accident and what happened and how you are healing."

Gaze aversion   Although rare during the intervention, the child or teen may look away from the therapist or the image and hold the averted gaze.

    Suggested response: "It is normal to want to look away when we are drawing and talking about the accident. You take as much time as you need to rest or relax. Just let me know if there is anything you want to say about what you are thinking or feeling about the shooting."

Feeling it is happening again   Sometimes children have physical sensations or pain as the event is elicited in the drawings or verbal narrative.

    Suggested response: "Your body is remembering, and that sometimes hap-pens. Take a deep breath and blow that feeling out of your body." Repeat two or three times slowly if necessary. If the child has physical sensations, it is important to assist him in transforming the image. For example, if a child yells, "My leg" and grabs his leg as if the event is occurring, I would first attempt the breathing technique, and then reframe the image with a drawing.

Emotional Responses

Smile Children and teens often smile upon learning they are not at fault for the event or when they suddenly realize they were brave or strong to have survived. Although rare, something humorous that occurred at the event, or during transport or treatment, may elicit a smile. Some children will laugh or smile throughout the intervention. This may represent anxiety or fear. The important thing to do is reassure the child that her reactions and responses are normal after a traumatic event. I do not point out incongruent affect and verbalizations, as the child may assume I have a preferred way for her to behave. It could confuse the child.

Suggested response: Reflective listening and smiling along with the child conveys understanding.

Anger Some children express significant affect along with physically throwing the markers or pencil, slamming a fist or marker on the table, or threatening to get even or hurt someone they perceive as responsible for the event (see revenge fantasies below).

Suggested response: "That is what happens when boys get hit by a car; they are really, really mad. It is normal to feel angry after being hurt. Tell me more about that feeling."

Anxiety This is very common because the child is required to address the event and his associated feelings and thoughts. Excessive laughter or talking, darting eyes, biting fingernails, and silliness can be visible signs of anxiety.

Suggested response: "Take a moment to take a deep breath. Try to relax your body a bit. It is normal to be anxious when we draw and talk about the accident. It is over, and the feelings are normal. We can help our bodies learn to be calm when we think or talk about the accident."

Yelling Some children become very animated and loud when talking symbolically to perpetrators depicted in their drawing.

Suggested response: "I can hear that you are really mad at that person. That is how kids feel when they get hurt. Tell me more."

Fear of dying This fear is very common. Most children are afraid of dying while hospitalized because they associate hospitalization with death. This happens even when the child has been admitted for something obviously nonfatal.

Suggested response: "It is normal to be afraid you might die when you have been injured or hurt in an accident. You are not going to die." You must know this for sure; if you are unsure, facilitating the CATTI is inappropriate at this time. "It is a normal worry. Many kids worry that they might die when they have been hurt and have to come to the hospital. The doctors and nurses are helping you get well and you will not die."

Fear a family member will die   This can occur if there are multiple victims in a motor vehicle accident, for example.

Suggested response: "It is normal to be afraid your brother/sister might die when you have been injured or hurt in an accident. It is normal to worry about that, but your brother/sister did not die in the accident."

Fear of loss of body parts   This is another common fear, even if obviously no body parts were affected. Children associate hospitalization with death and amputation.

Suggested response: "It is normal to worry that your hurt leg might have been cut off, but that did not happen and will not happen." You must know this; if you are unsure, facilitating the CATTI is inappropriate at this time. "The bone in your leg is broken, and the doctor has put it in a cast so it can heal so you can walk with your leg again."

Body integrity issues   Issues pertaining to the physical body are common, typically related to injured body parts or the injury itself. Children and teens want to know what happened to their body. It is important to answer questions but do not go beyond your scope of practice by including nursing or medical information. A child may want to know where the water in her lungs went. A teen who is a dancer may be devastated at the potential loss of that ability.

Suggested response: "It is normal to be worried about what happened to your body when you have been hurt in an accident. The water in your lungs will get absorbed into your body and become your pee. Your doctor knows what to do to help you heal, and he/she can answer any questions about your ability to dance, but it is normal to worry about that and to want to know if you can dance again."

Guilt   This feeling is very common, even when it is obvious that the event could not possibly be the fault of the child. This is true across the developmental spectrum. The most common guilt is associated with wrong-doing that caused the event. Others can feel guilt because they are taking up family time and resources because of their hospitalization. Some children feel guilt at not predicting the event or stopping the event.

Suggested responses:
     Toddlers and young children: "It is not your fault and you did not do anything bad to make it happen."
     School age: "It is normal to think you could have done something to cause it to happen, but it was not your fault, even if you don't believe that right now." If the child was hit by a car, you can address not only the importance of safety and paying attention but also the fact that the

law states that people who drive are supposed to slow down when they see children and go slow enough to be able to stop.

    Adolescents: "It is normal to think you could have done something to cause this to happen, but it is not your fault. It was an accident, and accidents happen in life." If the teen is involved in illegal or dangerous activity, address safety issues and the risk factors associated with their behavior.

Shame   Many children are embarrassed by injuries sustained on bicycles, skateboards, or sports injuries.

    Suggested response: "It is normal to feel as if you made a big mistake, or somehow caused the accident, but it was an accident, and these things happen in life. You did not do anything bad to cause it to happen, and you could not have done things differently in that moment to prevent or stop it."

Blame   In my clinical experience, most children blame themselves for causing their injuries, even when it is obvious they are not at fault. When a child or teen assigns blame to someone or something, I use the phrase "Tell me more" to learn the child or teen's perception about being at fault so I can correct the misperception. I may have him point to the person in the image that he blames for the event and ask the child to speak to the person even though he or she is not there. This generates strong affect.

    Suggested responses: "That is how kids feel when they are hurt. It is normal to be angry at the person or thing that injured you."

If a child is assigning blame to a person due to gender, race, or age, it is important to reassure the child that the person may have done the wrong thing but is not a bad person. It is the behavior that is wrong, not the person. Note: If the child secretly believes he is at fault, this can be very reassuring.

Feeling it may happen again   This is a common response. Children often expect to be reinjured if they find themselves in the same situation or setting again.

    Suggested response: "It is normal to think that the same thing would happen again, but that would be extremely unusual. When you go near the corner where you were hurt, your body may remember and you may have physical reminders such as your leg hurting. You may have sad and scared feelings and thoughts. All these are what we call traumatic reminders. It is normal. Your body is remembering. It is normal to think it may happen again. When you feel anxious, take a deep breath, and remind yourself that it is not happening again."

Rescue fantasies   Some children and teens have fantasies that if only they could have done a particular act or said something just right, the event could have been prevented.

Suggested response: "It is normal to wish you could have done something differently, but there is nothing you could do to get the gun from the person that shot you and your friend. You could have been hurt worse or killed. You did everything exactly right, because you survived and you will heal. It is normal to wish you could have prevented you and your friend from being shot."

Revenge fantasies   Very common for children and teens, revenge fantasies are a method of coping with the intense affect and feelings of helplessness generated by trauma, especially among violent teens. With young children, validating and reality testing often help abate their revenge fantasies toward those they perceive have hurt them, such as the car or the driver of the car. Violently injured teens openly want to seek revenge against those responsible for their injuries. Even though they are hospitalized, they may have friends to carry out these requests.

Suggested response: "That is how most teens feel. Tell me more. That is how any teen would feel. Tell me more. I am sure most teens would want to get back at those they hold responsible for injuries such as yours. Tell me more."

As teens are encouraged to express the revenge fantasies, the frontal cortex of the brain is accessed, and frequently they have a flash of insight about potential consequences. Although I have never had to make a report, if an individual is identified by name, reporting laws apply, and potential harm must be reported to the authorities.

Adaptive coping mechanisms   It is important to assess how the child or teen will cope with things when he returns home and then returns for follow-up care. While discussing the last drawing, I ask the child to imagine what a day will be like at home, in terms of attention, limitations on physical activity, pain, loneliness, and boredom. Once you have the child's perception of how things will be, you can correct misperceptions by helping the child develop adaptive ways of coping.

Suggested response: "Yes, it is a nice idea to think that everyone will be waiting on you and giving you lots of attention. That usually happens for a short time, and then everyone gets busy and they don't have as much time for you. Let's make a plan for things you can do when you are bored."

Maladaptive coping mechanisms   Some children imagine unhealthy or impossible ways of coping, such as staying at home forever or never going out in a car again. It is helpful to test this reality with them as to whether their idea is realistic and if not, what alternatives they might have.

Suggested response: "That may seem like a really easy way to avoid having to go in a car again, but do you really think it will be possible to never ride in a car? How can we solve that problem? What plans can we create to help you go in small steps so you feel safe but will eventually help you be able to ride in a car without being afraid?"

Cognitive Considerations

Traumatic reminders   Children may express fears of crossing a street, riding in a car, or other actions associated with the event. Ask the child what she imagines it will be like to cross the street or ride in the car. This gives you a chance to normalize the fears and assist with devising strategies for coping.

Suggested response: "It is normal to be afraid of going near where the accident happened, but it would be extremely rare for something to happen to you again there. Can you imagine some steps that would allow you to feel comfortable going to the park again?"

If the child comes up with a reasonable plan, wonderful. If not, helping the child problem solve is useful. For example, "A first step might be to walk to the park with your mom, not go into the park, but just look around. When you go home you can talk about all the feelings and body sensations you had at the park and remember that they are all normal. Then, go to the park again the next day with your mom and stay a bit longer, but do not go into the park. Then go home and talk about any feelings or body sensations you have about the experience and remind yourself they are normal." Usually with a menu of choice to get them thinking, patients will devise a plan that will work for them.

Treatment regimen   Some children and teens refuse to comply with their treatment plan. This may occur when the patient senses a loss of control or is fearful of medications or treatment procedures. I have also witnessed children's noncompliance with treatment in order to remain in the hospital to avoid child abuse in the home.

Suggested response: Most children do not like the hospital. Some dislike the prescribed medicine. Others may have a variety of other objections. "It is normal not to want to take a drink of something with a straw when you have had a tube in your nose. It is hard to do everything you are told to do when you are hurt and scared. I am sure they have explained why you have to drink some water, and the nurse has tried to make it easier. Sometimes none of that will help. Sometimes you just have to be the one to decide when you will take a drink. So, you wait, and when you are ready, let me tell you exactly what it will be like. It will be scary, and you will not want to do it once you begin, but the water will be cool on your tongue and you might feel it going down your throat. Then the scary first drink will be over. The most important thing is for you to decide when to take a drink."

Usually the child will comply when he is in control and has a description of the process and outcome.

Follow-up care plan   Children and teens have follow-up care appointments that often involve getting a scan or removal of stitches, staples, or a cast. It is important to stay within one's scope of practice and not discuss medical issues. It is important to reassure the child that her anxiety and fear are normal and that she can tell her doctor about her fears of pain or removal of stitches. Child Life staff are skilled at preparing the child or teen for medical procedures. That task is not a part of CATTI. Although extremely rare, if issues arise beyond the identified goals of the CATTI, the child or teen should be referred for an evaluation for additional therapy sessions.

Suggested response: "It is normal to be afraid of having the cast taken off your leg. I know you have been told the doctor will use a small saw. The saw does make a loud noise, but the saw will not cut skin. It only cuts super hard surfaces like a cast. All the kids I know who had their cast off said it was scary to think about, but it didn't hurt. Remember, you can ask the doctor any questions you have or ask the doctor to explain anything you want to know."

Reintegration strategies   This pertains to returning home or to school with bandages or medical devices, scars, crutches, or a colostomy. Children are often fearful of being teased, of going to school looking different in any way. Try to have the child identify his concern or a specific fear, then use role-play to practice limit setting.

Suggested response: "What do you think it will be like to go back to school? What do you think kids or teachers will say to you about your crutches? Sometimes when you go back to school or out in the world, everyone asks a lot of questions about what happened. You may want to talk about it, and you may not, or you may get tired of explaining what happened. Some kids like to know some things they can say when they don't want to talk. How about, 'I don't want to talk about it right now, but I'm okay, thanks.' There may be kids who say mean things, but it is usually because they are afraid. Do you have something you plan to say if someone is mean to you? Let's think of some ideas together and practice saying them so it will be easier later."

Cognitive understanding of event (linguistic coherent narrative)   The creation of a coherent narrative is one of the core elements of resolution (Siegel, 1999). To consider the intervention successful, the child should have a coherent linguistic narrative about the event. Usually this is accomplished in one session. When the patient becomes very verbal about his experience, he has achieved this goal.

Suggested response: "Thank you for sharing your very important story with me. It helped me to understand what happened, who helped, and about your time in the hospital. You did a great job being in the hospital, and I am glad I got to know you and your important story."

Future sporadic therapy The therapist needs to educate the child and family about the possible need for future therapy. PTSD symptoms should abate in a month, but if not, the child should be seen for follow-up treatment.

Suggested response: "For most kids, feeling worried, anxious, or jumpy and having pictures of different parts of the story pop into your mind will all go away shortly. If you are still feeing scared or worried or still have lots of visual images and fears associated with the accident, have your mom call me, and we can see about helping you more with your feelings about the accident. It is normal to have lots of feelings about what happened."

CHAPTER 3

A Neuro-developmental Model
of Art Therapy Treatment

Neuro-developmental Art Therapy (NDAT) is a mind/body approach to trauma resolution therapy designed to treat those with a history of relational trauma or exposure to child abuse, chronic neglect, or violence (Chapman 2002, 2003). Many of the children with whom I work require long-term treatment. They have experienced multiple forms of traumatic exposure, multiple transitions and losses, and often multiple living situations. Others have written about developmental approaches to art therapy (Malchiodi, et al., 2003; Aach-Feldman et al., 1987; Uhlin, 1972; Williams and Wood, 1977; Lowenfeld, 1957), and about the brain and art therapy (Haas-Cohen and Carr, 2008; Kaplan, 2000). The NDAT model was developed out of the earlier theoretical constructs of the short-term CATTI model. The unifying aspect is the focus on the right hemisphere of the brain to bring about healing. By engaging in the kinesthetic activity of art making, play, and other creative work involving the right hemisphere, the sensory nonverbal neural pathways are activated along with left-hemisphere verbal neural pathways, thus utilizing the integrative capacity of the brain toward achieving maximum therapeutic potential (Jones, 1994).

NDAT consists of four stages of treatment over an extended period of time. It is different from short-term, acute trauma treatment. Relational trauma and repeated exposure to child abuse and neglect are not single, one-time events. Long-term damage to the neural systems requires repeated exposure to treatment interventions to ameliorate the damage. To address sustained issues of grief and loss, maladjustment, and the inability to relate to others in a positive manner, a sense of trust has to be established. This chapter describes the practical application of the NDAT model for treatment of relational trauma, also referred to as chronic exposure to trauma.

There are other treatment models that take into consideration neural development and information processing. Dr. Bruce Perry developed the Neurosequential Model of Therapeutics (NMT), an assessment and treatment approach that incorporates child development, clinical traumatology, and developmental neuroscience (Perry & Hambrick, 2008). Specific problem areas in the limbic system and cerebral cortex are the focus of the interventions. The model is successful and being implemented in a variety of agencies and treatment facilities in the United States. The beginning of Perry's model incorporates massage, yoga, sensory-motor integration, and other body-based activities to stimulate the development of the midbrain and the higher structures of the brain.

Dr. Robert Melillo, author of *Disconnected Kids*, developed the Brain Balance Program based on Hemispheric Integration Therapy (HIT) (Melillo, 2009). His program assesses and treats imbalances between the right and left hemispheres using a series of specific sensory, physical, dietary, and academic exercises that address targeted areas of the brain to bring them back into synchronization. His treatment model has been successful with thousands of children with neurological disorders.

By contrast, NDAT serves to activate and develop the lower structures of the brain, where the relational trauma damage occurred, before integrating the treatment model to affect the limbic and cerebral cortex and bring balance to the functioning of the entire human organism. Many of the children referred to me for therapy have undiagnosed sensory, motor, vestibular, and/or proprioceptive delays that greatly affect their ability to sit, focus, move, and regulate their body. Beginning with art and play activities, NDAT offers specific interventions to correlate with different aspects of kinesthetic, emotional, and cognitive information processing. When the significant developmental task of attaching with a primary caregiver is missing or inadequate, the development of a child's concept of mind/body/self is compromised (Schore, 2012). Additionally, the child does not have the ability to develop the sensory and motor systems that normally occur through interaction with others and the environment—foundations for learning and behavior. Once the lower structures of the neural system are integrated, they will inform the higher structures (Perry, 2009) and move the individual toward a more normalized functional capacity.

THE NDAT TREATMENT MODEL FOR RELATIONAL TRAUMA

The NDAT model consists of the Self Phase, the Problem Phase, the Transformation Phase, and the Integration Phase. As seen in Table 3.1, there is vertical and horizontal correlation among aspects of neural activity, information processing, and reactions to trauma within the NDAT model. It is advantageous to conceptualize the stages as a continuum rather than as specific phases assigned by a number of sessions or as meeting specific measurable criteria. For example, children with sensory or visual motor delays begin with Self Phase art and play activities to strengthen and develop those deficiencies. As they make gains, the focus can shift to problematic behaviors or relationships, the second phase, but without abandoning sensory and visual activities.

There are four elements in each session: motivation, art making, exploration

Table 3.1 Neurodevelopmental Art Therapy: Treatment Model

Neural Activity	Cognition	Visual Information Processing	Psychological Reactions	CATTI	NDAT
Prefrontal	Abstract	Creative/ integration	Reconstruction	Symptom reduction	Integration Phase
Cerebrum	Abstract	Cognitive/ symbolic	Acknowledgment	Retelling with images	Transformation Phase
Limbic	Emotional	Affect/ perceptual	Retreat	Visual drawn narrative	Problem Phase
Brain stem	Reflexive	Kinesthetic/ sensory	Impact	Scribble	Self Phase

of images, and closure. To inspire the child to engage in art making, I use motivation to interest them in the topic or subject of the art project. For example, to encourage a child to make an animal totem I begin by asking her if she has ever wondered what it would be like to be a bird, or a cat, or a centipede. I might ask if she has a favorite animal or if she likes a particular animal. I have gathered a large collection of finely detailed, sculpted wild, farm, zoo, and domestic animals, to which I have added sea creatures, prehistoric animals, and insects. I invite the child to help me arrange the animals on a large table. When the figures are all in place, I ask which creature is interesting to the child, which one she might like to sculpt or to draw, and which one she would like to select as her totem for the day. Creating motivation usually requires only a few minutes of the session, but gradually introducing the activity helps the child become willing to proceed with the art making.

During art making, my role is one of helper. I get supplies, hold things, or do whatever the child or teen asks of me to facilitate the art making process. Safety and acceptance of the child are my focus of attention. I do not ask questions about content or process during the art making. As the end of the session nears, I say, twice, that the art-making time will be over in a few minutes. During the last several minutes, I comment that I will begin making space for the art. I put some supplies away to create a visual representation of the end of the art making. I arrange the worktable so there is a clear space for their art and pull up two chairs where we then sit to view and discuss their project.

Initially I reserve about 5 minutes for dialogue and discussion. As the therapy progresses and the child shows more willingness to explore the images together, the dialogue period lengthens. The manner in which I engage the child in this discussion about their imagery is fully described in Chapter 6, but I make a point of asking what was challenging or required problem solving, what was satisfying and enjoyable, and how the child saw herself reflected in her art. With the consistent and repetitive nature of the inquiry, even the most resistant teenager will eventually begin to answer the questions.

It is important to provide closure at the end of each session, to bring a sense of completion for the client and especially with regard to the artwork, which is a representation of self. We discuss whether to take the art home or to save it in her portfolio at the studio. If the child is still working on a particular project, I ask her if there is any particular media supply she needs for the next session. If not, I might ask if there is any media she would like or some medium she has never used that she would like to try. I do this so that when the child next arrives at the studio, the materials are out and waiting for her. If she voices no preference, I assure her I will have choices and ideas for the next session. I have found that talking about the next session increases the child's desire to return to therapy. Before we leave the studio, I always make a point of asking, "Can I tell you something I learned about you today?" Usually the child is curious. I point out a positive quality, behavior, or kindness I noticed during the session. For example, I make comments about courage; note the child's ability to express her wants, needs, thoughts, or feelings; or mention that she was fun, curious, or engaged with the art. This enables the child to leave with a feeling of having been noticed, accepted, and valued.

The NDAT model is both neurobiologically and developmentally based. Working within a framework of re-creating attachment and sensory-motor experiences requires a client-centered approach in order to foster developmental needs and experiences that the child lacks. Because many of the children and teens have behavior and emotional regulation problems, the sessions are highly structured in a variety of ways. The environment is free of clutter and distraction, and the décor and furnishings are predictable and consistent. My expectations for behavior and engagement with the art activity are offered at the beginning of each session. Within this highly structured environment, however, the client has total freedom as to the content of her art. As she moves forward in her development, I modify my child-centered approach to reflect her growth. The case studies illustrated this.

THE SELF PHASE

The Self Phase is the starting point of therapy. I assert that it is also the most critical time in therapy. Not until the client has a clear, concrete idea of who he is and is comfortable and confident in his ability to control his behavior and relate to others can it be said that he has achieved the goals of therapy.

During the first session, my focus is on assessing the development and regulation of the physical body. Can the child or teen be in the studio, sitting upright in a chair at a table, able to make eye contact, breathe normally, and engage in dialogue?

CASE NOTE: A 14-year-old girl was referred to therapy for truancy and problems controlling her behavior in the classroom. During the first session, she continually placed her head on her arm while drawing. She shifted her body frequently and would attempt to sit upright, but soon she placed her head back on her arm as she drew. I asked her if she could sit up. She looked at me and said, "I can never sit up, not at school, not at dinner, I just can't. I always sit like this, even in church I have to lean on my mom or dad." I mentioned that we could do some things to help her with that difficulty but also told her that it makes sense that she cannot pay attention in class and does not want to go to school when she can't sit up. She said tearfully, "Nobody else thinks it matters, but it is hard to be in the class when I can't concentrate."

Here was possible evidence of a 14-year-old with severe vestibular delays that were manifesting in behavior problems. The tearful teen was relieved to have the connection made between her delay and her difficulty focusing and learning in the classroom setting.

During the Self Phase there is often a high level of resistance. Behavior may be poorly controlled. Information processing may be slow or inconsistent, requiring the therapist to incorporate slower speech, movement, and transitions. Limits and boundaries are tested.

Attention to safety is critical. The beginning of rapport and trust building occurs on a physical level by making references to safety. I ask the child if he is comfortable, if the room temperature is all right, and whether he needs a snack or beverage. I watch for every opportunity to use the word *safety*. This creates a level of vigilance that matches his need for safety, containment, and boundaries and creates a mental representation that my attention is focused on safety at all times. Just as the infant is not cognitively aware of safety, the child's body will become used to a reduced state of hyperarousal.

Children with relational trauma and child abuse histories often lack a concept of their own mind/body/self. Sensory and motor delays are common. Typically, they are unable to make associations to, or distinctions between, body sensations and emotion. Dissociation is common and frequent as the body sensations activate the limbic structures and emotions arise. The client dissociates as an adaptive coping mechanism for detaching from their inner experience. Allen posits, "Dissociatively detached individuals are not only detached from their environment, but also from the self—their body, actions, and sense of identity" (Allen et al., 1999, p. 165).

Self Phase treatment interventions are all nonregressive and highly structured to provide the ego containment the child or teen may not have. I choose activities in which structure and limits are inherent in the art media. Presenting the media in this manner serves as a container for the child's anxiety and fear. For example, taping the drawing paper offers a mental representation of boundaries. Offering fingerpaints on a tray or cookie sheet creates physical boundaries for the media. The interventions begin with nonthreatening sensory experiences designed for assessment of physical development. No skill is required. The art directives are designed to be enlivening and fun, with a focus on exploring the media and physical mastery of the media. I make every effort to avoid regressive experiences that can be frightening to the client at this stage of therapy.

Self Phase Interventions

The interventions described here are typical of my art therapy practice, but they are not for session-to-session, step-by-step treatment. My directed sessions are mixed with nondirective art experiences chosen by the child or teen. As the child becomes involved in their preferred art media or becomes engrossed in a large project for which she has passion and in which she has found meaning, I join with her in her agenda for the art and the therapy. Beginning with Self Phase interventions appears to be successful and comfortable for children and teens. The interventions are described here in detail, often with case vignettes. Additional ways of utilizing these activities therapeutically are offered in the following chapters.

Sensory-Motor Art

Usually, the first art activity I offer is what I refer to as sensory-motor art. Others refer to it as bilateral scribbling and drawing (McNamee, 2003, 2004, 2006; Talwar, 2007; Tripp, 2007). This is a fun, no-skill, warm-up activity that I usually do at the beginning of each session with each client. I ask the child to sit across from me at a table covered with white butcher paper 4 feet long, 36 inches wide. I tape the paper to the table at both ends. We each select two different color markers, one for each hand. I choose colors that are different from the child or teen's selection. She is instructed to begin scribbling along with me. Once she is engaged, I give these instructions: "Make random marks, up and down vertically, back and forth horizontally, let the horizontal scribble evolve into a circle, then go back to vertically, horizontally, let the horizontal evolve into an arc, let the arc expand and cross your arms to scribble to the far edge of the page with both arms, make circles, make circles fast, make circles slow, make dots with both hands at once, make dots with alternative hands, make dots at the same time with both hands, return to scribbling a circle, go slower and smaller, slower and smaller, and slow to a stop and make a dot in the center." The paper is turned over and we take turns selecting items to draw with a marker in each hand. I remind the child that the images she draws with her nondominant hand will most likely be very different from those drawn with her dominant hand.

What I have done with this first activity is guide the child or teen through the developmental sequence of early, normal graphic development (Kellogg, 1969; Lindstrom, 1964; Lowenfeld, 1957). The scribbling sequence includes a repetitive crossing of the midline, and the scribble and two-handed drawings offer an opportunity to assess the child's gross and fine motor development, eye-hand coordination, and motor planning. The kinesthetic aspect of the scribbling activates the lower structures of the right brain and stimulates the formulation of imagery (Lusebrink, 1990). The bilateral stimulation and eye movements appear to bring the hemispheres of the brain into better synchrony.

It has been interesting to find that when children and teens engage in this activity at the beginning of each session, parents report improved school performance and an increase in focus of attention. One teen was failing all grades and three months later was a C student. After six months of therapy, the teen was a B student. Although I cannot credit such academic improvement to repetitive bilateral scribbling, when I wrote about the technique in my website newsletter, I encouraged art therapists to try it and welcomed feedback. I received many responses, all positive. Those who used the technique at the beginning of their sessions reported that clients demonstrated increased investment in the therapy session, showed increased ability to focus and attend, and increased their verbal interaction during the session. One art therapist wrote of a mute autistic child who began speaking. However, research is required before such improvements can be attributed directly to bilateral scribbling and drawing.

Following this brief warm-up experience, we move to a different table with one large and one medium piece of drawing paper, a spectrum of markers, a pencil with an eraser, scissors (unless otherwise indicated for safety precautions), acid-free glue, glue brush, and a wide variety of magazines. I explain to the child that I prefer to get to know him through art rather than asking questions. I invite him to select images or words from magazines for a collage to introduce himself (Wadeson, 1980). I assure him that he has full control over what he shares and what he does not, and that he can talk or not talk about any symbol or word he may include in the collage. If there is resistance, he is reassured he does not have to do any art activity he does not want to do. It is extremely rare for the child not to create a collage or part of a collage.

When the client indicates that he is finished, I invite him to comment on the collage. I listen carefully and note what he speaks about and what he does not. I do not ask any questions other than for clarification of what he has said. The collage is a way to learn about the child, but it also serves as a unique assessment tool that reveals the degree to which the child has developed a sense of self. I am able to note if the images and words are about self or other. I specifically note themes, such as protection, fear, or isolation, and whether the selected images are reflective of a personal self. I also note how much of the offered paper is used for the child's collage. Those with an underdeveloped sense of self typically use little of the page space, while those with a more fully developed self-concept typically use more of the page for their images.

When the child finishes describing the collage, I ask if he would be willing to look at the image in a different way to learn more about himself. I reassure the child or teen he does not have to talk about anything he doesn't want to talk about and does not have to answer any questions he prefers not to answer. Framed in this manner, with the opportunity to be in control of the dialogue and the experience, most readily agree. My questions are simple, designed to facilitate a positive, nonthreatening experience. Offering the client a choice to talk about himself, I ask, "Is there an image in the collage you like best? Is there one you like least? Is there one that you are surprised you selected, or one you wish you did not choose? Is there one that you could have included but did not?" If the collage requires two or more sessions, that is acceptable.

> CASE NOTE: A 15-year-old girl was asked to create a collage to intro-duce herself during the first session of therapy. She proceeded to look through magazines and included the following images from magazines in her collage: a car, a fish, a piece of jewelry, and letters that formed her middle name. She then took the paint and used all the colors, one by one, to paint a one-inch wide stripe, about two inches long, of each color next to each other on the page. She also painted a disembodied eyeball on the page. She indicated the collage was complete. I asked her if it was okay if I looked at the images and she agreed. I spent a few moments looking at the images. I then asked her if she had anything to say about the image or any part of the image. She looked at me bewildered and said, "What do you mean?" I said, "I was wondering if you wanted to make any comments about anything you made." She replied, "No. I just put things on the paper because you asked me to." I said, "You are right, I did ask you to put images or words on the collage, and I just wondered if these have any meaning for you or if they are about you in any way." She replied, "No. I just picked them because they were there. I don't even like fish. These are the letters of my middle name, but I don't go by that name."

Here is an example of a teen's apparent lack of the concept of a mind/body self. The directive for the collage was to select images or words that illustrate who you are, what you like, what you do, and anything you think would let me know a bit about you. The teen put whatever images she happened upon into the collage. It is important to consider resistance as a possible reason for this response to the art. However, it is usually those with a disorganized or traumatic attachment experience who create fragmented and disorganized introductory collages representing the self. Even the most resistant teens are able to represent some aspects of their personality along with their typical singular interest in sports, video games, fashion, or music. The ability of the therapist to gauge the level of self-development in the client is important in determining treatment goals and plans. With the teen mentioned in this vignette, I would proceed in therapy with art activities to develop metaphorical and symbolic attachment experiences and strengthen the sensory and motor systems that aid in the maturation of the right hemisphere to facilitate the creation of a mind/body concept of self.

Other sensory-motor interventions include stampings and rubbings, which offer the experience of immediate gratification plus cause and effect. More important, these activities create a visual representation of the self through the actions of the self. Most children begin by stamping randomly on the page, followed by wanting to put paint on the palm of their hand and stamp with their hands. After they do random stamping and hand stamping for a while, they shift to using the shapes to form patterns, designs, or artistic scenes. This shift is evidence of the movement from enjoying the sensory and motor aspects of the activity to more complex information processing by using the shapes to form patterns and designs. I offer precut sponge shapes for young children and use found objects and uncut sponges to be self-designed symbols with adolescents. The symbols are dipped in paint-soaked sponges in low bowls. A large paper is used for experimentation before the child is given drawing paper to make images of their choice. Rubbings are made with chalk or oil pastels rubbed onto drawing paper placed atop any surface the child or teen selects. Rubbings can be made on wood, tile, cement, rocks, trees, rugs—almost any surface. The activity is designed to foster tactile stimulation, eye-hand coordination, gross motor skill, and experimentation with the concept of cause and effect, an early developmental task.

A favorite tactile discrimination activity is to drop coins or beads into a shoebox filled with dried pinto beans. I invite the child or teen to feel for the objects in the beans, which requires fine motor skills to discriminate between the tactile surface and shape of the beans and the coins. They keep whatever they find. I reassure them that nothing in the box will trick them or hurt them.

Another activity to develop tactile discrimination is to fill a 12- to 16-inch deep nylon or fabric bag with fifteen small objects with various tactile surfaces: a small piece of wood, a small rubber ball, a large paper clip, a small matchbox with no matches, a 1-inch square piece of wet sponge, a small piece of sandpaper, a piece of soft plush fabric, etc. As I name each object, the child identifies the item inside using his sense of touch, removes the object, and places it in front of him. Some children can readily identify the object by touch, while others have great difficulty.

I incorporate self-soothing techniques to calm the child's physical body. This is a way to bring a focus of attention to the body and an opportunity to make connections between emotions and the body. We discuss how emotions are felt in the body and he learns to soothe the body and mind when stressed. Breathing and progressive relaxation exercises are examples. I may lead the child in a simple guided imagery process to elicit his perception of a safe or comforting place. After a brief period of breathing and relaxing the body, I ask the child to let his mind wander to a place that is completely safe and comforting, either real or imaginary. We practice using the safe place imagery to return to a state of physical homeostasis. This activity also demonstrates whether the child or teen is able to imagine a safe place. Some children cannot. I then take time to slow down the process and ask them to imagine, along with me, what a safe place might look like, what we might see, who might be there, what it would feel like to be there, the colors, shapes, and designs we would see. Then we create a representation of that image together on the paper. The mental representation created is that safety is important, that I can take time to focus on their safety, and that together, we can create a safe place for the child.

Fingerpainting offers tactile, kinesthetic and bilateral stimulation. I tape the paper down to imply a boundary. I place a small bucket of warm water, a wet washcloth, and a dry washcloth near the child, reminding her she can stop to clean her hands at any time. There is the potential for rapid regression at the beginning of a fingerpainting session. To control the experience I ask the child to cover the page with paint and smooth it out to make a drawing surface and then stop. When she has done so, I ask her to draw a ball then erase it, draw a ladder then erase it, draw an animal and erase it, then draw a vehicle. By this time, the child is engaged in the creative aspect of the painting and I tell her she can erase the vehicle and create any images that come to mind. When the child creates one she wants to keep, I place it aside and offer more paper.

To stimulate the auditory senses and motor planning, a handheld drum can be used. I invite the child or teen to play softly, play loudly, play fast then slow, and replicate his heartbeat. I ask him to play feeling states: mad, sad, fearful, and happy. To conclude I ask him to play how he is feeling at that moment.

It is important to watch for signs that the child or teen has become comfortable and accepting of the activities I have asked him to engage in. Once a solid rapport is established, I introduce body awareness activities. I ask the child to draw a person without looking at the paper, to draw himself by looking in a mirror, to sketch gesture drawings of an individual in different poses quickly, in 5 to 10 seconds. These body drawings are intended to lead to a level that allows me enough comfort to introduce a body tracing. I do not ask the child to lie on the floor. At this time in therapy, a prone position on the floor may stimulate a strong feeling of vulnerability, especially for abused children. Instead, I hang the paper on the wall and ask the child to assume a variety of poses, such as a robot, an animal, a dancer, an athlete, or a superhero. Then I ask him to select a pose he would like me to trace. Before I begin the drawing, I hold the pencil or marker in front of the child or teen so he can see it, and I describe where I will be drawing, indicating that I will not be touching his body at any time. I describe the intended route of the drawing implement. When I begin drawing, I repeat the route of the pencil as I draw.

When the tracing is finished, I find that offering a brief menu of choices facilitates completion of the project. I provide a choice of media and the child or teen is invited to add facial features, clothes, and accessories in order to transform the tracing into himself or as a superhero, rock star, athlete, or anything he wishes. This activity involves gross motor activity. Affect is elicited frequently. Some children add knives, guns, or other themes of protection to their body tracings. Others poke the drawing tool into the face drawn on the body, a metaphor for self-harm. I have seen regressed children and teens create themselves as much younger or infantile, and pseudosophisticated individuals create an image of themselves as an adult. All these observations are clues to the child's perception of self.

Symbolic Expression of the Self

As the child or teen becomes comfortable, I begin to include activities that elicit her perceptions about herself, her environment, and other interpersonal information. To assess metaphorically the themes related to the client's home environment and protection, the child or teen is invited to select from different styles of small, premade wooden birdhouses and to decorate it in a manner that would appeal to her if she were a bird or one that would attract the type of bird she would like to have come and live in her birdhouse. Themes of protection, comfort, and safety surface with this activity. Some birdhouses become completely camouflaged, an attempt to hide, while others are completely covered with sparkling jewels, and some have elaborate security systems. It is remarkable how the surface of the birdhouse often reflects the child's emotional state. Depressed children often use camouflage materials to decorate their birdhouse; those who demand attention often cover the birdhouse in jewels or glitter; and children with abuse histories often create elaborate security systems or houses with fences and little to no access. This activity also offers the child a larger repertoire of tactile sensations as she uses a variety of art media for the activity.

Continuing in this vein, I ask the child or teen if she would be willing to work with some symbols of her own choosing, and the client typically agrees. I place two 11- by 12-inch sheets of drawing paper side by side. At the top of one sheet I print the word WANTS and on the other I print NEEDS. I offer various colors of construction paper and scissors and invite the child to cut out four, five, or more symbols—more if she wishes—that represent her wants, or things she would like to have in her life, and place them on the paper titled WANTS. When she has finished, I invited her to create five, six, or more symbols that represent her own needs—the things she needs to survive and live in the world—and place them on the paper titled NEEDS. Then I invite her to comment on the symbols. Thus, an array of symbols that are unique to that child or teen is created.

I ask the child if she would be willing to explore the symbols in a different way, reassuring her that she has control over what she answers and talks about. Most clients agree. I move the papers apart so there is a 6- to 8-inch space between the sheets. I ask her to move the symbols that represent survival items into the middle space, and we discuss them and set them back on the NEEDS sheet. Then I ask her to place the symbols in the middle that have to do with pleasure or fun, and we discuss those before returning them to the WANTS sheet. I ask her to place the symbols in the middle that represent relationships, or interaction with others, and we discuss those. I then remove the ones that have to do with relationships and interaction with others and ask, "Would this be enough? Would these items be all you need?" The dialogue that results often leads to a discussion about important qualities of a friend or a family member. I may also ask what is the most important symbol in the three categories, or which is the least important, or which ones you can get from others, which ones you can find only within yourself. The client's response to these activities indicates whether she are ready to move on to the Problem Phase of therapy.

During the Self Phase, the activities and my prompts are designed to be emotionally safe and to strengthen the sensory and motor systems. This results in improved participation in therapy, affect regulation, and behavior. Readiness to move to the Problem Phase is indicated by clients' ability to engage in eye contact, to sit comfortably, and to have a basic level of comfort talking about art making and themselves. The change is gradual. The child is moving from enjoying the sensory and motor aspects of the activities to a focus on the art making or the art product. He can tolerate the attention directed toward himself and his thoughts and feelings associated with the art he has created. If the child resists moving forward to the new activities of the Problem Phase, I simply return to a place of psychological safety and continue with sensory and motor or, often, nondirective art where the child can choose the media and art task.

THE PROBLEM PHASE

Emotions are the focus in the Problem Phase. The goal is therapeutic emotional homeostasis. Evidence of emotional homeostasis occurs when the child has been able to participate in the development of a safe and secure therapeutic relationship that enables the exploration of the nonverbal symbolic affective communications that arise in the art or play. This does not necessarily mean engaging in verbal dialogue. A very young child may not articulate what has occurred in the play, but the repetition of replaying the trauma is evidence of mastery and can be seen in symptom reduction and changes in behavior or functioning. Emotional homeostasis also is evidenced in the absence of dissociative strategies in the service of warding off painful emotions (Schore, 2003a).

> CASE NOTE: A 16-year-old boy with a history of abuse and neglect was referred for therapy. He was becoming increasingly oppositional, defiant, and lethargic. He lived in a group home for severely disturbed teens. He attended art therapy regularly and dissociated during every session. As he began to explore the symbolic content of his art, he became aware of the visible empty space in his images. I brought to his attention that he sometimes seems to "space out" when we were talking about difficult subjects. He agreed, and began to refer to his dissociative episodes as "spacing." When he would do so, I offered him paper and pastels and asked him to put color and shape on the paper to represent the feeling he had just before he "spaced." He always drew a big black circle on the paper. During one of these exchanges, I asked him to draw what was behind the black spot, and he admitted, "It is all the stuff I try not to think about. You know. All the bad stuff that made me bad." I said, "You are not bad. You are behaving in a way that you learned to behave to survive. When you 'space,' it is another

way you protect yourself. If you can express the feelings in the art, you won't need to 'space.'" He said, "I doubt it."

He continued in art therapy and, over time, expressed and discussed his feelings of worthlessness, hopelessness, and fear portrayed in the art. He began to notice changes and a lessening of the empty space in his images. He was surprised, and although he did not stop dissociating, the frequency and duration of the episodes noticeably decreased during the therapy sessions.

The teen's ability to discuss and engage in dialogue about his inner experience is evidence of increased emotional homeostasis and affect tolerance. Although his dissociative episodes did not stop, he began to explore the meaning and content of the emotions that were walled off, or behind the "space."

As the art experiences shift and address PTSD symptoms or behavior problems more directly, it is common for a defensive behavioral pattern and psychological retreat to reappear. This can take the form of denial, minimization of the problems, a push for autonomy, ambivalence about therapy, or a desire to quit therapy. There may be heightened anxiety evidenced by difficulty regulating affect, increased resistance, and increased limit and boundary testing. Support is highly crucial at this time. When difficult feelings or thoughts arise during the Problem Phase, I reassure children and teens that they have control over what they talk about and when they want to talk. After they have disclosed abuse or violence in art or verbally, I explain that they may have sleep disturbances, with or without nightmares, or dreams about the trauma. They may have an increased awareness of traumatic reminders (Pynoos, Steinberg, & Goenjian, 1996), and they may have feelings or body sensations similar to those during the event. I let them know that grief responses or feelings of loss may reoccur more frequently during this time in therapy. I discuss these responses as normal reactions to making art about, talking about, or thinking about traumatic experiences. I establish trust by validating the responses as normal and by offering containment in the art and the opportunity for the child or teen to be in control of their own expression as tolerated.

Problem Phase Interventions

The focus during this stage of treatment is to utilize art as symbolic and metaphorical expression. Rather than address his issues by raising questions, I engage the child in art-making experiences that allow for the gradual unfolding of his story. It is highly probable that he will be defensive and resistant. To counter this normal reaction, I offer many nondirective art-making opportunities along with the Problem Phase interventions. By engaging in a state of attunement (Schore, 2012) with the child or teen, his level of comfort, resistance, and participation guide me as we co-create the pacing of the art therapy.

A good place to begin Problem Phase interventions is with a directive I learned from neuropsychologist and art therapist John Jones (1994). The child is invited to try something new and fun that involves combining different media within a single project. The point of using different media is to elicit a preference, but more important, the activity moves from the highly structured markers to paint, a very fluid media.

The properties of media have the ability to elicit or contain primary process material, or affect. Structured media such as pencils, markers, collage, and wood and glue all utilize fine motor movement and are easy to control. These types of media have firm boundaries. What I refer to as expressive media are things that are commonly used by children and teens that elicit a mild to moderate amount of affect for most children. Oil pastels, chalk pastels, painting on medium-size paper with medium to small brushes, and modeling clay all have boundaries that are more flexible and therefore elicit a moderate amount of affect. What I refer to as unstructured media include watercolors, clay with water, large paper and paint with large brushes, and media requiring ripping, tearing, or pounding. These media all have fluid boundaries and are more difficult to control. They will elicit deeper affect quickly and should be used with caution by those not trained in their use, especially when working with disturbed individuals. A child or teen may go very deeply into the body and affect very fast, become afraid, and refuse to participate in art in the future. An art therapist never randomly selects media. The properties of the media are a primary consideration in determining which media to use with a client. Combining several media in one activity offers me a safe and contained way to assess how quickly a child will regress or become dysregulated as we move from structured to unstructured media.

For the art making, a sheet of good-quality 18- by 24-inch piece of drawing paper is placed horizontally. A spectrum of eight or more markers, a set of sixteen or twenty-four oil pastels, a set of sixteen or twenty-four chalk pastels, acrylic paint in assorted colors, paint brushes, water in a container for rinsing paint brushes, and a small wet towel are placed within reach. The child or teen is invited to pick one marker, any color. I ask her to scribble all over the paper until I tell her what to do next. After about 15 to 20 seconds of random scribbling, she is instructed to turn the paper over and write her initials, however she wishes, with the same large movement. The next step is to enhance or decorate the initials with only markers, any colors. After 2 to 3 minutes, I tell her to stop using markers and continue to enhance or decorate her initials using only oil pastels, any colors. After another 2 to 3 minutes, I tell her to stop using the oil pastels, switch to the chalk pastels, and continue to enhance or decorate the initials using any colors. Next, 2 to 3 minutes later, I tell her to switch to the paints and continue to enhance her initials with any paint colors. After several more minutes I let her know she should finish and be ready to stop soon. I wait and then remind her again to finish up in the next minute.

After the child or teen has stopped, I invite her to look at the image and notice the colors and shapes. Directing her attention to her creative product is a safe place to begin. I may ask whether she noticed that she liked one medium better than another, or which medium she liked or did not like as she was combining it with others. I may ask if the task was hard or easy, and what she liked or disliked about the experience. These nonintrusive questions provide a mental representation of shared exploration as a nonthreatening procedure.

I ask if she would be willing to look at the image in different ways and, optionally, to respond to questions about the way the image looks, which is also a nonthreatening request. While she is engaged in looking at the image, I ask her to think about what she is seeing and respond to the following questions if she would like to comment. I let her know it is all right if she doesn't have anything to say. I ask her to take as much time as she needs before responding and offer a long pause to give her time to reflect on the image and formulate a response. If no response is given, I simply ask a different question. I ask some or all of the following questions (based on what the image looks like):

1.Which letter is most developed?
2.Which letter is least developed?
3.Which letter do you like best based on the way it looks?
4.Which letter do you like least based on the way it looks?
5.Which letter is most familiar?
6.Which letter is least familiar?
7.Which letter is most powerful?
8.Which letter is most vulnerable?
9.Which letter is protected?
10.Which letter needs protection?
11.Can you give the image a title?
12.Does the image have any positive parting advice for you?

This activity is a great way to begin to deepen the exploration of self that was initiated during the Self Phase when the child introduced herself with her collage. Without being intrusive, I am giving her a chance to take a step closer to her "self" and "feeling" states. She can answer the questions or not. It is up to her. The child or teen usually has a strong opinion about the mixed use of various media in rapid succession. She discovers immediate likes and dislikes, which, when expressed, are met with validation and acceptance. This multimedia activity invites curiosity and discovery.

Exploring Feelings

Another beginning Problem Phase intervention is to explore emotions with various colors in a tissue paper collage of feelings. This activity allows me to determine how much the child or teen is aware of his feelings and his perception of his emotional self. I offer a choice of Bristol board in different sizes and ask the child to select the paper that will hold all his feelings, reassuring him he does not have to talk about anything he does not wish to. I give him Mod-Podge in a cup with a brush and various colors of tissue paper. I ask him to select a tissue color that represents each feeling he has, tear the appropriate size, and place it on the Bristol board, then brush it with the Mod-Podge to secure it. I remind him he can layer feelings—for instance, the sadness color on part or all of the anger color, the anger color and the hate color together, or the fear color with the mean color. The use of strong words and the kinesthetic aspect of ripping the tissue activate right-hemisphere nonverbal feelings. Again, the child or teen is invited to comment rather than being asked a direct question about the image. This activity enables the child or teen to view internal feelings in concrete form. I invite him to ponder the image as he thinks about the following questions (based on what the image looks like):

1. What color is largest? If it had a voice, what might the color say?
2. What color is smallest? If it had a voice, what might the color say?
3. What color has some advice for the largest color?
4. What color has some advice for the smallest color?
5. Which color is in charge?
6. Which color would like to be in charge?
7. Which color would like to hide?
8. Which color would protect the hiding color?
9. Which color is most satisfied?
10. Which color is least satisfied?
11. Is there anything you would like to change about the image?

This line of questioning is safe and nonthreatening. We are using the symbolic colors elicited from the right hemisphere as a tool for dialogue. With metaphor and mental representation, the child or teen is identifying, expressing, protecting, and controlling feelings. The child or teen accesses the right-hemisphere nonverbal feelings through the kinesthetic activity. The represented externalized feelings, in concrete form, can be explored safely and validated, and the child or teen has the experience of controlling and managing affect. The resulting mental representation is that feelings can be transformative and change can occur.

Moving more directly to the exploration of feelings, I offer polarity drawings, Riley's term for art directives that look at both sides of an issue (Riley, 1999). These are particularly useful with teens. The ambivalent adolescent is able to evaluate both sides of an issue and formulate an opinion, developing autonomy. An 11- by 14-inch paper is divided with a line down the middle, or two sheets of paper are used. The client is invited to use art media or collage to express "Who I Was When I Was Little/Who I Am Now" (Riley, 1999); "How Others See Me/ How I See Myself" (Riley, 1999); "How I Am Valued/How I Am Criticized" (Riley, 1999); "The Light Part of Me/The Shadow Part of Me"; "The Angry Part of Me/The Happy Part of Me"; "My Strengths/My Vulnerabilities." Moving deeper, I may ask them to portray "How I Act Out My Anger/How I Act In My Anger."

> CASE NOTE: B. is a 15-year-old boy referred for therapy because he quit school and was drinking excessively with friends. He lived with his mother, 18-year-old twin sisters, and 12-year-old brother. During one session, I asked him to depict "How I Act In My Anger" on one half of an 11- by 17-inch piece of paper along with "How I Act Out My Anger" on the other half (see Figure 3.1). He depicted acting in his anger with an image of alcohol and a reclining figure in the dark. He depicted how he acted out when he was angry with images of screaming people. I asked B. if he had anything to say about the image. He said, "Well, I act in my anger by drinking and passing out. I act out my anger by screaming and yelling at home and then my mom starts screaming and then everybody is screaming at each other. That is how my family is."
>
> I then suggested to B. that he make an image of how he would like it to be. I asked if he wanted to cut the image vertically and place it in the middle of the paper, but he chose to work separately. He depicted himself in a home with various family members doing things together. I asked B. if he had anything to say about his image and he replied, "Well, see, here we are all getting along and everyone is home. Nobody is home at my house much, so I just hang out with my friends." After a long pause, he said sadly, "Yes, I really do drink to get away from it all." He took the picture of his family "together" with him when he left the session.

In addition to exploring affect, the use of two sides of a single issue broadens the child's repertoire of intellectual concepts, allows for the expression of negative or angry affect, and often elicits surprising insight. The structured media and containment of the small paper serves to contain and limit expression of affect so it is less likely to frighten him. Nonthreatening doses of self-exploration allow the child or teen to gradually become aware of and sensitive to his affect and not become anxious or fearful. Many children and teens can go too far too fast if the art therapist does not carefully facilitate the depth and breadth of expression. An art therapist will not push the child to reveal the content of his art. Often, the content is not visible to the child or teen right away because he is not yet able to bring the unconscious content of the art to consciousness.

Family Issues

Exploring the child or teen's relationship with family members and addressing family issues is a significant aspect of the Problem Phase of therapy. Rather than discuss family members directly, it is safer for the child or teen to speak of family members metaphorically, such as identifying them as animals. I begin with my collection of over 100 carefully sculpted animals, bugs, fish, insects, dinosaurs, and other creatures. Together we arrange all of them in a standing position on a table. I ask the child to select one for each member of the family including herself. After she makes her choices, I ask her to arrange them from oldest to youngest. Beginning with the youngest animal, I ask her to tell me everything she know about that animal: what it looks like, what it eats, where it sleeps, how it plays, where it lives. I ask about personality traits: Is it friendly or mean, domestic or wild, small or large, cute, funny, friendly, elusive, scary? I write down all the comments she makes to describe that animal. We repeat the descriptive process for each of the remaining animals. I invite her to listen as I read back each description aloud and ask her to tell me if it reminds her of the person or not. I comment that some descriptions will be neutral, some will be funny, and some may reveal something true or serious about the individual. This is a great way to begin exploring family members, their personalities and their behaviors. It is remarkable how many of the projections match the associated family member.

This activity neutralizes the negative and often embarrassing associations held by some children about their family members and their behavior. The symbolic associations to the animal are often quite profound and direct, humorous or sad. The child or teen is able to tolerate the affect associated with the animal as a first step toward expressing negative thoughts and feelings about family members directly.

Expanding on this concept, I invite the client to create an environment for each creature family member, a place where the animal family member can reside, deserves to reside, or should reside. It is surprising how much aggression is expressed metaphorically toward the family member when the child is offered an opportunity to sublimate the aggression. This gives her an opportunity to have metaphorical control over the animal family member. The therapeutic goal is to allow a time and place for negative emotions to arise in a safe way that gradually increases affect tolerance and reduces dissociative coping.

> CASE NOTE: I asked a 14-year-old boy to select a creature for each family member. He chose a tarantula to represent his mother. When asked to tell what he knew about the tarantula, he said, "Everybody is afraid of it, they are scary, they are poison, and they are mean." I asked if any of these descriptions fit his mother or her behavior, and he replied, "Yes, she is all those things. She can kill you. She says it." His eyes began to fill with tears. I quietly asked, "Does your mother ever tell you she will kill you?" With tears rolling down his cheeks, he replied, "Yes, and I think she is joking, but sometimes when she is really mad at me, I am not sure. I get really scared."

This is an example of the depth of emotion that can be activated when the physical self has been strengthened and developed to tolerate the surfacing affect. The art allows the affect to become visible in a metaphorical and symbolic way that can then be tolerated. In my clinical experience, dissociation is not as common in art therapy, because the image serves as a visible reference point for the affective experience. It is as if the person is connected to the image and it holds them to the here and now.

Moving forward to explore family members and relationships in more depth, I provide materials to create dolls to represent family members. This activity takes many sessions, but it has proven to be very successful by nonverbally eliciting deep thoughts and feelings about family members. To get started, I offer an assortment of commercially made, small wooden dowel figures that range in size from 1 to 2½ inches in height, including the head. I invite the child to select one for each family member, including himself, and to select the one he wants to create first. Often the child starts with himself. I ask what he would like the "self" doll to wear—what type of hair, shoes or boots, etc. We usually spend one or two hour-long sessions on each doll. Fine-tip markers are usually used to draw the face, but some children have used small beads to create facial features. I offer a large collection of fabrics and Model Magic for shoes or boots or for arms, hands, or legs. I provide artificial flowers that can be taken apart to make skirts or shirts, and small wood pieces for making hands, ribbons, and hair. Cut feathers can also be used for hair. My role is to facilitate. The child makes the doll just as he wants. I have been asked to purchase special fabrics, yarn of a specific color, and other supplies.

If what I have on hand does not provide the accuracy the child wants to achieve, I willingly provide these items or make them. I knit a tiny cap and shawl for one child. My focus is on the creation of the dolls, but my participation deepens the connection with the child or teen's family for both of us. I begin to use the family member's name. We talk about personality traits. Because the figures are small and manageable, children and teens become comfortable discussing their family members. The child has made the family member as perceived, and the small figures take on significant meaning. Many times I have asked a child or teen to speak to a particular doll about a particular issue. This can elicit deep feelings, especially if the family member has passed away or is no longer a part of the child's life.

Exploring the Unspeakable

Some particularly difficult issues involve shame and secrets. I have found that children and teens are often willing to explore such issues when they are given a safe way to externalize them. It fulfills their need to protect themselves from disclosure or a verbal dialogue about an especially sensitive issue. Some art therapists use what are commonly referred to as "secret boxes." Symbols or images of things to be kept secret are placed or glued inside the box, while symbols or images of what others are permitted to know are arranged on the outside of the box. My method is different. I invite the child or teen to select a box from a bin containing many boxes of various sizes, but all smaller than a shoebox. I provide several 2-inch-square pieces of paper, markers, and a pencil. I ask the child to write a word or make a symbol privately on as few or as many papers as he desires. These are to represent experiences or feelings he would like to contain or get rid of, or at least hold outside himself. The child folds the papers, puts them in the box, and tapes it shut.

I then offer strips of precut plaster casting and a small bowl of water. I ask the child to encase the box in plaster so it can never be opened. The box casting requires three or more layers of casting material. After the plaster is dry, I invite the child or teen to transform the box completely, to make it something that reminds him of what he likes about himself, or something he's thankful for. I offer paint, fabric, wood, jewels, beads, buttons, flowers, decorative papers, ribbons, and other art media.

Although I never ask children to reveal what is inside, I do encourage dialogue about their response to each step of the process, what it feels like to have the material contained, and what they now think and feel about the transformed object. Children must feel safe to reveal or dialogue about uncomfortable issues. These small, safe steps create a mental representation of safety, control, and containment that serves as the scaffolding for the increasing revelation of deeper feelings.

Traumatic reminders of the event are also explored (Pynoos, Steinberg & Goenjian, 1996). Typically, these reminders create physical or emotional states of hypoarousal or hyperarousal. This often occurs through the activation of related sensory reminders, such as smells, tastes, sounds, or sights. The reminders can surface unexpectedly throughout a lifespan. I like to address these reminders by exploring feeling states through art. For example, I may introduce a topic for an image "Last Time I Felt Sad" or "Last Time I Felt Lonely" or "Last Time I Felt Angry." I offer collage or other drawing and painting media. When the image is complete, I invite the child or teen to comment if desired. Then I ask if she can recall what elicited the feelings and if she felt them in her body and, if so, where. These body sensations will elicit affect, and I stay with the affect. I normalize the child's response by gently reminding her that her body holds her emotions and that our bodies are designed to release emotions. I reassure her that her response is a normal reaction to what she has experienced. If the child does not want to respond or participate in the dialogue, I do not pursue it at this time. Her mental representation is that we can talk about painful feelings and she has control over the pacing for doing so.

By accessing the right-hemisphere nonverbal body sensations and memories through the containment of the art, the child or teen is able to tolerate the affect first in the image and then in herself. Eventually, the linking of body sensations to behavior to cognition enables the child or teen to recognize the traumatic reminders (Pynoos, Steinberg, & Goenjian, 1996) and respond nonreactively with cognition-driven behavior.

Grief and Loss

It is usually during the Problem Phase of therapy that grief and loss issues arise. Art can serve as a method of expressing what is often too overwhelming for words. Prayer flags, memorials, and memory books are all useful for memorializing those who have passed away.

Before beginning, I bring up the topic of art as a memorial and briefly describe the Reverend Martin Luther King Jr. Memorial, the Vietnam Veteran's Memorial, and the Lincoln Memorial. We then discuss the particular personality of the person in the child's life who is deceased, what the person liked and disliked, and any other information about the person that the child knows and wants to share. I take note of the words that are used. As I read back the words, the child or teen can think about that person and how he might want to create a small memorial for that individual. If he seems interested in doing so, I suggest prayer flags, a memorial sculpture, or a memory book, but if he offers a different idea, I welcome it. One child chose to create a diorama of him and his father fishing near a lake and said that was how he wanted to remember his dad.

Prayer flags are made by cutting various colors of good-quality 8½- by 11-inch paper in half vertically, folding each strip in half, and firmly creasing the folded edge. I provide scissors, glue, glue brush, glue gun, markers, color pencils, paint, pastels, origami and other decorative papers, jewels, ribbons and cording, buttons, and yarn. I include words or groups of words from used greeting cards that have sentiments of sympathy, caring, and hope and family words such as mother, father, brother, sister, and grandmother. The child or teen creates prayer flags for the deceased, as many as desired, using the materials arrayed around him. He can write his own sentiments on the inside of the prayer flag if desired. If he wants to keep the contents private, he can glue the prayer flag shut.

Prayer flags can also be made for nonfamily individuals the child or teen has lost, including pets. This activity can be extended to include prayer flags for anyone to whom the child wishes to send good wishes, encouragement, or healing thoughts. A cord, ribbon, or string is threaded through the folded flag and held in place with tape or glue so they do not slide together. Ample extra cord or ribbon is left on the ends for hanging and tying.

Memorial sculptures can be made from any media. A typical method is to select a base from a variety of boxes, picture frames, and wood scraps. Many children and teens make an altar-shaped form and install a photo of the deceased on the altar space. They often include artificial flowers and images reflecting the personality or special preferences of the deceased. Some children add a poem. Sometimes they write words on the sculpture. I do discuss with them that eventually the glue will dry, the boxes will fade or get dusty, and they most likely will not have the sculpture forever. We take a photo or make a detailed drawing of the memorial for safekeeping.

It may take several sessions to create a memory book. I invite clients to start by thinking of all the things they know about the deceased person and write them down. To get them started, I ask if they know the person's favorite food, television show, flower, or article of clothing and his or her favorite activities, such as reading or gardening or fishing. I then introduce more interpersonal topics, both positive and negative: what you liked best about the person, the last time you did something fun together, the last time you had a disagreement, the last time the person made you feel bad, and the last time the person made you feel good. I also introduce issues pertaining to their personal loss: what I miss most and what I wish I could say that I did not get to say. To facilitate closure, I introduce concepts of moving forward: what the person would want me to do now that they are gone, how I can honor the life of the person, and how I want to always remember the person. Whether or not the child utilizes my suggestion is not as important as the mental representation that it is all right to discuss these topics. Parents report that their children seldom give up the memory books even though they no longer look at them.

At the end of each session in the Problem Phase, I offer a few words of recap. Special consideration is given to the closing minutes of the session. I ask the child or teen if there are any uncomfortable feelings, thoughts, or images he would like to leave behind at the studio. I have at the ready 18- by 24-inch paper and oil pastels. Using gross motor movements, the child can scribble shapes and color to illustrate "Leaving the Worry Behind." If the child resists, I simply ask him to use the art media to get out any extra energy that may have been stirred up. Once he begins, the motor movements increase, the pressure on the pastel intensifies, and the body engages. Following this activity, the child or teen is typically in a calm state. I also use this technique for specific issues that arise. Sleep problems are a good example. I ask the child or teen to think about being awake at night and to scribble with oil pastels whatever had come to mind. I also suggest that he will be able to sleep. Children and teens are amazed that this technique works.

A reduction in symptoms indicates the child has moved through the Problem Phase of therapy. Changes in behavior and functioning are evident. The child demonstrates behavioral improvement at home and school, including academically, and he usually has satisfying relationships with peers.

TRANSFORMATION PHASE

The Transformation Phase is one of redefining, reclaiming, and practicing. There is stability of affect and behavior, but a temporary retreat to earlier problematic behavior is not uncommon. The goal is cognitive homeostasis, having a cognitive understanding of the past, and utilizing cognition-driven behavior. Symbolic exploration of the nonverbal affect-laden content of the art provides access to the higher structures for contemplation. Erroneously held negative beliefs about the self are explored and redefined. Fragments of the self, memory, and experience have become integrated through creative acts that reclaim and revitalize the self. Behavior problems are not extinguished, but they are no longer denied, and there is an effort to improve.

CASE NOTE: A 15-year-old girl with a history of neglect was seen in
therapy for many months for a substance abuse problem. She had been
mostly free from substance abuse but was relapsing occasionally. During
the Transformation Phase, I asked her to make an image that depicted
where she was and where she was going and to indicate where she saw
herself in the image. She painted an image along the Pacific Coast
Highway of Southern California. She stated she was on the road. When I
pointed out that I could not see her on the road, she said, "Well, I guess
you are right that I didn't put myself on the road. I don't know where I am
on the road because I am still using. I have not really totally quit."

Although this is not good news, it is a good example of a Transformation
Phase image. She is no longer in denial, and she is honest about the fact that she
has not quit her substance abuse. We may return to earlier Problem Phase
approaches to explore symbolically more of the painful emotions being dissociated via her substance abuse.

The Transformation and Integration Phases are typically shorter than the Self
and Problem Phases. A gradual shift begins when there is evidence of psychic relief
from trauma, which is observed as a nearly total abatement of symptoms. The presenting behaviors are no longer as evident or frequent and mainly appear during
times of extreme stress, if at all. The reports from home and school are consistent
with the positive changes in behavior and functioning seen in the therapy setting.

The child or teen has addressed aspects of his traumatic experience, grief, and
losses in various symbolic ways over time and now has a realistic self-concept and a
coherent narrative of his life experience. He exhibits primarily cognition-driven
behavior and is not as reactive to stimuli related to his trauma or loss. As in development and healing, there may be steps forward and steps back, but the child or teen
is developmentally on track and has replaced his maladaptive coping with life-
affirming coping.

Because the client has been responsible for his own interpretation of his art,
he has developed the level of skill that allows him to use symbolic and metaphorical content in new ways. Many who have used art as the focus of their healing now use the metaphorical and symbolic content to help them discover
deeper aspects of themselves, their relationships, and their future goals.

Working with art media to portray their life story creates a visual autobiographical life narrative. Creating their life story from birth to the present offers an
opportunity to visually represent past experiences and recall the states of mind
associated with those visual representations that open new forms of information
processing (Siegel, 2002). Children now have a context for their life trauma and
can see that the trauma was a part of their life but that it does not define their life.

Transformation Phase Interventions

Creating an autobiographical life narrative is a process that will take many sessions. To begin, I provide a 12-inch by 5-foot scroll of drawing paper. The left

side is taped to the table, with about 3 feet of paper exposed. The additional paper remains rolled and held in place with a heavy object such as a metal ruler. Placing my hands on the smooth surface, moving them with an easy sweeping motion, I invite the child or teen to imagine that this paper will be a map of her life. A variety of drawing media and collage media, including toy catalogs and stickers, are available so she can create the beginning of her life story with images. For motivation, I ask whether she knows if she was born in a hospital or somewhere else. I ask if she was told who was there to celebrate. I ask if she has ever been told about her early days as a baby, what toys or activities she liked, or if she remembers a special toy. I offer a selection of baby stickers and baby accessory stickers to make it easy and fun to get started. The child adds drawings and images from magazines as she works. In toy catalogues, the child or teen sometimes find pictures of toys she had in the past. In many cases, this part of the narrative brings up feelings of loss, such as loss of a favorite toy, or the loss of a family member or pet.

I have consistently found that the end of participation in the creation of the narrative corresponds with the arrest in the child's development due to traumatic events, diagnoses of chronic illness, or other life-changing experiences. I neither insist on nor encourage further work on development of the narrative. Rather, I refocus the child or teen with nondirective art making to elicit the nonverbal, right-hemisphere, body-based memories so they can be expressed and integrated. I reintroduce the narrative project from time to time, and the child works on it as desired.

Another reason children may stop work on the narrative project is that they have reached the chronological point at which they were removed from their home, became homeless, or experienced another traumatic event. Justifiably, they may be resistant to the idea of including those events in the narrative. I reassure them that they do not have to complete this part of the narrative. I suggest that if they wish, they can leave a space and revisit this part of their life at another time. They are taking control of their own expression and pacing, an important part of the Transformation Phase of art therapy. Usually, they are able to go back and fill in the empty spaces once they have a context for the experience in their life. It is not uncommon to return to Problem Phase interventions to address issues that arise in the creation of the autobiographical life story.

To aid in the process of transformation, opportunities for transformational art experiences are a focus of the treatment. A mental representation is created that change can occur, can occur in therapy, and can occur with the help of another. I offer transition tasks such as "Complete a Picture." I glue some part of a transformational image to a sheet of drawing paper and ask the child to draw the rest of the image. Another approach is to divide paper vertically and ask him to create an image with collage or other media in response to the prompt "The Best Person I Could Be/The Worst Person I Could Be" (Riley, 1999). Then I divide that paper and put a new sheet of drawing paper between the polarity drawings and ask the child to create a representation of "Who I Want to Be." With older children and teens, I include "Where I Have Been/Where I Am Going." Many draw a bridge or open road in response. I may ask, "Where are you on this journey today?" I am sometimes surprised at the honesty children convey in their answers, but it tells me they have become comfortable about revealing their backward steps, resistance, or experimentation with old or risky behavior patterns. I validate this as a normal, healthy part of their progress in therapy and thank them for their honesty about their art. I instill feelings of hope and forward thinking rather than failure, disappointment, or worse, shame.

To encourage creative, forward-leaning thoughts, I include "invention art" projects during the Transformation Phase. By now, the client has a very good idea of the variety of media available and how they are manipulated. I invite her to invent something teens (or children) need that no one has yet created. I may suggest she invent a new method of cooking or invent an ideal self. The invention tasks are fun and enlivening. They engage the full use of one's imagination. When the invention is complete, we describe the invention according to what it looks like and compare the descriptions to the child or teen. They are often amusing, sometimes neutral, and sometimes poignant.

Creating "A Room of One's Own" is another favorite Transformation Phase intervention. For motivation, I ask the child or teen to imagine having a room that is his alone. He can decorate and furnish it however he wishes. I tell him he has complete control over who is allowed into the room and who is excluded. I ask him to think about sensory comforts, about necessities for living, and about how he would spend his time in the room. I offer an assortment of shoe and boot boxes and invite the client to pick the size and shape he would like his room to be. Using any media they wish, children are encouraged to create their own space, the décor, the furniture, and such accessories as a computer, a television, or a fish tank. The room creation typically takes several sessions.

Clients are asked to consider how they would use the space. They can divide it, change the shape of the box, or alter the roofline. I offer fabric, balsawood, paint, decorative papers, collage magazines for pictures of appliances, and various sizes of plastic shapes for skylights and windows. Some children glue images from magazines to the windows to create scenery they would like to see from inside their room. When the room is complete, I ask them to describe a few hours spent in it, elaborate on who is allowed to visit and who is not, and tell how they will take care of the room. I also ask what they could do if they become bored or lonely. Children and teens very much enjoy imagining and creating a place to be in control of themselves and their own personal space.

In many families, there are no visual records of the child or teen as an infant or child. Many of the young people with whom I have worked have never seen a photograph of themselves as a small child. Some may have a photograph, but only one. Although not as desirable as an actual image of the child or teen, we can create a visual representation of his life that provides a context for their existence and life experiences.

It is during the Transformation Phase that the autobiographical visual narrative scroll is completed. As clients bring the narrative to the present time, I ask them to imagine three possible futures for themselves. I suggest they may want to continue adding to their life story as time passes and offer to add as much paper to the scroll as they desire for future entries.

INTEGRATION PHASE

During the fourth phase, the Integration Phase, symptoms have reduced, adaptive coping skills are developed, and the goal is termination of treatment. We have identified the child or teen's support system and reviewed and practiced coping skills. He is becoming future oriented and has the ability to separate past experiences from who he is now. There is symptom reduction, a continued refinement of self-regulation, and emotional processing. By this time in art therapy, the child or teen has an affinity for the creative process or creative activity.

Art is often used not only as a coping mechanism but also for pleasure. In the last chapters of Daniel Siegel's book *The Developing Mind* (1999), he writes of his integrated patients having a desire to be creative. I posit that having some form of creative endeavor is a component of a healthy and integrated mind. I do not mean to imply that one must make art to be healthy. If one has had an experience of safe self-expression, exploration, and healing, then creativity can be seen as a tool rather than a pastime. Creativity serves as a way to express and contain thoughts, feelings, and ideas and as a pathway for further knowing.

> CASE NOTE: A 13-year-old boy came to art therapy because he was skipping school, stealing, and exhibiting disruptive behavior at school. During many months of therapy, he had explored his adoption history, abandonment by his parents, and a difficult adjustment to the culture of his adoptive home that was different from his own. As the boy neared the end of therapy, he told me that he thought he did not need to come anymore because he was not getting in trouble and was busy: He and his friends had formed a band. He was thrilled that he had earned his share of money for the bass guitar that he wanted to buy. His parents required him to earn half the cost of the guitar by doing extra household chores and helping with his younger sister. I agreed that he had made many changes in his behavior, that he was engaged with his music, and that therapy was getting in the way of his life. He laughed and asked, "How about if I go a certain time with no trouble at home or at school and then I can quit therapy?" I asked, "What amount of time would you think would be fair—a week, or what?" He replied, "No, a week is not long enough. I think a month would show that I really don't get in trouble anymore, not just for a week." I agreed. He made a series of small sculptures that reminded him of his progress in therapy and had plans to have sculpture material at home in order, he said, "to make art when I am not making music."

This example of a teen demonstrating confidence in his ability to refrain from getting in trouble at home or at school was evidence of his readiness to terminate therapy. He had transformed his negative behaviors and was now engaged in creative and social endeavors that occupied his time and served as a method of creative expression.

The Integration Phase is a positive stage because the child or teen is experiencing the relief of symptom reduction and gaining the ability to regulate her affect. She experiences a sense of satisfaction with her usual activities and is able to have meaningful social interaction with peers. She demonstrates a developed and accurate self-concept by knowing her strengths and vulnerabilities. She is able to regulate her affect in the face of traumatic reminders (Pynoos, Steinberg, & Goenjian, 1996) or while experiencing stress. The child or teen is able to utilize cognition-driven behavior demonstrated in thinking before acting, evaluating risk, and considering consequences. Coping mechanisms are adaptive and life affirming. The child or teen has identified her support system and is comfortable with her level of safety. Psycho-education is useful to explain to the child or teen the possible developmental need for future therapy (Pynoos, 1996), as the symptoms may reoccur at significant times in the future. A young girl, for example, may have to revisit her issues of sexual molestation when she becomes interested in dating.

Bringing art therapy to closure takes place over several sessions if possible. Once teens decide to terminate, it is hard to get them to return for more than a few sessions. This phase of therapy includes the opportunity for clients to review their art portfolio. It is often a surprise to them to see where they began and the content and quality of their images early in therapy. The portfolio provides a visual record of their progress, setbacks, and movement forward in the art therapy. Children are often surprised to see themselves reflected in earlier "self states." They select the art they want to keep, and I explain that the rest will be discarded after six months. I express that it was an honor to be a part of their life journey and to witness the art and stories they have created. I let them know my door is always open and that they are free to visit or return to art therapy at any time.

Integration Interventions

A major task of the Integration Phase of therapy is to create new methods of coping, living, and relating to others. A useful tool for this activity is to ask children to create an image that represents their "Inner Advisor" (Rossman, 2000, p. 216) by suggesting they use color and shapes or an image to put their inner healer or advisor into visual form. Another option I offer is a large circle approximately 15 inches in diameter made from good-quality drawing paper. I invite them to use collage or other art media to depict "My World." This allows for a visual representation of their perceived and/or imagined future.

It is during the Integration Phase that the child or teen is encouraged to identify and activate his support system. They do so by letting a family member, a trusted family friend, or another trusted adult know how to be of help when called upon to listen, comfort, or help problem-solve in times of stress. I offer community resources that may be available to the child, such as theater, dance, or art groups, the library, and youth centers.

The Integration Phase is also a time of reviewing relationships. Children create art with collage media or drawings to represent the qualities they find appealing in a friend and those qualities they find irritating or dissatisfying. Once they have completed the image, we discuss which ones they can tolerate, those that could be discussed with the friend, and those that are deal breakers. There are times when the child may want to establish new boundaries. For instance, a child or teen may not want to attend a traditional family holiday event that requires her to be around a perpetrator who hurt her in the past. Helping the child or teen communicate the need for these changes to parents and caregivers is an important way to support her during her transition toward emotional self-care, boundaries, and physical and psychological safety.

Another transitional technique is to create symbols and rituals for new ways of coping and living. I particularly like the use of animal totems for this art project. Together we use my collection to arrange a large variety of sculpted wild, domestic, farm, and zoo animals, insects, sea creatures, amphibians, and reptiles on the table. After looking at and thinking about the choices in front of her, she picks the one that could serve as her protector or guide during times of trouble, doubt, or fear. When she has selected the totem, I ask her to sculpt it from clay or Model Magic. Following the modeling of the creature, the child is invited to build a safe environment for her totem. While she is doing this, we discuss the similarities between her animal — its qualities and characteristics — and her. I ask the child to imagine a mild problem the animal could have and then imagine how the animal could solve that problem. Then I ask her to imagine an even more severe problem the animal might have and how the animal would solve that problem. This offers an opportunity to address the fact that everyone has both positive and adverse times in life, including losses. I reinforce that these are normal life experiences and that they are unavoidable, but how we respond is a choice. This imparts a mental representation that these experiences are normal and occur throughout a lifetime and that now the child can cope and will be able to handle new challenges.

One of the last activities in NDAT therapy is to create "Boundary Bowls." I begin by introducing children to the idea that in many cultures, a bowl or vessel is used for many things. A vessel can be a symbol for offering, giving, ritual, harvest, bounty, fulfillment, holding, or beauty. I explain that I would like them to make a bowl that represents boundaries and giving. To create a bowl, a balloon is blown to 4 to 6 inches in diameter. Mod-Podge is brushed on the bottom half of the balloon. Strips of newspaper approximately 1 inch by 5 inches are layered on top of the Mod-Podge and then more Mod-Podge is brushed on the newspapers. This is repeated until there are eight to ten layers on the bottom half of the balloons. The edge can be left irregular or gently folded toward the balloon to form a smooth edge. Let the material rest until it is at least dry to the touch. This part of the project can usually be completed in one session.

When the material is dry or nearly dry, pop the balloon. I provide assorted tissue paper and magazines and ask the child or teen to decorate the outside of the bowl with layers of tissue and images that represent things he needs to keep at bay, his personal boundaries. On the inside of the bowl, the client uses tissue and images or symbols to represent what he wishes to protect or nurture, his self-protection symbols. Mod-Podge is used to adhere the tissue layers and/or magazine images. When completed, the bowls have utility and beauty, but they should not be used for serving food.

SUMMARY

The NDAT model is one that begins with building and strengthening the physical body and the sensory and motor systems. This allows the system to develop the mind/body/self that is the scaffolding for the next phases of therapy. In my clinical experience, children and teens are often unwilling or unable to talk about themselves or their trauma. They do not like to answer questions, or they do so with minimal participation. Activating the right hemisphere with visual and sensory experiences allows children to portray their experiences in nonverbal formats that enable them to externalize the images and the affect associated with them. The neural systems will move the information processing to the higher structures and left-hemisphere explicit memory, as evidenced in the ability to engage in verbal dialogue about the experience.

The NDAT approach is a working model. I hope that others will expand on these concepts to create other effective PTSD treatment models. The ability to heal from adversity is one of life's challenges. Giving children and teens the opportunity to recover from their traumatic and neglectful histories offers them the potential for a happy and fulfilling life.

PART II

NEUROBIOLOGICAL DEVELOPMENT AND THERAPEUTIC CONTEXT

The development of a secure attachment with a primary caregiver is described as the essential task of development during the first year of life (Schore & Schore, 2008). An infant is born with only partially developed peripheral and central nervous systems, and it is widely accepted that both genetics and experience interact to shape postnatal brain development (Cozolino, 2002; Schore, 2003a; Siegel, 1999). Attachment—parent to child, child to parent—is the context for the growth of the nervous system. The genetically programmed development of the brain is optimized by an attuned caregiver. When the attachment process breaks down in situations of deprivation or trauma, development of the nervous system is compromised, necessitating a therapeutic context for treatment and repair.

The process of creating attachment between mother and child begins at birth and is central to their relationship throughout the first year of life. The infant is completely dependent on his caregiver for survival. Infant and caregiver share repeated interactions in which the infant signals needs and the caregiver responds. This give-and-take places the infant in close proximity to the mother as they share repetitive visual, tactile, olfactory, and auditory experiences. These early sensory sensations stimulate the infant's brain and facilitate attachment behavior (Schore, 2001).

In an ideal world, new mothers would have the resources, support, and preference to be with their infant at least during the first year of life and optimally for the first 3 years. In addition to having the opportunity to create a secure attachment during this time, it is within this specific interactional pattern that the matrix for optimal emotional and social development forms. The mother's presence and caregiving behaviors allow the infant's sensory systems to adapt comfortably to the increasing stimulation within the relationship. However, our current socioeconomic structure places heavy demands on parents, mothers in particular, to return to the workplace to provide financial support for their children. Many children are placed with multiple caregivers many days and hours per week in environments that may be overstimulating or mismatched to the infant's developmental needs. Many day-care facilities offer high-quality care, but there is no substitute for the infant's consistent contact with his mother and her ability to develop a specific interactional pattern with her child (Schore, 1996).

Embedded in these attachment experiences is the mother's opportunity to develop a state of attunement that allows her an extremely nuanced sensitivity to her infant's internal states and to subtle changes in growth, development, and information processing. Infant right-brain development occurs in a dyadic relationship with another person's right brain and body (Schore, 2012). Without either language or cognition, the infant conveys internal states of arousal to the mother via right-brain-to-right-brain sensory communication, and the mother responds in these modalities: "Through visual-facial, auditory-prosodic, and tactile-gestural communication, caregiver and infant learn the rhythmic structure of the other and modify their behavior to fit that structure, thereby co-creating a specifically fitted interaction" (Schore, 2012, p. 75).

Within this dynamic relationship, the infant and mother have experiences of affective resonance and ensuing states of positive arousal. If the mother is not attuned, the infant will signal his negative arousal by crying, arching his back, averting his gaze. The mother can repair this situation by responding in a way that meets the needs of the child and calms the infant, restoring the synchrony between them. This is successful attachment at work. Schore asserts that this regulatory process of affect synchrony is the "fundamental building block of attachment and its associated emotions, and resilience in the face of stress and novelty is an ultimate indicator of attachment security" (Schore, 2012, p. 76).

If the infant remains in a state of negative arousal and a prolonged period of misattunement, the result is the failure of the development of a self. This stressful state, if repeated frequently and sustained, is damaging to brain cells and constricts brain development. Securely attached infants experience themselves as worthy of care and effective at obtaining care in a nurturing world. As a result, infants with secure attachments demonstrate good developmental outcomes and resiliency (Waters, Wippman, & Sroufe,1979). Those with insecure or especially disorganized attachments exhibit more psychopathology, and in many cases their sensory-motor functioning is compromised (Green & Goldwyn, 2002; Solomon, George, & De Jong, 1995).

Just as attachment occurs in genetically determined sequential experiences with a primary attachment figure (Schore, 2001; Siegel, 2002), the infant's sensory and motor systems develop through sequential and repetitive interaction with the primary caregiver and eventually the infant's extended environment. Piaget (1964) refers to this as the sensory-motor stage of cognitive development. Cognition is demonstrated through motor activity during infancy. Learning about the world occurs during physical interaction with the parent and the environment. These early sensory experiences also contribute to the maturation of the developing right brain.

The right hemisphere develops before the left and is more mature and more functional than the left (Schleussner et al., 2004; Schore, 2012). Right-brain activity begins immediately after birth. For example, the infant's olfactory and hearing systems can discriminate between the mother and another individual. The earliest communication between mother and child is nonverbal collaborative communication, inherent in the early dyadic relationship (Siegel, 1999). The mother and infant engage in right-hemisphere-to-right-hemisphere communication that is essential for the maturation of the developing right brain. The communications are sensory, body-based communications of the right brain: voice, body gestures, touch, facial expression, muscle tone and movement, tactile sensations, eye contact, and mutual gaze (Bowlby, 1969; Schore, 2012):

> In sustained mutual gaze transactions, the mother's facial expression stimulates and amplifies positive affect in the infant. The child's internally pleasurable state is communicated back to the mother, and in this interactive system of reciprocal communication, both members of the dyad enter into a symbiotic state of heightened positive affect. This psychoneurobiological mechanism is essential to an imprinting phenomenon in the child's developing right hemisphere, thereby enabling the maturation of limbic areas in the cortex that are involved in socioemotional functions. (Schore, 1994, p. 71)

Based on the repetitive postnatal interaction with the attachment figure, the sensory systems develop from primitive to complex. These experiences allow for a gradual increase in the ability to process incoming sensory information. While the infant is exploring the world through sensory modes, the neural networks are being formed that are the foundation of cognitive, emotional, and social development (Schore, 2003a). Because the brain develops from the base forward, lower areas of the brain develop and organize before the limbic and cortical structures. As the infant's brain develops in this sequential, hierarchical fashion, the increasingly complex limbic and cortical areas develop and organize and begin controlling reactive portions of the brain (Perry, 1995). The development of the higher structures is dependent on the optimal development and organization of the lower structures (Fisher & Murray, 1991):

> Just as common sense shows that the first year of an infant's life must be devoted to the development of a functional sensory-motor system in order for the child to take in the information needed to develop his emotional-cognitive system, so at each stage of development each new system is dependent upon the full function of the system that developmentally preceded it. (Pearce, 2002, p. 50)

Mahler and colleagues (1975) propose that the development of motor skills, language, and the ensuing cognition plays a role in the child's ability to decrease his dependence on the mother's physical proximity. Fred Pine refers to the necessary tools required for learning:

> For learning to take place, the *basic tools* for the process must be biologically and
> psychologically intact and must have developed in age-appropriate ways . . . Tools
> such as the capacity for intake of information through visual, auditory, and tactile
> channels (and output through all channels as well), perceptual discrimination,
> visual organization, visual and auditory short and long-term memory, sequencing of
> concepts, and sustained attention. (Pine, 1985, p. 186)

Those infants who do not have an opportunity to develop a secure attachment
with a primary caregiver have not had optimal development of their fragile sensory systems. The negative effects of the lack of maturation of the right hemisphere, and consequently the lack of an attachment with a primary caregiver and
the opportunity to develop sensory and motor systems gradually, affects all future
development and functioning:

> Deficits in function must be associated with defects in dynamic structural systems,
> and a theory of the genesis of psychopathology needs to be tied to current develop-
> mental neurobiological models of the experience-dependent anatomical matura-
> tion of brain systems, especially those involved in socioemotional functioning.
> (Schore, 2003b, p. 32)

Many children referred to therapy for emotional and behavior problems are
operating with reactive cognition. They are unable to tolerate affect or regulate
their emotions and often present with an inability to control their behavior.
Many of these children are not able to participate in therapy initially because
they are not able to form a therapeutic relationship. Often they dissociate to
avoid emotions. Many cannot focus for more than a few moments before becoming distracted or anxious. Therefore, it is advantageous to revisit early critical
periods in development in the context of the therapy setting in order to replicate
missed opportunities for the optimal development of the systems that process
information. Only then will the child be able to access the middle and higher
structures of the brain and participate fully in therapy.

Describing their neurosequential model of therapeutics, Perry and Hambrick
(2008) assert:

> The more the therapeutic process can replicate the normal sequential process of
> development, the more effective the interventions are. Simply stated, the idea is to
> start with the lowest (in the brain) undeveloped/abnormally functioning set of
> problems and move sequentially up the brain as improvements are seen. This may
> involve initially focusing on a poorly organized brainstem/diencephalon and the
> related self-regulation, attention, arousal, and impulsivity by using any variety of
> patterned, repetitive somatosensory activities. . . . Once there is improvement in
> self-regulation, the therapeutic work can move to more relations-related problems
> (limbic) using more traditional play or arts therapies and ultimately, once funda-
> mental dyadic relational skills have improved, the therapeutic techniques can be
> more verbal and insight oriented (cortical) using any variety of cognitive-behavioral
> or psychodynamic approaches. (p. 42)

The next three chapters are devoted to development and functioning of the right hemisphere, based on my clinical practice. I have observed, consistently, that the pathways for sensory information processing and attachment can be fostered at later ages in development. Chapter 4 offers ways to develop and strengthen the sensory and information-processing systems in infants and toddlers. Activities for children and teens are also provided. Chapter 5 describes ways to replicate attachment behavior in the therapy setting. Chapter 6 presents ways to facilitate expression from the unconscious right hemisphere and describes how the therapist and client remain in right-hemisphere information processing during art and play.

CHAPTER 4

Development of the Right Brain:
An Essential Task of the
First Year of Life

This chapter offers ways for therapists to help parents and caregivers develop and strengthen an infant's sensory system and engage in attachment behaviors with the child as he moves from infancy (birth to 18 months) and into toddlerhood (18 months to 36 months). The simple, short play activities engage the parent and child in safe, enjoyable, growth-enhancing activities not only for the child who is developing on a typical trajectory but also for the child whose functioning is compromised either by genetics or from a lack of attunement with a caregiver during early development. The activities can be done by parents, therapists, teachers, and foster parents. All enhance development and strengthen attachment behavior between the caregiver and the child. The chapter also offers a variety of suggested activities for the same purpose for older children and teens who experienced adverse conditions in early life that prevented optimal development.

Sensory and motor delays can be caused by genetics, by prenatal and postnatal experiences, and by the interaction between biology and environment. The presenting symptoms that arise as a result of these delays can overlap with other childhood disorders. Studies suggest that children and teens with attention deficit hyperactivity disorder (ADHD) may have underdiagnosed sensory problems (Mangeot et al., 2007) and that particular sensory deficits may account for specific subgroups in populations of those with ADHD (Reynolds & Lane, 2009). In my clinical experience, many children and teens diagnosed with attention deficit and mood disorders have been denied the opportunity to develop a secure attachment with a primary caregiver. These patients often have tactile, auditory, fine motor, gross motor, visual/perceptual, vestibular, or proprioceptive delays. Many have receptive or expressive language delays. They may present with hyperactivity, inability to focus, distractibility, and inability to sit upright for more than a few moments without fidgeting or changing position.

The Neuro-developmental Art Therapy (NDAT) model of treatment can help repair these early deficits of attachment and sensory and motor delays by providing an opportunity to revisit critical periods in development. This model promotes a relationship in which the child has interactive sensory and motor experiences that were inadequate or totally missing in their early years. These experiences provide the necessary scaffolding for the development of the sensory-motor systems, restoring the developmental trajectory that leads to competent behavioral management, learning, and social interaction. The process of engaging in these early missed experiences offers an opportunity to develop a core concept of mind/body/self that was not developed during the initial primary relationship with a caregiver (Schore, 2012).

I have compiled a variety of developmentally sensitive interventions that facilitate cortical development and that offer the caregiver and the infant/toddler/ child/teen novel and developmentally consistent parent-child interactions. Many sensory and motor experiences are inherent in art making. However, understanding and using specifically focused interventions for specific delays can lead to rapid improvement.

> **CASE NOTE:** A 14-year-old boy was referred for art therapy following his arrest for stealing a bicycle from a neighbor's garage. I noticed immediately that his initial drawings contained indicators of neurological impairment: gross asymmetry, lack of closure at corners or circles, forms or objects that slanted 15 degrees or more, and visual-spatial difficulty. I offered this young teen a variety of sensory, bilateral, and gross motor art activities at the beginning of each session for a period of ten sessions. He was highly resistant to any dialogue, so for most of the remaining time in each of the ten sessions, he made art in silence. I offered a variety of textured media for three-dimensional sculpture. We dialogued about his art as much as he was able to tolerate, and he was able to see aspects of himself reflected in his art process and product.
>
> After ten weeks of art therapy, his father reported that the teen was doing much better at controlling his behavior at home and in school. One day, I asked the teen if he noticed anything different about himself after coming to art therapy for the past couple of months. He replied, "I notice that I think more before I do things."

This example clearly illustrates the benefit of recognizing and addressing sensory-motor delays rather than focusing only on the problematic behavior. Here is evidence that once the teen is able to be in greater control physically by strengthening his sensory-motor skills, the lower structures are able to inform the higher structures that are the locus of control of more complex information processing and behaviors, including social behaviors.

RIGHT-BRAIN DEVELOPMENT

Infants primarily sleep and eat during the first few days of life. Their central nervous system and sensory system are not fully developed, and initially they can tolerate very little stimulation as they begin to adjust to an environment much more complex than the womb. Optimally, they are in a state of physical safety and security, with their attachment figure in close proximity providing food, smiles, and hygiene care. A newborn infant's highly sensitive and underdeveloped sensory system requires gentle movement, soft voices or music, and low-stimulus environments.

As children mature and are awake for longer periods of time, their sensory systems strengthen and they are able to tolerate more stimulation. Engaging in safe and fun sensory-motor activities will aid neurological development. Activities for older children may also be taught to parents and caregivers, as they offer ways parents can play and interact with their children as they grow, reinforcing the parent-child relationship while promoting the maturation of the child's capacities. Some parents intuitively stimulate and play with infants and children, but others need support and concrete suggestions. One parent reported she had never played with her child until she learned activities that could guide her interaction with him.

When the activities between the child and caregiver are facilitated by a therapist, it is imperative to let parents know that both infants and toddlers with delays require very short periods of stimulation, measured in seconds or minutes. As the child matures, he can gradually increase the time spent on each activity. The therapist should help the caregiver become attuned to how her child signals that it is time for a break. Such signals include apathy, fussiness, or irritability. Some children continue an activity even when they are too tired or frustrated and provide only subtle cues that parents may miss but the therapist can help them recognize. I remind parents and caregivers that babies require constant supervision and should never be left alone, with or without toys. Never assume a baby will not do something he has not done before.

When I use these interventions with older children in the therapy setting, I begin with 10 or 15 minutes of remedial activity. The remainder of the session is devoted to art therapy or play therapy. The introductory activities may be either novel or familiar. If there is evidence of a significant delay, I repeat activities that will strengthen particular skills to reinforce the newly developed neural pathways.

VISUAL DEVELOPMENT

In the earliest stages of infancy, the visual system is limited to attend to the human eyes and face at a distance of 6 to 12 inches (Fantz 1961). The caregiver's face and eyes are the optimal source of visual stimuli for the infant. They are the pathway for nonverbal communication between caregiver and infant. Mothers instinctively cradle newborns on the left side of their body to nurse, a position that results in a cessation of adrenal hormone production in the infant, activates the sense of taste, aids in the successful adaptation to the new environment, and facilitates the attachment experience (Kennell & Klaus, 1979; Klaus, 1970, 1972; Pearce, 1992). Left placement of the infant also stimulates visual senses not activated before birth. Placing the infant in the left-breast position puts him in close proximity to the mother's face, activating the visual circuits that respond to that stimulus, promoting visual development. Because the right hemisphere receives input from the left side of the body, when the mother turns the infant to feed at the left breast, the mother's left eye looks directly into the left eye of the infant, facilitating right-brain-to-right-brain communication (Schore, 2012).

Techniques for Visual Development in Infants and Toddlers

Simple techniques aid in the development of the visual system of infants and toddlers. Those recommended by the American Optometric Association (AOA) include changing the position of the crib or the child's position in the crib from time to time, using a dim night light, hanging mobiles, talking to the baby when walking around the room, and keeping the baby's toys within his visual field of 10–12 inches (www.aoa.org).

One of the earliest ways to stimulate visual strengthening is to engage in mirror play using a wall-mounted mirror. Holding the baby so he can see himself and his mother and repeating the child's name or making friendly faces will promote attachment as well as strengthen the visual system. Placing a toy under a cloth and then revealing it helps promote visual memory. Blowing a large bubble for the infant to see and watch or rolling a ball back and forth in front of the infant will aid in visual tracking skills. With a toddler, batting a balloon back and forth or rolling a ball back and forth strengthens visual tracking and eye-hand coordination.

When working with a mother and infant, I encourage them to engage in these activities together, facilitating their attachment. For example, in ball rolling, I do not become a third participant in the activity. Instead, I may get the stray ball and return it to the dyad, offer encouragement, or help the mother recognize the child's nonverbal communication such as fatigue or boredom with the activity. When blowing bubbles, I blow them so the mother and infant have the shared experience of tracking them.

Techniques for Visual Development in Children and Teens

Problems with visual perceptual development and visual motor development are often evident in children's drawings. Circles lacking closure, distortion of forms, gross asymmetry, slanting of images 15 degrees or more, drawing and redrawing or excessive erasures, and lack of spatial depth in drawing or painting are all possible indicators of visual difficulties (Uhlin, 1972). Children with these difficulties frequently announce they "hate to draw."

To aid children and teens with visual perceptual development, eye-hand coordination, and visual discrimination skills, I usually begin with bilateral scribbling and drawing. This is an excellent way to engage with the client in a safe, fun, and no-fail experience, activating the lower structures of the brain and stimulating the formulation of images (Lusebrink, 1990). Another reason for beginning therapy sessions with a kinesthetic activity is to release tension in the body to facilitate physical comfort in the therapy setting.

Bilateral scribbling, described in Chapter 2, is excellent for fostering bilateral coordination and bilateral integration by strengthening the connections between hemispheres via the corpus callosum. Bilateral integration involves the ability to use both sides of the body at once, eye-hand coordination, and visual motor skills. Bilateral integration is "assumed to be basic to cognitive structures related to body awareness and spatial orientation" (Morrison, 1985, p. 95). Bilateral cooperation involves crossing the midline of the body, an imaginary line that divides the body vertically into equal halves. The ability to move the hands across both sides of the body is associated with the development of manipulation skills and manual coordination (Bruner, 1973) such as writing. Children who cannot cross their midline often turn their writing or drawing paper so they do not have to cross the midline of their body with their hand. Some will switch hands to perform tasks on the opposite side of the body. Children with bilateral coordination problems may not have crawled as an infant, may have difficulty with tasks that involve two hands, and may have trouble using drawing materials or eating utensils.

Bilateral scribbling and drawing facilitate crossing the midline. While they are scribbling, I ask children to draw an arc with both markers and then ask them to draw two arcs that go across the entire page, crossing their arms while drawing. At first, many children cannot do this, but with a bit of practice, they are able to do so with an increasing range of motion each time.

For visual perceptual, visual motor, and motor-planning skills, I offer the child or teen tracing paper and ask him to trace a favorite image. He may be asked to copy various simple shapes drawn across a paper or to draw around various objects such as a ruler, upside-down bowl or plate, or small box. I may also suggest that the child draw a self-portrait by looking at his image in a mirror placed next to the drawing paper.

A game I call "Whack the Balloon" is designed to foster eye-hand coordination and motor planning. It also helps children sublimate their aggression (Kramer, 1979). I sit across from the child with a balloon 18 inches long. The child has a heavy cardboard tube about 1 inch in diameter and 18 inches long. As I move the balloon back and forth horizontally about 2 to 3 inches above the table, the child attempts to whack the balloon with the tube. In the beginning, I move slowly and do the activity for only a short time if the child has difficulty. As his skill level improves, I move the balloon faster.

Another activity to develop eye-hand coordination and motor planning is "Marker Wars." I sit across from the child at a table covered with a large piece of taped-down butcher paper. A line is drawn horizontally across the middle of the paper. With a marker in each hand, I attempt to cross the line with my markers while the child, also with a marker in each hand, uses his two markers to try to stop me before I cross the line. I move the markers parallel a few inches apart and not too quickly. After the child's motor control has improved, I move faster and more freely.

To aid the development of visual discrimination, I often have children and teens reverse the figure and ground in their drawings (Uhlin, 1972). Instead of using dark drawing implements on white paper, I have them use white pencil, chalks, pastels, or paint on black paper. Children with visual discrimination delays can draw better using white on black (Uhlin, 1972). Reversing the figure and ground offers them a novel visual perceptual experience. (Uhlin, 1972).

Another fun way to aid visual perceptual development is to create drawings together. I provide a sheet of paper and drawing implements for both of us. We each draw one line or shape on our paper and then pass it to the other person, add to the other's drawing, and then give it back. We repeat this until we both decide the drawing is complete or want to start a new round. A variation is to take turns following each other's lines around a large piece of paper.

TACTILE DEVELOPMENT

The infant's skin is the earliest organ to develop in utero, and responsiveness to touch appears at approximately eight weeks of gestation (Hepper & Shahidullah, 1994). Tactile input postnatally contributes to attachment behavior, brain development, and physical and emotional development (Caulfield, 2000; Schore, 2003a). A study of institutionalized infants who received an extra 1,000 minutes of tactile stimulation administered over a ten-week period rated them at a higher functional level on the Gesell Developmental Schedule than those who did not receive extra stimulation (Casler, 1965). Infants use touch to explore people and objects, they soothe themselves with sucking, and they are soothed by gentle stroking.

Hypersensitivity and undersensitivity to touch are signs of underactivity in the right brain (Melillo, 2009). Many children are *tactile defensive*, a term describing those who avoid physical contact because they do not like to be touched. They may also have sensitivity to certain fabric textures or to the constriction of elastic or belts. It is important to remember that highly tactile-defensive children can tolerate only small amounts of tactile stimulation at first.

Techniques for Tactile Development in Infants and Toddlers

Strengthening the neural pathways to respond to tactile sensations occurs in everyday experiences when touching textures: skin, a blanket, paper, plastic, wood, water, and other safe objects. Many infant toys are designed with this in mind. For a toddler, filling a tote bag with objects such as a washcloth, a plastic or wooden toy, a Styrofoam cup, a sponge, a tennis ball, and an aluminum foil ball delights them as they dump the contents and return them to the bag. Supervised water play with a plastic funnel, cups, rubber toys, and boats is an enjoyable tactile experience for young children. Having the child taste a variety of textures, such as a cracker, a banana, an apple, pudding, or jelly, increases oral tactile awareness.

Young children can fingerpaint safely with pudding, whipped cream, or yogurt. I may add a bit of juice for color. Sometimes I add cereal, blueberries, raisins, or cracker crumbs for a variety of textures for a baby to touch and taste. Young infants and toddlers explore by putting things in their mouth, so using edible items provides a safe medium for experiencing tactile sensations with both fingers and mouths.

Techniques for Tactile Development in Children and Teens

When children are able to listen and respond to directions and no longer put objects into their mouth, they are developmentally ready for fingerpainting. Since this is inherently a messy activity, I use a cookiesheet or tape the paper to the table to define a boundary. I may add a small amount of sand or sugar to the paint, mist it with water to make it more fluid, or add thick condensed milk to offer a variety of tactile sensations. For a three-dimensional experience, I have children build sculptures with a variety of media, including wire, chenille stems, feathers, ribbons, string, cork, Styrofoam, plastic windows from packaging, wood, nuts, bolts, and various papers, including construction paper, Saran wrap, wax paper, aluminum foil, gift paper scraps, sandpaper, and glue and tape.

Creating hats, costumes, or puppets is an excellent way to stimulate tactile awareness and tolerance. Tactile-defensive children will often tolerate touching when another is providing assistance while making or trying on hats or costumes or learning to use a puppet.

Mask making is another activity that offers various types of tactile stimulation. I use preformed papier-mâché masks and offer a variety of materials, including paint, ribbons, tapes, feathers, jewels, beads, glitter, sequins, and various textured papers such as tissue paper, foil paper, rice paper, and handmade paper. I may ask children to create the mask of an ancestor or of their future self or to decorate the mask however they would like.

I sometimes ask children to collect items from outside the studio to make a nature collage. The outdoor environment offers a different set of stimuli: different air temperature, different smells, and different light. They gather pinecones, stones, grasses, twigs, moss, dirt, leaves, and other natural textures. This is followed by another tactile experience, assembling these items on paper or into a sculpture on cardboard secured with glue or tape. Some children make nature mandalas by arranging the natural items on a precut circular shape of medium or heavy cardboard or mat board.

To strengthen tactile discrimination, I drop coins or beads into a shoebox filled with dried pinto beans and invite clients to feel for the objects in the beans. They may keep whatever they find. I reassure them that nothing in the box will trick them or hurt them. Similarly, I keep a 12- to 16-inch long nylon or fabric bag containing fifteen small objects with various tactile surfaces: a small piece of wood, a small rubber ball, a large paper clip, a small matchbox with no matches, a 1-inch-square piece of wet sponge, a small piece of sandpaper, a piece of soft plush fabric, and so forth. As I name each object, the child identifies the item inside the bag using his sense of touch, removes it, and places it in front of him. Some children can readily identify an object by touch, while others have great difficulty.

Clay is also an excellent tool for tactile awareness. The cool, wet clay manipulates easily. Adding various textures such as rice, flour, salt, crushed cereal, sand, or small pebbles changes and expands the tactile experiences. It is important to remember that the tactile-defensive child may not want to touch some items. Clay is often one such medium. I assure the child that her response is not unusual or unexpected and offer plastic gloves for comfort. After a time, she may let me cut the tip off one finger of the glove so she can feel the clay. As tolerance is developed, the child often wants more of her hands exposed and eventually, the gloves are removed entirely.

GROSS MOTOR DEVELOPMENT

Gross motor development refers to the use of the large muscles in the body, particularly arms and legs and torso. Children must be active to develop these large muscles, and they are able to be more active as the muscles develop. Gross motor movement requires space. In earlier times, children were safe playing outside for extended periods of time. Now, outdoor play mainly consists of organized activities such as sports, which do develop large muscles but provide little opportunity for imaginative free play and exploration. As technology has afforded children the opportunity to be entertained passively and continuously, many children rarely play out of doors. Instead, they spend their discretionary time indoors playing video games, watching movies, and texting, none of which uses large muscles. Many schools have cut back on physical education classes, further limiting gross motor experiences.

Infants and toddlers with gross motor delays usually have low muscle tone. Their muscles appear limp, they may be late to crawl or to walk, or they appear to favor one side of the body, as revealed when they reach for a rattle or bottle or in body movement. Children and teens with gross motor deficiencies are often labeled "clumsy" for they often run into furniture or walls and have difficulty walking up and down stairs, jumping, climbing, or riding a bike. Some children are very lethargic and appear depressed at times.

Techniques for Gross Motor Development in Infants and Toddlers

While holding a baby firmly under the arms, the caregiver can gently bounce the baby on her lap for 5 to 10 seconds, then rest. She can repeat this a few times, being sure to rest after each interval. The baby, because of underdeveloped muscles, cannot tolerate longer periods of stimulation. As the muscles develop, bouncing time can be gradually increased to 10 to 15 seconds.

I have heard someone mention that holding a baby firmly and rocking him back and forth on a beach ball develops balance. I do not recommend this. I am careful not to expose a baby to anything I would not want him to try independently. The baby may try to sit on the ball and could be injured, because babies have not yet developed the protective extension reflex—the term for putting one's arms out to prevent falling. This protective extension develops in stages. At six months, an infant will put his arms out in front to break a fall. At eight months, he will stretch the arms out sideways, and at ten months, he can put his arms behind him to catch himself.

Ball play, however, is useful in developing gross motor skills. I begin with a balloon, since it is slow moving and easy to see. As the child develops better visual motor skills, I change to a soft ball about 4 to 6 inches in diameter. I encourage children to kick, bat, or roll the ball. Sometimes they just want to hold onto the ball until they learn to enjoy the interactive aspect of ball play. When the toddler can walk and has balance, he can be invited to kick the ball.

Lying on the floor and encouraging the baby to crawl over you to reach a toy is a safe and multisensory way to use large muscles. In addition to the strength and dexterity developed, this activity offers the baby an opportunity to practice motor planning, eye-hand coordination, visual skills, and tactile stimulation.

Techniques for Gross Motor Development in Children and Teens

Once the child is walking and has balance, blow bubbles for him to chase, catch with his hands, or step on. Avoid blowing bubbles at the child. It is better for him to have to move to catch or step on the bubbles. Be sure to have the child wash up after this activity, as he will have slippery soap residue on his hands and feet or shoes.

Children delight in crawling through tunnels made from large cartons or blankets arranged over straight-backed chairs. Young children will spend considerable time doing this activity. It develops leg and back muscles, as well as visual motor skills.

Pounding or pulling clay, tearing cardboard or heavy paper, and painting on large paper with large brushes are ways to build large muscles with art media. Children like to make rubbings by placing paper on a variety of surfaces and rubbing across the paper with an oil or chalk pastel. Stampings can be made by using precut sponge shapes or found objects. In a large open bowl, place a sponge soaked with paint. Press the object onto the wet sponge and then press the object on paper. Do not be surprised when children want to paint their hands and stamp their hands on the paper. I am prepared with a small bucket of water and a towel for easy clean-up.

Many opportunities for gross motor muscle building occur in outdoor play. Crawling, jumping, climbing, running, carrying, pounding, stretching, holding, pulling, and balancing occur in many structured and unstructured activities. Jumprope, hopscotch, wagon pulling and riding, kite flying, and bicycle riding all use large muscles and help develop balance.

FINE MOTOR DEVELOPMENT

Fine motor activities include writing, drawing, and manipulating small objects. These skills rely on development of the small muscles, especially the fingers, and they improve as the muscles are used. By the time the children reach about 1 year of age, they usually have a pincer grasp that enables them to pick up objects, and they are able to transfer items from one hand to another. Children with fine motor delays often have difficulty printing, writing, drawing, and cutting with scissors. They tend to avoid these activities. They may have difficulty managing a fork or spoon, building with small blocks, or playing games that require fine motor facility.

Techniques for Fine Motor Development in Infants and Toddlers

With infants, simply varying the size of objects to grasp is a good beginning. All objects should be large enough that they can't be swallowed, soft and smooth enough that they can't hurt skin or eyes, and unbreakable. Rattles, blocks, and stuffed animals in different sizes are examples of objects that help develop fine motor skills, and incidentally provide tactile stimulation.

As they grow and develop, babies practice fine motor skills when they pick up cereal, raisins, or other small foods. To develop finger and hand manipulation, give the baby toys that have buttons to push, beads to slide, or rings to stack. Placing a variety of small toys in a low open box will intrigue infants. They like to take the toys out of the box and put them back. Stacking items such as blocks and nesting toys is an excellent activity, as is pinching, poking, or rolling clay. All these fine motor activities also promote the development of eye-hand coordination, one of the most important skills for the baby to master.

Techniques for Fine Motor Development in Children and Teens

Art offers many opportunities for fine motor development. Drawing or painting with small brushes on small paper, making tracings, and creating sculpture from small items such as toothpicks, Styrofoam packing shapes, marshmallows, buttons, nuts, bolts, and string all require fine motor skills. Lacing beads, pasta, or cereal onto a shoestring, cutting with scissors, and sorting buttons or beads also aid fine motor functioning. Other examples include small mosaic tile projects, sculpting with small amounts of clay, origami, sewing, knitting, sticker art, and soap carving. Board games, card games, pick-up sticks, and puzzles also engage fine motor skills.

AUDITORY DEVELOPMENT

The first cells to develop in the embryo are thought to be sound sensitive, perhaps to pick up the stimulus of the mother's heartbeat as a template for the development of the infant heart (Tomatis, 1991). Just after birth, infants are able to hear and respond to voices by turning their heads in the direction of the sound. Children do not learn to hear, but they do learn to make meaning of sounds by paying attention to them, processing the source of the sound, and identifying voices.

Children with auditory delays often cannot do these things. If they do not have a physical hearing loss, they may have auditory processing delays. They may have trouble listening, be sensitive to loud noises, have difficulty speaking and articulating, and ask to have things repeated. Some children must look at the speaker or look at others before responding to a question. They may have difficulty staying with the topic of conversation. Some children may have auditory discrimination problems or an inability to hear and process words; sometimes these children are accused of not listening or not paying attention. Other children may have auditory visual memory problems or an inability to visualize a sequence of things they are told to do. Although they may be trying, these children, too, may be told they do not listen.

Techniques for Auditory Development in Infants and Toddlers

When music is used for auditory stimulation with babies, soft music is essential. Their underdeveloped auditory system is highly sensitive and easily startled or overstimulated. Soft sounds of the mother's voice, rhythmic nursery rhymes, or lullabies stimulate auditory processing. Moving a rattle or noisemaker to different places within the infant's field of vision or allowing the infant to shake small film cans (lids securely taped closed) filled with various sounding items such as buttons, rice, or beads enhances sound seeking. Even if the infant does not understand the words, identifying outdoor sounds such as a dog barking, birds singing, and horns honking helps him learn the predictable rhythm of adult speech, tone, and articulation. To give the infant a variety of sensory sounds, crinkle paper, ring a small bell, or talk in a whisper to promote auditory development. Giving toddlers musical instruments such as small maracas or small homemade drums, bells, and rattles will increase their repertoire of sounds.

Techniques for Auditory Development in Children and Teens

Although I do not work on auditory skills in art therapy, when I become aware of a client's lag in auditory processing, I speak more slowly and use a simple style of speech. I check to be certain she has understood what I have said. I usually encourage caregivers to work on these skills with their child or teen by listening to and naming sounds in noisy places and playing games such as "Name That Tune," where one person hums or claps the beginning of a song and the other tries to guess the tune. Taking turns creating stories is another useful technique. I remind parents that in the beginning, short stories are best. As the auditory functioning improves, the length of the story can be extended.

Another technique is "Matching Sounds." I work with the child to half-fill ten pairs of identical containers (film cans, margarine tubs) with small objects such as rice, beans, kosher salt, paper clips, pennies, or buttons. The containers are placed randomly in front of the child and she is asked to shake the containers and find the two that sound the same. These containers can also be used to create different rhythms and sounds by shaking, rolling, or tapping them.

VESTIBULAR DEVELOPMENT

Located in the inner ear, the vestibular system is the first system to develop fully during gestation. It detects movement and gravity and works with other sensory systems to determine space and locate where the person is in that space. As infants become toddlers, they develop the musculature and balance to sit upright. The trunk muscles develop tone along with the neck and head to create equilibrium and balance. This is a precursor to locomotion. Children with vestibular delays often cannot sit upright, fidget, and have difficulty focusing. It is hard for them to listen for extended periods without moving or rocking.

Techniques for Vestibular Development in Infants and Toddlers

Changing the baby's position while holding him, from over the shoulder to a cradle position and back, moving slowly in space while holding him upright, or balancing him on your lap for a brief period will aid in vestibular development.

As the infant matures, giving him horsey rides on the back of one person while he is held firmly by another adult, bouncing him on the knee while holding both hands, gently swinging him in a bucket swing, or rocking him in your arms will help strengthen the vestibular system.

Techniques for Vestibular Development in Children and Teens

Although I do not work on these skills directly in art therapy practice, I am sensitive to the problems caused by delays in vestibular functions. I am careful to pay close attention to signs of fatigue when children are sitting upright and offer them opportunities to move or change position.

Sitting on a large exercise ball or a T-stool for short periods will help strengthen the vestibular system. Kranowicz (2003) recommends the T-stool be made from a 12-inch long, 2- by 4-inch piece of wood for the seat, and a 10- to 12-inch tall, 2- by 4-inch piece of wood for the leg. Children will enjoy trying to sit, balanced, on the one-legged stool but will find it difficult depending on the severity of the delay. It is recommended that this activity be limited to very short periods of sitting at first as it may be challenging for some children.

Having children try to walk on a trail of masking tape arranged in a line and turns on the floor will also help develop balance, as will having them crawl on their hands and knees with a small bag of rice or beans on their backs. Kranowicz (2003) also recommends a standing teeter-totter, created by resting a 3-foot by 3-foot plywood sheet on a 4- to 6-inch beam, which allows children to safely practice balancing as they rock back and forth in a standing position on the plywood surface.

Riding in a wagon, riding a tricycle, and games such as leapfrog, hopscotch, and jumping on a low trampoline also strengthen the vestibular system.

PROPRIOCEPTIVE DEVELOPMENT

Proprioception refers to awareness of the position of the body in relationship to gravity, self, and others (Melillo, 2009). Proprioceptive ability aids in the tasks of running and walking smoothly, climbing, carrying, sitting, stretching, and lying down (Kranowicz, 2003). Children who have poor balance or exhibit an unsteady gait when walking may have delays in proprioception. They may keep a hand or shoulder near or on the wall when they walk down a hallway. I have seen children with proprioceptive delays draw the human figure balancing on one foot. Children who experience delays in motor planning often have problems with bilateral integration (Morrison, 1985).

Techniques for Proprioceptive Development in Infants and Toddlers

In early infancy, simply making O shapes with the lips, smiles, and other friendly faces will encourage the child to imitate facial movements, a beginning place for controlling motor movements. Also helpful are nursery rhymes with hand movements or clapping and finger play. Switching positions of the baby while being held, from one side to the other, and gentle movement or slow dancing with the baby held upright firmly will also help him to orient in space. Avoid quick movements. These activities should be done for only brief periods of time, with pauses for rest.

Toddlers like playing patty-cake, playing clapping songs, throwing beanbags, and batting a balloon. All aid in the development of motor planning.

Techniques for Proprioceptive Development in Children and Teens

Young children can practice controlling body movements and motor planning by playing with a pounding bench, shapes-in-holes toys, building toys that snap together, and toys propelled with wheels.

I encourage children to walk like a turtle for a few moments. Then I ask them to switch to moving like a frog, then a penguin, a snake, a bunny, and others. This activity involves listening, moving, stopping, and switching movements, all of which are aspects of motor planning.

Other activities for motor planning include Music/Freeze, a game in which someone sings or plays music and when the music stops, the child stops moving until the music begins again. In place of freeze, you can substitute: walk with hands in air, take big steps, take little steps, crouch low to the ground, reach high to the ceiling. You can ask children to skip, jump, or hop, but only for short periods as they may not have good balance and will tire easily.

Using both sides of the body at once is helpful for proprioceptive development, such as catching a large, soft ball with two hands. Throwing the ball slightly to one side and then the other will use both arms and legs, as will batting a balloon with two hands. Throwing beanbags with one hand and then the other and riding a tricycle or bicycle also use both sides of the body. These activities aid in the development of muscle tone for gross motor development, bilateral integration, and increased joint stability (Morrison, 1985).

IS IT PSYCHOTHERAPY?

Many therapists have found that utilizing these activities at the beginning of therapy sessions is beneficial. I have been asked, "Is it therapy?" or "How do I chart these activities as therapy?" These are astute questions that warrant comment. It may seem to be out of the scope of psychotherapy practice to be working on developing sensory skills with a client. However, if the child is not able to sit, focus, or attend to conversation, play, or art, the therapy is compromised.

These activities can be described initially as assessment and rapport-building activities that engage the child with the therapist in nonthreatening, safe, and easy ways. Engaging in some of these activities at the beginning of each session will afford the therapist the opportunity to learn if there may be sensory development and processing problems, clarifying the possible need for a comprehensive assessment by an occupational therapist trained in sensory processing and sensory integration techniques. When there is improvement, it can be charted.

The activities, described neurobiologically, are those that strengthen the child's ability for information processing, affect tolerance, and physical control. And, these skills are related to the child's ability to function satisfactorily emotionally and socially.

Children suffer greatly when they cannot process incoming information and cannot understand what is being said in a classroom, or when it is obvious that

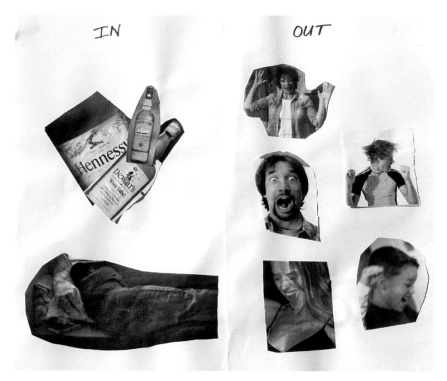

Figure 3.1 How I Act In My Anger/How I Act Out My Anger.

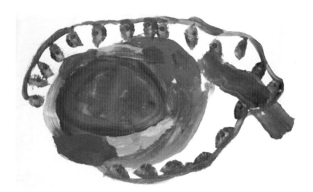

Figure 5.1 Fear.

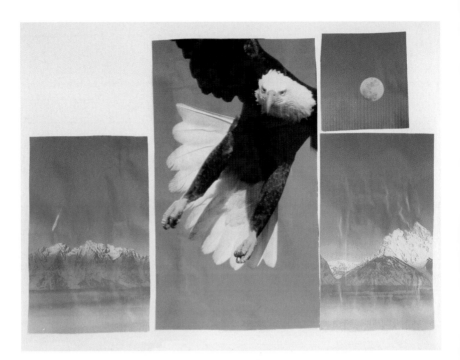

Figure 6.1 Animal Totem.

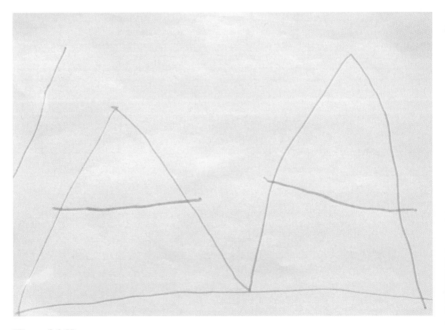

Figure 8.1 House.

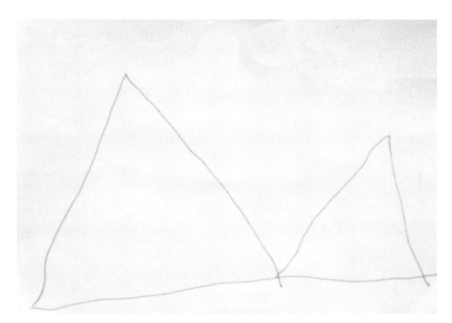

Figure 8.2 House #2.

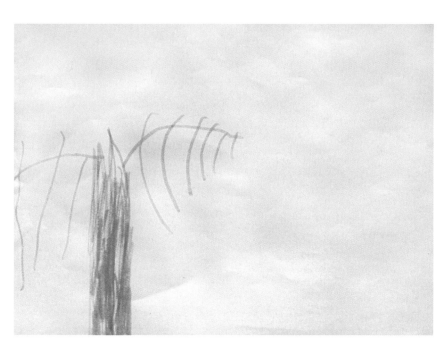

Figure 8.3 Tree.

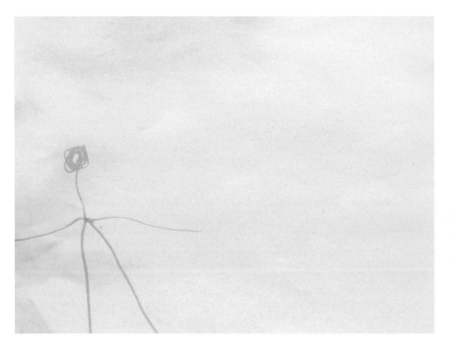

Figure 8.4 Person.

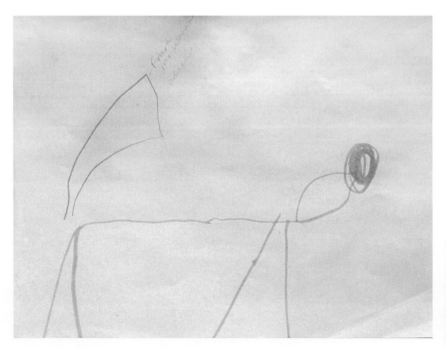

Figure 8.5 Animal.

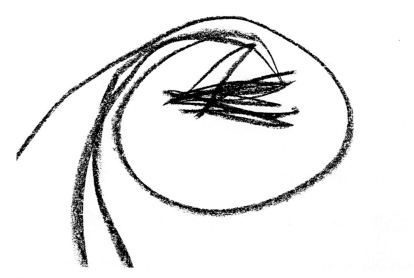

Figure 8.6 Black Drawn on White.

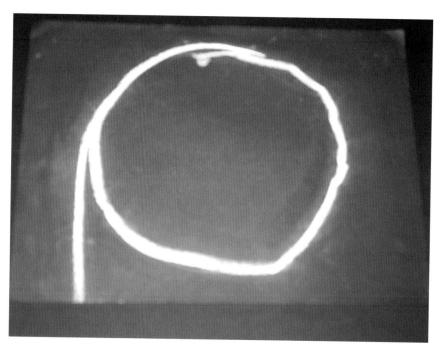

Figure 8.7 White Drawn on Black.

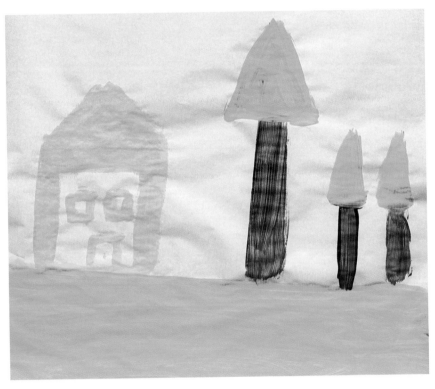

Figure 9.1 House and Trees.

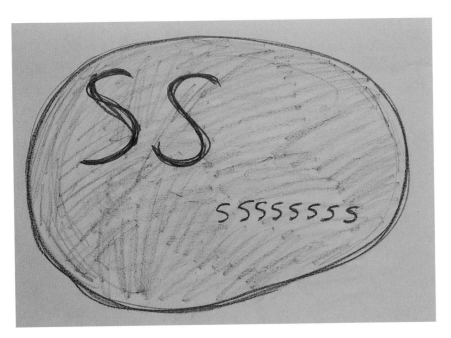

Figure 9.2 Enhanced Initials.

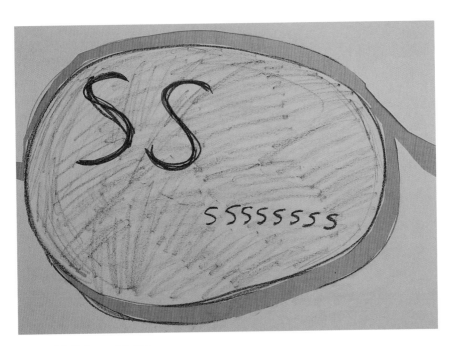

Figure 9.3 Enhanced Initials.

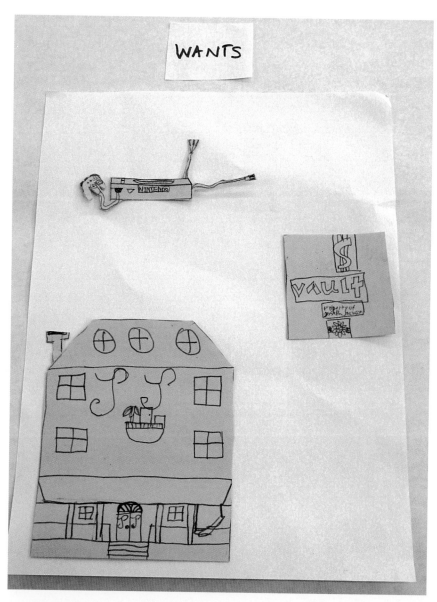

Figure 9.4 Wants.

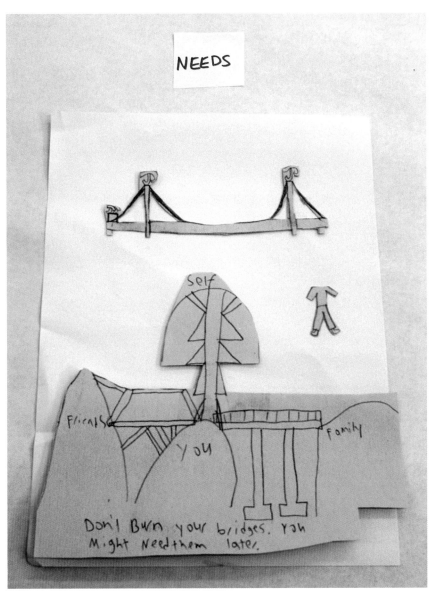

Figure 9.5 Needs.

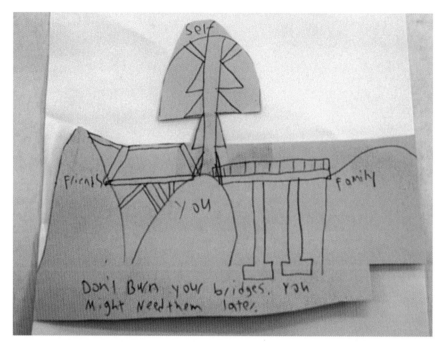

Figure 9.6 Bridge with Self.

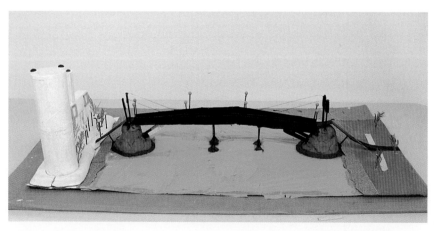

Figure 9.7 Bridge Sculpture.

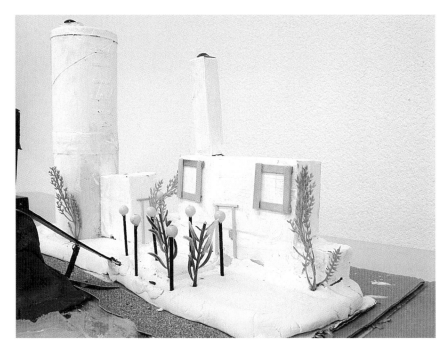

Figure 9.8 Bridge Sculpture.

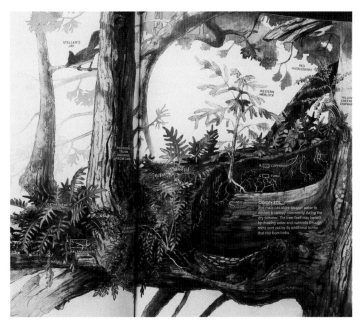

Figure 9.9 New Growth.

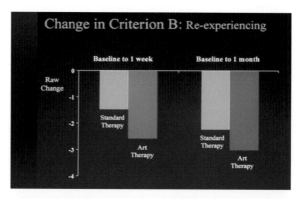

Figure A.1 CATTI—Reduction in Re-experiencing Symptoms.

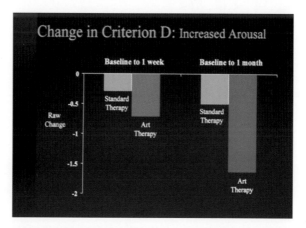

Figure A.2 CATTI—Reduction in Increased Arousal Symptoms.

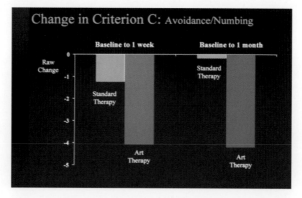

Figure A.3 CATTI—Reduction in Avoidance Symptoms.

they cannot run or are uncoordinated compared to their peers. Feelings of shame, incompetence, and hopelessness from these experiences undermine the self-confidence needed for social and academic activities. Children who are able to make improvements are proud of the development of new skills and demonstrate improved self-esteem and self-confidence in other areas of their lives.

Those who have implemented the inclusion of these activities at the beginning of art therapy sessions have reported improvement in the client's ability to participate in therapy, a greater ability to focus and attend to tasks, and increased verbal dialogue during the sessions. Over time, there are reports of improved behavior and academic performance.

CHAPTER 5

Right-Hemisphere Communications: Right Mind to Right Mind

The right hemisphere is the current interest in psychoanalytic PTSD treatment for relational trauma. The brain first encodes information in the right hemisphere visually, followed by sensory and other somatic memory (Ogden & Minton, 2000; van der Kolk et al., 1996). The most common recall of traumatic material is in visual form (Cohn, 1993; Terr, 1991; Tower, 1983). Positron emission tomographic (PET) scans show PTSD patients, when presented with transcripts of their own accounts of their traumatic experiences, demonstrate heightened activity in the right amygdala, areas of the temporal and frontal cortex, and the right visual cortex (Rausch et al., 1996), demonstrating that the right hemisphere is involved in the storage and retrieval of traumatic memory. According to Fosha (2003), "Right brain functioning, the quality of the right mind, so to speak, involves processes that are emotional, visual/linguistic, and somatosensory; the language in which emotional experience is encoded is non-linear and not linguistic, and somatosensory" (p. 3).

Accessing traumatic memory with images or other nonverbal right-hemisphere means is logical as the right hemisphere body-based memories are primarily nonverbal. Lanius and colleagues found "the differences in brain connectivity between PTSD and comparison subjects may account for the nonverbal nature of traumatic memory recall in PTSD subjects" (2004, p. 36). Videotapes were recorded during the process of documenting my outcome research using the Chapman Art Therapy Treatment Intervention. I observed that when a child was asked to "draw what happened, why you had to come to the hospital," nearly every child spontaneously looked up and to the left, an indication that he or she was accessing the images of the right hemisphere.

Considering that the right hemisphere is dominant for implicit processes (Arizmendi, 2008), therapies that use implicit communication and nonverbal methods to access implicit memory may be indicated. As Uddin and colleagues (2006) conclude: "The emerging picture from the current literature seems to suggest a special role of the right hemisphere in self-regulated cognition, body perception, self-awareness, and autobiographical memories" (p. 65).

These right-hemisphere processes afford maximum opportunity for cortical consolidation and the integration of memory into explicit memory that is no longer dependent on hippocampal retrieval (Siegel, 2012). The corpus callosum serves as a method of information transfer between hemispheres, yet primarily as an inhibitor of one or the other hemispheres:

> We must inhibit one in order to inhabit the other. If one thinks of the relationship between the two hemispheres as like that of being the two hands of the pianist (whose two hemispheres do indeed have to cooperate, but equally must remain independent), one can see that the task of the corpus callosum has to be as much to do with inhibition of process as it is with facilitation of information transfer and cooperation requires the correct balance to be maintained. (McGilchrist, 2009, p. 210)

Cortical consolidation involves both hemispheres. The lower right hemisphere is activated as the memories emerge from sensory modes, and the left hemisphere is involved in narratives and language of experience. Then the right hemisphere is again involved as change continues with the restructuring of the high right hemisphere.

This chapter describes ways to apply neurobiology, interpersonal neurobiology, and attachment dynamics implicitly in the clinical setting. I address specific issues and include case vignettes to demonstrate the implementation of a two-person therapy with the use of mutual co-regulation in an intersubjective space as a mechanism for change through therapy.

THE BEGINNING OF THERAPY:
MEETING OF THE RIGHT HEMISPHERES

Neurological research has informed my approach to the beginning of therapy with abused and violent clients. I have found that I need to be flexible. Seldom do clients with histories of relational trauma have the ability to settle into a structured therapy session at the beginning of treatment. I keep in mind several considerations as I prepare to meet a client for the first time: Is there a chance that meeting with a stranger in a private setting will be a traumatic reminder (Pynoos, Steinberg, & Goenjian, 1996)? Are there signs of cognitive delays that may have been caused by prolonged periods of hypervigilance (Perry, 1995)? Do I see evidence of sensory-motor delay, auditory processing delay, expressive or receptive speech delay? In the art therapy setting specifically, is the client anxious about a perceived lack of drawing or artistic skill? Any of these considerations can create a sense of dread, shame, or terror in many children and teens to the point that they refuse to attend therapy.

As I begin, my primary goal is to create a sense of safety and comfort. When the child or teen arrives, I let him see me at the door so he can get a sense of what I look like from a distance. I wave and smile, then step inside the door to allow him to enter at his own pace. In the waiting area, I greet the parent/caregiver and the child individually and then direct my attention to the adult first so the client is able to take cues from the adult's reactions and behavior (Chapman, 2001).

I do not expect nor suggest that a young child should separate from the parent during the first few sessions. I invite them into the studio and simply point out or describe the toys and art media. I am careful not to place my body between the mother and the child. I sit in a child-size chair, slightly in the background, and observe as the child begins to explore the toys, sticker box, markers, and paper. Once the child and adult are engaged in an activity, I ask permission to bring my chair closer to see what they are creating. My focus is on the image or the play, not the child. Gradually, as the child becomes more comfortable in the new environment, he begins to explore independently. I do not encourage a particular activity nor give directions to the child. I wait to be invited into the play, but use very little conversation. Prior to the session, I have made contact with the parent and arranged that she leave and return to the studio for short periods until she feels the child is comfortable and then remain in the waiting area. I reassure the child that he can leave the playroom to visit the parent at any time.

School-age children and teens are invited to explore the studio with or without a parent. I describe the various media in general terms and remain quiet while they explore. Once a client indicates he is ready to move on, I simply invite him to sit at a table with art supplies arranged in an inviting and self-explanatory manner. Parents of school-age children and teens are asked to wait in the waiting area, and the client is told he can visit the parent at any time. I direct the client to a simple, safe, nonthreatening art activity that requires no drawing or art ability and only one sentence of instruction.

My focus in the beginning of therapy is first, the client's physical safety, and second, any nonverbal expression that indicates resistance, frustration, apathy, or anxiety. I respond by offering comfort on a physical level. For example, if I notice tension in the child's body, I might suggest she take a break and stretch, have a drink of water, or move around for a few minutes.

> CASE NOTE: An extremely resistant teen was already 15 minutes late for the first appointment when the group home leader called and said the teen would not get in the car and did not want to come to therapy. I suggested he tell the teen that he did not have to come today, but maybe he would be willing to drive to the facility and check it out. I offered that the teen was welcome to come inside and just look around, that doing so would be fine for today, and that I would not expect any art making or talking.
>
> Thirty minutes later they arrived. The teen remained in the vehicle another 10 minutes before, very slowly, walking to the studio with the group home staff person. He stood in the waiting room refusing to move

when invited into the art studio. I looked at the teen with my left eye on his left eye and introduced myself. He met me with a silent stare (I had been told ahead of time that art therapy had been requested as a last resort, since all attempts at therapy had been unsuccessful. I was told the client liked art.) Rather than encourage the teen, I waited for several minutes before quietly stating, "I learned from the group home staff that you like art." The teen replied in a surly tone, "Well, I don't."

My response was sincere when I said I had completely misunderstood the message. I apologized for assuming the wrong thing and offered that perhaps he would like to just look at the art studio space today, and I reiterated there was no pressure. He stood for 10 more minutes before silently entering the studio. He stood away from me for another few minutes, then sat down in front of the paper, scissors, magazines, glue, and glue brush arranged for him at the table.

I sat to his left, on the same side of the table, and made a two-sentence comment. "If you would like to know what I was going to invite you to do today, I planned to ask if you would like to introduce yourself with collage, just pictures and words, no talking. You don't have to do this or anything else, but I am glad you came into the studio." He sat for another 5 minutes, then quietly began to glance through a magazine. He put it down, pushed it away and said, "There is nothing I like in these magazines." I went to the magazine shelf and focused my attention on finding an image he might like.

I did not know L., and yet I found an image he immediately wanted. He sat down and began a collage. When he indicated he was finished, I said only, "Would you like to comment on the collage?" His comments were strikingly personal and said in the voice of a much younger child. My response was, "I can see how you are able to see [his identified emotion] in the images." The semantic nuance of my comment is important. I did not want to appear to merge with him in any way by saying, for example, "I see that, too," as if I could see what he saw or experience the images as he did. One must be mindful that the image is reflecting the unconscious affect of the client. I did not offer any interpretations or comment on my perspective of the image. My second question was whether he would be willing to come back the next week. He replied, "I think so, yes." The session had lasted 110 minutes. He was in therapy for 2 years before successfully terminating treatment.

As you can see, the 50-minute hour is not possible with extremely resistant clients. Just as flexibility is required for meeting the needs of an infant, it is required to create a state of attunement (Schore, 2012) with an older client. My goal is to create an environment of unconditional acceptance. I do not know, nor am I able to know, specifically what to do from theory or practice. My responses emerge from my own body-based affective cues. I have found them to be reliable because I am in a state of attunement with the client and in the moment.

THE THERAPIST'S ROLE IN
RIGHT-HEMISPHERE COMMUNICATION

Just as early mother and infant communication is not verbal, in the beginning of therapy I begin my interaction at the first level of information processing in post-natal development. I re-create the physical sense of "being with" uncondition-ally, and without expectation of dialogue. The client learns through sensory information processing how I move and behave. I do not mean to imply that I do not speak during the session. If the child initiates conversation, I respond. Typically, by the second or third sessions, most clients are conversational, but not always, and especially teens.

Repetition of experience also serves as right-hemisphere–to–right-hemisphere communication. My visual presence at the beginning of each session as I greet clients at the door serves as a consistent visual transitional image. Similarly, I always walk with them to the door at the end of every session and wave goodbye as they leave. The session day and time is always consistent unless changed by the client.

My demeanor is similar each session. I welcome them back and I am warm, friendly, and cordial, but not chatty, or inquisitive. Prior to each session I place the portfolio containing their art from previous sessions in the studio. The studio is always clean and clutter-free. We both always sit in the same place at the table. Consistency in as many ways possible helps to organize the body. It also has an effect on behavior.

My attire is repetitious. Early in development, the infant's vision is capable of attending to the face and eyes of the mother, the main sources of affective engagement within the dyad. Similarly, I wear the same clothes, jewelry, hair style, and shoes for the first six months to a year of treatment; I dress in black so the source of affect is my face and eyes. As the client moves forward in their development, I make subtle changes in my appearance. Not one child or teen has commented on my clothing choices.

I primarily use my left eye to look at the left eye of the client when speaking to him while making eye contact. This re-creates the early attachment experience of the mother's right-hemisphere–to–right-hemisphere communication with the infant. Mothers instinctively cradle infants on the left side, as this "facilitates the flow of information from the infant via the left ear and eye to the center for emo-tional decoding, that is, the right hemisphere of the mother" (Manning et al., 1997, p. 327).

Using the left eye to left eye during communication in therapy is a remarkable tool. It takes only one or two sessions before many clients look at me primarily with their left eye on my left eye. When we are engaged in sensitive verbal dia-logue, I find we are both looking at each other left eye to left eye. I use this technique with highly resistant teens and they become noticeably less resistant. After a time, some children consistently use their left eye to look at my left eye whenever they make eye contact with me.

Finally, meeting needs is a form of right-hemisphere communication. Having preferred snacks and beverages on hand and having the client's preferred art media out and ready are ways to validate their choices and imply that their needs are important. Early in the therapy if something is spilled, I clean up the mess. If the child dumps things over, I pick them up. When a child needs technical help with art making, such as holding something while being glued or help with tools, I am there for him.

Art making also presents many challenges and opportunities for problem solving. Helping the child solve problems or offering technical help creates a mental representation that things can be changed and that the therapist can help them do so.

ART AS RIGHT-HEMISPHERE COMMUNICATION

In making art, the kinesthetic activation of the lower structures is followed by activation of the limbic structures that express the emotional fragments of the self in visual, concrete form. Through the client's own creative act, representations of the self are reflected in the image. The visual experience of self-recognition, in even a slightly new form, alters the perception of the self in the mind:

> Objective brain processes knit the subjectivity of the conscious mind out of the cloth of sensory mapping, and because the most fundamental sensory mapping pertains to body states and is imaged as feelings, the sense of self in the act of knowing emerges as a special kind of feeling—the feeling of what happens in an organism caught in the act of interacting with an object. (Damasio, 2002, p. 9)

The inherent novelty of creation and self-discovery is life affirming and enlivening. While making art, helplessness is replaced with action and apathy is replaced with curiosity. Art engages sensory, kinesthetic, affective, perceptual, and visual systems through color, line, form, shape, symbol, and imagination.

There is an interesting difference between the way the right brain and the left brain approach problem solving. According to Schutz:

> The right brain possesses special capabilities for processing novel stimuli. . . . Right-brain problem solving generates a matrix of alternative solutions, as contrasted with the left brain's single solution of best fit. The answer matrix remains active while alternative solutions are explored, a method suitable for the open-ended possibilities inherent in a novel situation. (2005, p. 13)

Speaking the right-hemisphere language of images and symbols speeds up the therapeutic process as the therapist removes personal ego, biases, and projections by focusing on the art. This focus is advantageous to the client as well, as the right hemisphere is apparently a better historian of actual experience. According to Gazzaniga, "The left brain weaves its story in order to convince itself and you that it is in full control," and the "creative output of the right brain as a more reliable expression of experience or emotion" (1998, p. 25).

The art produced in therapy serves as a pathway to an intersubjective space. The art therapist prepares the path by providing the media, a safe space to create, and unconditional acceptance of the content of the images produced. The client and therapist view the art together and respond to it individually, but with a shared experience of viewing the image therapeutically. Rather than make interpretations about the image, the therapist responds to the internal affective states of the child. This is described by Schore (2012) as amygdala-to-amygdala communication that shifts from a cognitive unconscious to an affective unconscious (Schore, 2012).

> CASE NOTE: A 9-year-old boy had lost his 6-year-old brother several months earlier. His brother had been killed in a crosswalk. During his second therapy session, the boy requested drawing materials and said he wanted to make a drawing. He looked at the paper before he began to draw. He became tearful and pushed the empty paper away. He said, "I don't know why, but I just can't draw." I assured him he did not have to draw and he became calm. After a long pause, I asked if he would be willing to look at the image. He stated, "I didn't draw anything." I replied, "I know, but let's look at it anyway." As I held the blank paper up for him to see, he sobbed, "It's so empty. Just like my brother's room last week when we took all his things out for my baby sister. It was so empty."

The created image, in this instance even though there is no image, contains and reflects the emotional content to the creator. As illustrated here, the affect preceded cognitive information processing. The role of the art therapist is to facilitate the dialogue that will engage the client to reflect upon and discover the meaning of the symbolic content of the image. The art serves as a container for the elicited symbolic affect and as an intersubjective space where we can have a shared experience.

> CASE NOTE: S. is an 8-year-old girl referred for therapy for behavioral problems at home. She is a bright, creative child from an intact family. S. does well in school; however, when told to do something at home she becomes oppositional, defiant, and physically aggressive and demanding with others. I saw S. in therapy for a few sessions, and my assessment provided no clues to her behavior. She did not appear to have any delays, anxiety, or problems with frustration and delaying gratification. She was able to focus, she exhibited good self-esteem and social skills, and her affect was bright during the therapy sessions.

In one session, without knowing why, I asked S. to paint a picture of fear. I gave her a large piece of butcher paper and fluid paint media and said, "If fear had a color and a shape, what would it look like?" She happily agreed and painted a large purple circle and added some red paint, added two shapes in two colors of blue, and drew a large blue and purple line around the perimeter of the painting. She then added purple dots in the empty space between the circle and the outer circle (see Figure 5.1).

When she finished painting, I asked S. if she had anything to say about the image, and she replied, "It looks like teeth." I agreed, and we talked a bit more about the colors in the image, and then our time was up for the session. As they left her mother handed me the intake form she had completed. The form contains basic questions about the child's developmental history; a history of any hospitalizations, illnesses, or injuries; and a place for parents to provide any other information that may be useful for me to know. After S. and her mother left, I read the form and was surprised to see what the mother had written.

At age 3, S. had been injured at preschool, impaled in her gum and tooth by an object, requiring her parents to drive her to a dentist over an hour away so the object could be removed. She had to be held down for the procedure, had a severe reaction to the medication, and was very ill. She was terrified and in pain during the transport and procedure.

When S. returned to therapy for the next session, I had her painting of the teeth available and asked her if she recalled the incident in her preschool. She could not recall anything about the incident. When I mentioned that she had to ride in the car to the dentist, she remembered aspects of the ride and the dentist. I invited S. to participate in the CATTI to create a narrative of the event, which she did. We invited her mother into the session to help her with the parts of the narrative that she could not remember. Once the narrative was complete and the event retold with the images, I offered, "I think sometimes when your mom and dad tell you what to do at home, your body remembers that hard day, and you immediately rebel now because you can. When you were little, and being held down, you could not do anything, and it made you afraid and mad. Now, when you're told what to do, your body becomes afraid and you become angry and fight. S. said, "You know, I think you might be right." I offered, "So, next time you are asked to do something, maybe you can remind yourself that this is not the same as the time your teeth were hurt." S. said, "Yes, I can do that. I think I can remember it now."

Before the next session, S.'s mother called to report that S. was no long defiant and fighting and did not need more therapy. We had one session for closure.

This case note illustrates that the right-hemisphere–to–right-hemisphere communication was happening below the level of conscious awareness. I do not recall previously asking a child to paint fear unless he or she brought up the topic. The affect (fear) was communicated in nonverbal, body-based, right-hemisphere cues by the client to the therapist attuned to receive them.

MUTUAL CO-REGULATION

Mutual co-regulation occurs within an intersubjective space with a right-hemisphere–to–right-hemisphere transfer of affect between the client and therapist. Schore (2012) refers to this as a two-person biology model of treatment:

> I have asserted that the right hemisphere is dominant for "subjective emotional experiences," and that the interactive "transfer of affect" between the right brains of the members of the therapeutic dyad is therefore best described as "intersubjectivity." An intersubjective field is more than just an interaction of two minds, but also that of two bodies, which—when in affective resonance—elicit an amplification and integration of both CNS and ANS arousal. (p. 91)

Art therapy and play therapy provide many opportunities for mutual co-regulation that are inherent in the mutual interaction that occurs in the therapist-child dyad. Body-to-body regulation occurs with young children as they communicate with their body and the therapist responds with body communication.

> CASE NOTE: M. was a 2-year-old boy hospitalized for severe child abuse including a direct trauma to the abdomen. He was in a crib, and no family members were present. He thrashed about the crib and screamed and cried. I approached him with a few small toys held in my outstretched arm and placed them in his crib. He stopped crying and placed his body over the toys in a protective posture. Later, I returned with a few toys, presented them in the same manner, and stayed a bit longer and a bit closer to the crib. He accepted the toys and did not appear as fearful. Later, I returned with toys that were a bit larger and stayed nearer the crib. He dropped a toy from the crib and I returned it to him. He dropped another toy. Again I returned it to him. Soon, he began to drop toys from the crib, and as I returned them, M. took several deep breaths, an indication that his body was relaxing.
>
> Later, in the playroom, M. apparently experienced abdominal pain. He stopped playing, cried, and stomped his feet while pointing to his abdomen. In an attempt to convey empathy and to offer coping, I went directly in front of him, knelt to his eye level, and took three shallow, short breaths and stopped. He watched as I did it again, then he joined me in doing the same, and stopped. After the pain subsided, he returned to play. Whenever I noticed he was experiencing pain, I repeated the breathing at eye level. During future pain episodes, he sought me out to breathe with him. This became a coping device for other medical procedures as well.

I did not describe or converse with M. about what I was doing. We were engaged in a mutually shared experience with two minds and two bodies in the imaginal realm, attuned and co-regulating within an intersubjective space.

> **CASE NOTE:** T. is a 6-year-old boy who was having difficulty at home and school. He was oppositional and defiant, had temper tantrums that lasted for long periods, and was mean to his younger sibling. T. arrived for the first session and began to explore the art studio and supplies. He decided to build a structure from wood sticks and began gluing them together. After working for a few moments, he flung the entire box of wooden sticks in the air with both hands. I said, "You moved fast. I did not know you were going to toss these sticks in the air." He said, "I want to do it again." I said, "These sticks are for building, not throwing. If you want to make something to throw, we can do that."
>
> As I began to pick up the sticks, he ran in and out of the studio twice, and then ran around the perimeter of the studio, perhaps a form of dissociation in a young child. As I continued to pick up the sticks, he stopped running and walked around the room. As I continued, he walked over and stood watching me. He then leaned his head on his elbow on the table and sighed loudly. I calmly and quietly picked up all the sticks. He looked at me sadly. I asked, "Are you sad because you cannot throw the sticks?" He said, "No, I wish I could build something, but now you won't let me." I said, "I will let you if you remember these are not for throwing." He looked at me surprised and said, "I won't throw them." I said, "Okay." I put the box of sticks in the same place it was on the table before he threw it. I did not remind him about the rule, and I did not behave as if he would throw the sticks by sitting slightly farther away from the box and a bit back from the table. Quietly, he completed his stick art.

T. was able to get into a state of regulation because I was in a state of regulation. The affect was expressed through his body by a sad face with a big frown. He thought he would not be trusted with the sticks again. Given the opportunity to be in a state of co-regulation, he was able to be in control and did not throw the sticks a second time.

> **CASE NOTE:** J. was a 16-year-old boy with a history of severe child abuse and neglect. He resided in a group home for most of his life. He was oppositional and defiant and hoarded food. He was bright and creative but did not do well academically. J. arrived for his first individual session and I offered him a snack. He asked if I had a bagel and cream cheese. I offered him a bagel and a small container of cream cheese. He carefully used the utensil to take the entire carton of cream cheese out of the carton in one motion. I sat quietly as he spread a pile of cream cheese on each side of the

bagel. He looked at me and I smiled. He smiled back. He ate the bagel and we went to the studio. The next week, he asked for the same snack. He put some cream cheese on his bagel but did not use an excessive amount. He put the lid on the container and returned it to the refrigerator.

My cognitive temptation was to "teach" J. not to use so much cream cheese for his health and his manners. Instead, I sat quietly and focused on the feeling of need that arose in me. I became curious and happy as I watched him enjoy his snack.

By being fully in the moment with J., I was able to move into a state of affect synchrony. I try to stay fully present in the moment of time. My state of regulation created a mental representation of unconditional acceptance. By allowing J. symbolically to have his primitive need met by taking it all, he was satisfied emotionally. By meeting the need, information processing was moved to the higher structures for behavioral control, the structures that have the neuroplasticity to change in psychotherapy (Schore, 2012).

DISSOCIATION AS UNCONSCIOUS COMMUNICATION

For those clients with histories of child abuse, neglect, and relational trauma, affect is often dissociated in the service of defending against the emotions that are sensed in the body in right-hemisphere information processing. In response to perceived threat, the autonomic nervous system serves as a warning system to signal the need for the formation of different self states (Bromberg, 2003).

Bromberg (2006) distinguishes dissociation from the defense mechanism of repression:

> Repression defines a process that is designed to avoid disavowed mental content that may lead to unpleasant intrapsychic conflict. Dissociation shows its signature not by disavowing aspects of mental *contents* per se, but through the patient's alienation from aspects of *self* that are inconsistent with his experience of "me" at a given moment. It functions because the content is *unbearable* to the mind, not because it is *unpleasant*. (p. 7) (his italics)

Dissociation is described by Schore (2012) as an avoidant defense mechanism: "The right brain is fundamentally involved in an avoidant defense mechanism for coping with emotional stress, including the passive survival strategy of dissociation" (p. 62).

Pathological dissociation, a parasympathetic state of withdrawal, is a metabolic regulatory process to disengage in the face of threat. This results in a collapse of the implicit self:

> Dissociation thus reflects the inability of the vertical axis of the right brain cortical-subcortical implicit self system to recognize and process external stimulus (extero-

ceptive information coming from the relational) and on a moment-to-moment basis integrate them with internal stimuli (interoceptive) information from the body, somatic markers, the "felt experience." This failure of integration of the higher right hemisphere with the lower right brain induces an instant collapse of both subjectivity and intersubjectivity. Stressful and painful emotional states associated with intensely high or low levels of arousal are not experienced in consciousness, but remain in implicit memory as dysregulated dissociated unconscious affects. (Schore, 2009b, p. 126)

The dissociative alteration in perception and awareness has been described in children and teens as being "detached," "spaced" and "checked out." The right vagal circuit generates a state of psychobiological dissociation. Allen and colleagues (1999) assert that "dissociative detached individuals are not only detached from the environment, but also from the self—their body, their own actions, and their sense of identity" (p. 165).

CASE NOTE: D., a 14-year-old girl, was referred for art therapy after being removed from her home where she had suffered child abuse. She resided in a group home for many months until her behaviors modified somewhat and she was placed in an adoptive foster home. She exhibited poor school performance and withdrew from peers and activities. D. had very high anxiety that included panic attacks during which she shook uncontrollably. During therapy, she dissociated frequently, was withdrawn and nonverbal, and only minimally participated in art.

I engaged D. in a variety of sensory activities at the beginning of each session. Her interest in art making gradually increased, and she had better social interaction with peers at school. Her academic performance increased in some areas, but not in others. D. was very resistant to talking and said little during the sessions. I felt ineffective, a sense of lethargy, and at a loss as to how to proceed. As time progressed, I felt anxious before she arrived for her session. I also felt rather bored. It seemed as if we were in a perpetual "holding pattern" in her therapy.

During one session, I let D. know that her foster mother had told me she had a panic attack that day and was shaking uncontrollably. She replied, "I did, but I am fine now." She commented that her foster mother had asked what may have caused the attack and added, "I really don't know what caused it." I told D. that I believed her. I informed her that her body was shaking because it could not contain some emotion or fear. At the mention of the word fear, she said, "I think it is a fear." I asked if she would be willing to look at the fear in art so we could learn more about the fear from her unconscious mind. She agreed.

I gave her various colors of construction paper and scissors and asked her to create a symbol of fear, whatever came to mind. She created the shape of a house. I said, "If the house could speak, what would it say?" She dissociated for a few moments and I gently asked her to look at the house, sit with the image of the house for a moment, and let it come to her what the house had to say. She sat for a few moments looking at the house and then said, "You maybe won't be here." I asked, "D., are you worried that you will not live in the house?" A tear rolled down her cheek and she said, "Yes, I worry about that all the time. I am afraid of being adopted because what if they change their mind?" I validated her fear as normal. I then asked her to create another symbol for another fear associated with her adoption. She dissociated for a long period. I quietly said, "Here is the house symbol. Can you make another symbol for a fear about your adoption?" She shrugged her shoulders. I asked, "Can I tell you some of the things other kids tell me they worry about when being adopted?" She agreed.

I offered that some kids worry they will have no place to go if something happens to the foster family. D. dissociated again for a long period of time. I asked if she worried about that and she said, "I worry about that all the time, every day." I validated her feelings as normal. I asked if she could depict a symbol for that worry, and she made two crosses on two gravestones, depicting the death of the foster parents.

I then said that some kids feel disloyal to their biological parents and siblings, and she offered, "I really worry that I will lose track of my siblings. I want to see my siblings." I again validated her feelings as normal. She created four red hearts to symbolize her wanting to be in contact with her brother and sisters. Lastly, I offered that some kids are worried they will do something wrong and the foster parents won't want them. She said, "I worry about that too. Although, I think I won't do anything bad." I assured her she probably would not, just like her foster parents will probably not die, but that the feelings are important and real whether it will happen or not. She glued all the symbols to a piece of paper, let out a loud sigh, stood up, and said, "It feels great to have all these things outside of me to look at. They don't seem so big on this piece of paper."

Bucci's (2007) multiple code theory of three modes of information processing contributes to the understanding of the symbolic information processing with art. The art allowed D. access to the dissociated affect with subsymbolic, nonverbal information processing from the subcortical right amygdala. Then with symbolic nonverbal information processing, she moved to the right orbital frontal processing and was able to create symbols to represent her affect. The information then transferred to the left hemisphere for verbal access to the emotions (Bucci, 2003). By responding to her body-based dissociative states, I was able to reengage her with the symbolic representation of her affect in the art, which she was able to tolerate. The art served as a bridge between that which is dissociated and affective tolerance:

The linking of the nonsymbolic and symbolic modes occurs via the symbolic non-verbal mode that refers to images. Images are the key referents connecting the sub-symbolic nonverbal affective cues (e.g., sensory information, motoric action, etc.) to words that can be used in treatment. Emotions may be communicated, for example, in verbal form using images, stories, metaphors, and so forth that can be shared and identified with by another and may even evoke a similar experience in the other. (Arizmendi, 2008, p. 449)

The material had been transitioned from implicit to explicit knowing. Her body, loud sigh, and comments indicated that she had some relief and had integrated some of the overwhelming and debilitating dissociated affect. Eventually, and with the use of her created symbols, D. was able to talk with her foster parents about her fears.

> CASE NOTE: K. was a 16-year-old girl with a history of child abuse and neglect who resided in a group home. She was oppositional, impulsive, and explosive at times. I asked K. to draw her initials and enhance them with different media. When she completed enhancing her initials as directed, she painted out all three of her initials with black paint. I asked K. if she would be willing to look at the image in a different way, and she shrugged her shoulders. I held the image in front of her, about 5 feet away, offering distance. I asked K., "What do you see in the image?" She replied, "I'm gone." I did not say anything but continued to hold the image. She continued to look at it for a few moments and then appeared to dissociate. I quietly continued to hold the image, and she eventually looked at it again, turned away, and appeared to be dissociating. I continued to hold the image in silence and she looked at the image a third time. With tears falling from her eyes, she said, "I think about killing myself sometimes, but I never tell anybody. I never really realized that I would be gone until I saw myself gone in the painting."

Staying in the right hemisphere long enough for the affect to arise and be tolerated can be done safely with images. The image is a reflection of the self. While she was dissociating, the image remained in constant concrete form. As K. continued to focus on the concrete image, she gradually tolerated the affective content, thus allowing it to move up to higher forms of information processing. This was reflected in her use of language to explain her internal state. Her perception about herself had changed.

CHAPTER 6

Discovering the Self:
Symbol, Image, and Metaphor

The symbolic and metaphorical content of the image is not found; it is revealed through the interactive process between client, therapist, and image. The therapist and client bring creativity to the therapy (Wadeson, 1980). The client creates with art media, and the therapist with in-the-moment responses facilitates an opportunity for the client to see beyond the obvious content to the symbols and metaphors in the image. McNiff (1992) writes about the artist and art making in the following quote, yet it applies equally to the role of the therapist: "If you are able to watch and respond to thresholds that emerge in their time, the process offers unending depth, surprises, and challenges. Creation is a sentient and instinctual flow that determines where to go and what to change or omit" (p. 13).

Art therapy is both a right-hemisphere and a left-hemisphere process. Art therapy utilizes the unconscious emotional content along with verbal dialogue. The art allows for symbolic expressions that often precede verbal association (Cohn, 1993; Lowenfeld, 1957). The art media, besides being the facilitator of expression, allow for the creation of symbols and metaphors beyond the limitations of language. In the process of facilitating the client's own discovery of the meaning of the symbols in their art, the therapist lays aside his own ego, biases, and projections:

> Thus, the symbol can never be a mere form . . . nor can it be understood except in the context of its religious, cultural, or metaphysical background—the soil from which it grew. The symbol reveals an essential part of the subject to be understood. It contains the vast ever-expanding realm of possibilities. (Cooper, 1978, p. 1)

It is human nature to try to identify and bring symbolic or metaphorical content in images or art products to consciousness in an attempt to impart insight.

This requires left-hemisphere cognition and linguistic dialogue. Engaging in a visual dialogue with the symbolic and metaphorical content of the image sustains right-hemisphere access. It is safer for clients when they offer their own perceptions about the image. As the client views the image, he will begin to experience affect. Those emotions precede "knowing" as the meaning of the image finds its way into consciousness: "Staying in the metaphor is necessary because often what is expressed in the art is not ready to be acknowledged or verbalized consciously" (Klorer, 2000, pp. 17–18).

This chapter consists of case vignettes that illustrate ways to help clients move below conscious and linguistic discourse to access the deeper meaning of symbols and metaphors and to remain with right-hemisphere information processing while exploring images and play. The act of altering images during therapy is given special attention.

PROJECTION AS A SELF-DISCOVERY TECHNIQUE

One of the most useful tools for facilitating self-discovery is to have the client describe the image he has created in terms of line, form, color, shape, and other visible aspects of the drawing. In the process of doing so, he subconsciously projects and describes himself, his behavior, his misperceptions, and his troubling issues and worries. The following three case examples illustrate ways to use projections as a mechanism of change in therapy.

Animal Totems

Most children and teens have an affinity for animals, so they usually enjoy being asked to select an animal totem for the hour of the session. I start by asking clients to name all the domestic animals they can think of. We continue with zoo animals, farm animals, and wild animals. Then I ask them to think of the one animal that they would like to have as their animal totem. It could be an animal they like, one they dislike, or one they don't know much about. I invite them to draw, sculpt, or use collage material to represent their chosen animal totem. Sometimes I ask them to create an environment in which to place their animal.

> CASE NOTE: T., a 15-year-old boy, was referred to therapy for substance abuse. During a session in the Transformation Phase of the NDAT model, I asked him to create a collage that included his animal totem and to place it in its environment. T. found a large eagle and put it in the blue sky (see Figure 6.1). When the image was completed, I asked him to look at it and pretend I could not see the collage and describe to me what it looked like. I told him I would write down the words or phrases he mentioned.
>
> He said enthusiastically, "The eagle is bad action!" I wrote that down, followed by his other projections: "It is intense, its wings are clipped, it is

high, it is cool looking, it is strong." I asked him to tell me if any of the words I read back to him reminded him of anything about himself. We had the following exchange:

Therapist: "Are you bad action?"
Client: (Sitting up taller): "Yeah. I am bad action."
Therapist: "Are you intense?"
Client: "Yeah, I guess I am intense most of the time."
Therapist: "Are your wings clipped?"
Client: "No. Well maybe when I smoke weed and ride my skateboard, I feel like that eagle with his wings clipped because I am always crashing."

I waited for a moment and he added:

Client: "I can't believe it. That is just like me; he is going to crash with those wings."

After a few moments, I continued to read from the list:

Therapist: "Are you high?"
Client: "Oh, I can't believe I said that! I have been smoking weed lately, and I made the eagle high with those clipped wings like me when I'm high. It's like me. Damn! I can't believe that."

I waited a few moments before continuing.

Therapist: "Are you cool looking?"
Client: "Yeah, I guess I am okay, pretty cool, yeah."
Therapist: "Are you strong?"
Client: "Yes, I am strong. Very strong."
Therapist: "You seem surprised at what your art revealed to you about yourself today."
Client: "I think that is unreal. I can't believe I made the eagle just where I'm at."
Therapist: "I would like to say that I am proud of you for being honest. It takes courage to admit where you are and not pretend you are somewhere else."
Client: (sadly): "Yeah, I guess I can't hide it in my art."
Therapist: "No, your art is a part of you. The metaphors of the high eagle with clipped wings that will crash are from your image and your words. If you would like to tell me, I would like to know what you learned about yourself today with your art."
Client: "That I am going to crash if I keep smoking weed."

By staying with the metaphorical content of the image, I do not have to guess at meaning. Many of the words projected onto the image are directly related to the client or presenting issue in some way. Asking a client to pretend you cannot see the image or three-dimensional art and having him describe the image in terms of color, line, and form is safe because you are avoiding asking for content about the image. The right-hemisphere responses are a reliable source of experience and affect.

Filling up the Paper with Paint

CASE NOTE: R., a 16-year-old male, was referred to therapy for skipping school and refusing to obey curfew. He was curious about art therapy and asked me during the second session, "How does art therapy work?" I suggested that if he wanted, he could engage in an easy and safe activity that would let him discover how art therapy works. I reassured R. that he would not have to talk about anything he did not want to talk about. I covered the 5-foot by 2-foot tabletop with white paper and taped it to the table. I offered him various colors of tempera paint and brushes and invited him simply to fill up the paper with the paint. I said he could use colors, shapes, whatever he wanted, but just fill up the paper with paint. He did so. Then I asked him to pretend I could not see it and to tell me what it looked like based on the colors, lines, shapes, forms, anything he could see about the image. I offered an example by stating, "It looks green, or it looks round." R. immediately said, "It is messy." I wrote the word *messy* on a piece of paper. I said, "It is . . . ?" He replied, "Confusing." I wrote that also. I said, "It is . . . ?" and he replied, "Strange."

After writing down his response, I said, "This will show you how your art can help you learn about yourself. You can answer my questions or not. Are you messy?" R. smiled and said, "Well, yes. Since I have been out of my house a lot lately I don't always have clean clothes on and stuff. That is amazing." I then asked, "Are you confused?" He said adamantly, "I can't believe it. I can't believe it because I am confused all the time." I then asked, "Do you ever feel strange?" R. replied, "I can't believe it. Yes, I always feel weird. I can't believe you know me from this."

In this example, the fluid quality of the media combined with gross motor activity elicited tolerable affect. A word of caution: I would not do this with a child who has distressing or severe behavior problems or a trauma history, or was in any way dysregulated. The fluid aspect of the media can then cause regression, and psychologically the client may access too much affect, causing him to become overwhelmed with affect and switch to states of hypoarousal and dissociation or hyperarousal. Clients who are in a state of hyperarousal may become overstimulated and behave accordingly—by, for example, trying to put paint on their body or throwing paint.

If a child uses a potentially shameful word during her description of the image, I change my pattern for all of the words. For example, instead of asking, "Are you ugly?" I would ask, "Does this word have any meaning for you now or in the past or a way you have felt about yourself or anyone else?" It is important to allow children and teens to save face, to have a way out for psychological safety. Otherwise, their defenses activate and resistance ensues.

R.'s fascination with the unconscious content of his images continued. During another session, I asked him to pick the one word he was most curious to learn more about. Right away he picked *confused*. I asked him to paint what *confused* looked like, and he painted the image of a head with many colors around it and in it. As we explored the colors, he revealed that he was confused because he missed his father and the things they used to do together before the father began working away from the home frequently. R. discovered that he was trying to fill that void by hanging out with friends. He was able to talk to his father, and they began to spend more time together. The father called after the therapy to say thank you for reconnecting him to his son. He said he had known there was a problem but did not know what to do.

> **CASE NOTE:** E. is a 15-year-old girl referred to therapy for depression. She had been hospitalized many times in the past for a congenital heart problem and had undergone two surgeries to correct the problem. E. was withdrawn, nearly mute, and lethargic most of the time. She was doing poorly in school, often refusing to go because she did not feel well. During one therapy session, E. indicated that she wanted to paint but did not know how. I offered her art media and paper and suggested she first fill up the medium-sized sheet of paper with shapes and colors to see how she liked the paint and to get a feel for how the paint spread on the paper. She used several colors and shapes and eventually the paper was covered.

I asked E. if she would be willing to look at the image together and she agreed. I asked if she had something to say about the image, but she did not. I asked if she would be willing to answer some questions about the colors and shapes, and she agreed.

> *Therapist:* "What is the brown?"
> *Client:* "That is my skin."
> *Therapist:* "What is the red?"
> *Client:* "That is my blood."
> *Therapist:* "What is the gray?"
> *Client:* "That is my madness."
> *Therapist:* "What is the yellow?"
> *Client:* "That is my room."
> *Therapist:* "What is the green?"
> *Client:* "That is my yard."

Therapist: "What is the white?"
Client: "That is my happiness."

After she had identified each color, I asked if she would be willing to continue looking at the image focusing on the colors and shapes. She agreed.

Therapist: "If the brown [skin] could talk to the red [blood], what would it say?"
Client: "You are inside me." (indicating her blood is inside her skin)
Therapist: "If the red [blood] could talk to the brown [skin],what would it say?"
Client: "You probably have AIDS."
Therapist (quietly and with eye contact): "Do you ever worry that you have AIDS?"
Client (tearfully): "Yes, I probably have AIDS because I have had so many blood transfusions."
Therapist: "I am sorry you are worried. It is good that you are telling me of your worry because we can talk to your doctor to get information and help with your fear. They do test blood before transfusions, so it is unlikely. Thank you for telling me about your worry because now I know you need help with your question."

She stopped crying, and after a few moments, I continued.

Therapist: "If the gray [madness] could talk to the brown [skin], what would it say?"
Client: "Stop burning me."
Therapist (quietly): "Do you ever burn your skin?"
Client (showing small scars on the inside of her arm): "Yes, here is where I burn on myself. I do it because I am different."
Therapist: "I am sorry you burn on your skin. You are very brave and it is good that you told me because that is not safe. Thank you for telling me you are hurting yourself."

I continued to have her imagine conversations between the various colors. As we prepared to end the session, she offered to help me clean up the paintbrushes and she began to tap the paintbrush on the paper to remove paint. As she hit the paper, she used increasing force until she was banging the brush on the paper, leaving large orange brush marks. Knowing that kinesthetic activity will elicit affect, I watched. She picked up another brush with blue paint and dribbled it over the orange brush marks on the paper.

Therapist: "What does that orange paint have to say to the blue paint?"
Client: "Stop it."

Therapist: "What does the orange paint say back?"
Client: "Shut up." (She dribbled more blue paint on the orange brush marks.)
Therapist: "What does the orange paint have to say to that blue paint?"
Client: "Get off me."
Therapist: "What does blue paint say back?"
Client: "Shut up, you just have to take it."
Therapist: "What does the orange paint say back?"
Client (loudly): "Get off me and stop it."
Client: "Shut up. You just have to take it and so shut up."
Therapist (quietly and with eye contact): "Are you telling me about something that is happening to you?"
Client: "Yes."

The client then disclosed that a family friend staying in the home had been sexually abusing her. She admitted the problems had been occurring for a long time but she was not able to talk with anyone about them.

It is unlikely E.'s fear, self-harm, and abuse would have been revealed through conversation. Though she has a loving and supportive family and extended family, she had not found a way to speak of the abuse. By activating right-hemisphere visual neural pathways, the brain creates a visual narrative that can then be translated into a coherent linguistic narrative (Chapman et al., 2001). Information processing occurs according to the organizational structure of the brain, that is, from the kinesthetic activity to the limbic structures, and then lateralizes to the left hemisphere, where language is accessible.

Altering Images

While exploring an image, a client will often refer to a part of the image that is unsatisfying or that turned out differently than expected. This is an opportunity for the therapist to say, "How can we change it to how you want it to be?" and work with the child or teen to problem-solve and figure out a solution.

Altering the image affects the body and mind. Clients may have psychobiological reactions during the altering of the image. They may experience pain unexpectedly, have chills or hot flashes, experience nausea, or express the need to go to the bathroom. On the other hand, altering the image may offer a solution to a problem. It can create pleasurable somatic responses and can lower pain. I let clients know this before they begin to alter images. I reassure them that it is normal to have body sensations or feelings and to let me know, as they make changes to their art, if they notice such things happening in their body.

CASE NOTE: N., a 12-year-old boy, painted an image with a skyline that he did not like. I asked if there was a way to change the image to his satisfaction. He slumped in his chair and said, "I can't. It is messed up and all this work is ruined because of the messed-up sky." I asked, "Can you imagine any way you could fix the sky?" He became angry and said, "I told you it is messed up and ruined now. I can't fix it because I can't paint over the dark with lighter paint and I don't want the sky dark." I said, "I have an idea. What if you were to cut carefully along the horizon line of the image and glue it to a new piece of paper? Then the sky area would be white paper for you to start over and paint the sky again." He looked at me with amazement and said, "Thank you for helping me save this. That is how I can fix the sky! You saved this from the trash." As a representation of self, the metaphor of saving the image from the trash was poignant.

I know that their art is a representation of self and I treat it as such. Suggesting a change invites problem solving, and fixing an image is a mental representation and a possible metaphor for healing the self. Together we are healing the image. The act of doing so leaves the client with a mental representation that change can occur and the therapist can help change happen.

> **CASE NOTE:** J., an 18-year-old girl, graduated from high school and was planning to attend college. As the summer progressed, her parents noticed that she was increasingly anxious and appeared depressed. They referred her for therapy.
>
> J. willingly came to the studio and participated in a few sessions of self-exploration. During one session, I asked her to depict an image of herself now with all her fears, doubts, and anxiety. She painted a very small, walnut size image on a large piece of paper. The image was dark with a heavy darker boundary line around the perimeter. She showed me the image and said, "That's me." I asked her to alter that image into what she wanted her self-image to look like. Without hesitation, she picked up colorful pastels and transformed the seed into a beautiful drawing of a blooming plant with color, grace, and beauty. She stood back and said, "That's it. I can't thank you enough for what you have done for me. Now I have my answers. I am going to frame this and keep it on my wall at college."
>
> J. shared little about the meaning of the image. She said she could not really put into words what the image was about. She returned for one more session for closure and said she was busy getting ready to go to college.

The image is a representation of a self that can be altered, and correspondingly, it alters the physical body, perception, and reality. Altering the image is a mechanism of change. The therapy is found in the act of doing. Although writing about enactments in therapy, Lyons-Ruth's commentary also applies to altering images created in therapy: "The organization of memory and meaning in the implicit or enactive domain only becomes manifest in the doing" (2013, p. 578).

THE LEFT HEMISPHERE AND LANGUAGE IN THERAPY

There are some things of importance that are better addressed with left-hemisphere verbal dialogue in PTSD treatment with children and teens than through right-hemisphere communication. One is the conversation that pertains to the purpose of therapy.

To children I say: "This is a place for children hurt by someone, who have been in an accident, have lost someone special, or have some hard things going on in their life. You don't have to talk about anything you don't want to, and I am not going to ask you lots of questions. My job is to be sure you are safe, to help you make art, to help us have a good time together, and to learn about you and how I can help you with your worries and your problems."

To teens I say: "This is a place for teens who have been hurt by someone, been in an accident, have lost someone special, or have problems in life. You don't have to talk about anything you don't want to, and I am not going to ask you a lot of questions. With art, I can help you figure out your plan for your life and heal the things that may be getting in the way of your plan. You are in control of the content and pacing of the therapy because this is for you. I will make sure you are safe and help you enjoy making art while you are learning about yourself and help you with your worries and your problems."

When children are offered basic information about therapy, they are better able to conceptualize it in the context of their life. I offered this explanation when describing art therapy to a group of juvenile inmates. One youth jumped out of his chair and hollered, "Can you be my counselor? I have been waiting a long time for someone like you to be my counselor." As Sandler and colleagues (1980) note:

> An essential element in introducing a child to treatment is making contact with the patient and his problem. If this can be done, the patient will feel he can be understood and the idea of treatment may then make sense to him. It is important that the therapist always say that she is there to help the child with his worries. Even if the child does not respond to the reassurance immediately, putting this stance into words helps to structure the therapeutic situation. (p. 157)

If not at the first session, by the second session, I discuss reporting laws and confidentiality. In addition to the confidentiality of verbal dialogue, I let clients know that their art is also confidential. I reassure them that I will not talk to a parent or caregiver about anything they have said or show their art without first discussing it with them.

FORMING A CONNECTION THROUGH LANGUAGE

Children use language in therapy in unique ways. Many times, communication opportunities are missed because one is expecting words. Sometimes highly resistant or dysregulated clients communicate with noises such as growls, exasperated sighs, extended periods of clearing their throat, or silence. Sometimes the only way they know how to connect verbally is with an insult, humor, or gang talk, but a negative comment can also be effective as a point of connection.

> CASE NOTE: A 17-year-old male, T., was hospitalized for a gunshot wound. He was mute and withdrawn, typical for an individual in the psychological stage of retreat (Lee, 1970). All attempts to engage him in conversation were unsuccessful. A student intern reported that she had tried to talk to him, but he would not talk. All he said was, "The food here sucks." I would have responded, "Tell me how bad the food is here."

With some children and teens, you may have very little background information on which to build a connection and must watch for openings. When a child or teen complains, I find a way to validate their perception without necessarily agreeing with them.

> CASE NOTE: A., a 16-year-old girl with a history of child abuse, multiple foster placements, and evidence of self-harm was referred for art therapy. I had been told that she had not utilized therapy well in the past and that art therapy was the "last resort." A. walked in and said, "I think therapy is a waste of time because all therapists think they can understand me, and absolutely nobody can understand me." I responded, "Thank you for telling me that nobody can understand you, because I believe you can feel that way." She looked at me with skepticism and said, "What do you mean?" I replied, "Well, in art therapy, it is not important for me to understand you. What is important is for me to help you understand yourself. What you choose to share with me is up to you." A. sat quietly for a few moments and said, "Well, actually I have never tried art therapy before, just crafts and stuff." I invited her into the studio and said, "Well, why don't we try something easy and fun that requires no art skill. You will be in complete control over what you share and what you don't." A. agreed, and made an introductory collage. We spent four sessions exploring the many images.

I also do not use teen language in an attempt to build rapport with teen clients. I use adult speech to avoid the mental representation of appearing to be like them or to merge with them. If I attempt to be like them, there might be confusion about me or my role. Similarly, I avoid self-disclosure, do not offer my opinions, and do not try to impart insight.

PERPETRATORS, JAIL, AND BLAME

It is not unusual to avoid discussion of sensitive topics such as the perpetrator of a crime, a parent in jail, or feelings of shame and blame, whether in the home or in therapy. Children may experience traumatic reminders or may become neu-rochemically dysregulated from a stress response during posttraumatic art or play. The activation of the stress system often makes language difficult to access. When I do talk about these issues, I am mindful not to rephrase my comments. Therefore, the child hears the same message and is not confused about content as he struggles to understand and integrate what is being said.

> CASE NOTE: V., a six-year-old boy, witnessed domestic violence in his home and had been physically abused by his father. V. had played and replayed aspects of his abuse in the play therapy sessions during which he focused primarily on the small, pliable, multicultural family figures and the wooden house. While holding the father doll, V. said, "My daddy is bad." I replied, "Your daddy might not be a bad daddy, but he did very bad things." Later in play V. said, "My daddy is not bad but he did bad things."

Using simple words helps the child comprehend what is being communicated and allows him to focus on the nuance of the dialogue.

I separate the person from the behavior. It is the behavior that is bad, not the person. Whatever positive aspects of the parent that can be salvaged will allow the child to be more accepting of the negative. For example, telling a child that his parent is bad will often result in a strong defense of the good in the parent and negate an ability to consider otherwise. The child must hold onto as much of the good as possible in order to integrate the negative. Most children appear loyal to a parent, even an abusive one. This may be because they do not experience the parent only as an abuser or because they fear further harm.

Children may not pose questions about a jailed perpetrator, but when the subject does come up, many are relieved to have an opportunity to talk about the person in jail or to ask questions. They may fantasize that the person is being hurt, has moved far away, or will reappear at any moment. I do make a point of discussing this with the child when it surfaces in the play or art.

> CASE NOTE: Mentioned in the previous case note, V. was playing dur-ing another session with the small pliable family figures and the dollhouse. He put the male family figure in a toy wooden dresser. He said, "My daddy was bad and he is in jail." I said, "Your daddy may not be a bad daddy, but he did do something very bad. He hurt you, and that is a very bad thing to do." V. corrected his response, "My daddy did a bad thing and he is in jail." I said, "Your daddy did a bad thing and he is in jail." Then V. took the father figure out of the box and tossed it in the window of the wooden doll-house and said, "He's back." I said, "No, your daddy will not be able to come back so soon. He will have to stay in jail until he learns not to hurt people." V. took the father figure out of the house, put him in a small bucket near the dollhouse, and said, "You are in jail." After a long pause, the child asked, "What is in jail?" I said, "Jail is where your daddy has a bed

and food. He is not being hurt but he has to stay there to learn not to hurt people." After a long pause, I added, "Were you worried about your daddy in jail?" V. replied, "Yes, I wondered what it was like in jail." I said, "Your daddy did a bad thing and is in jail and he is safe. And, it is not your fault even if you don't believe it right now."

It is important for the therapist to avoid making judgments about the perpetrator and to convey acceptance of the range of feelings the child may have about the perpetrator (Gil, 1991). It is advantageous for the child to retain as much of the positive qualities of his father as possible. He may strongly identify with his father, and if the father is said to be bad, the child may believe that he himself is susceptible to being bad, or is bad. Maintaining as much of the good object in the form of the father allows him to be less defensive and to accept that his father's behavior is bad. Also, children may secretly believe they were at fault. Adding the caveat "even if you don't believe it right now" addresses the fact that they may believe they are at fault for their abuse and for the fact that the perpetrator is out of the home and in jail.

SESSION CLOSURE

As with all psychotherapy, providing a sense of closure is important. In art therapy, the therapist facilitates closure among the therapist, the client, and the image or art produced in the session.

One way to begin closure with an image is to ask clients if they feel comfortable stopping the discussion about the image for the day. If not, I continue by asking, "What does the image need to be able to stop for today?" and "What do you need from the image to be able to stop for today?"

With children who have been affected by the session content, I offer a way for them to symbolically discharge the negative feelings or sensations they may be experiencing. One way to do so is with a brief guided-imagery technique. I ask the client to sit quietly and notice where she feels any stress (or worry) in her body. Then I ask her to ascribe a color to the feeling and see her stress in her body as that color. I ask her to take a breath of air of white light and mix it up with some of the stress color in her body. I say that when she exhales, she will be exhaling some of the color mixed with the white light. I repeat this, asking her to take another deep breath of white light, pick up more of the stress color, and exhale it. The third time, I ask her to take a deep breath of white light and mix it with the very last bits of stress and exhale it. Then, I have her take a breath of white light and breathe normally.

Another technique for this purpose I refer to as "The Load I Am Carrying." Before the end of the session, I have the client sit before a large sheet of paper taped to the table and offer him oil pastels, which require pressure to apply. I simply ask him to use the pastels to draw, with color and shape, the load he is carrying. Many clients start out slowly but become very engaged making huge marks all over the paper. When they indicate they are finished, I tell them to leave it all in the studio so they can leave without carrying the load.

Because art created during therapy is a representation of self, the image requires care and attention. When the art is complete, I give clients the choice of taking their art home or placing it in their portfolio that I keep at the studio. If the art is incomplete, I let them know I will take good care of it for them and that it will be here when they return.

IN SUMMARY

The use of art therapy is effective in fostering bilateral integration, or coopera-tion between the two hemispheres. The following quotes, the first from child psychiatrist Daniel Siegel and the second from art therapist and neuropsycholo-gist John Jones, refer to the mechanism of change inherent in art therapy:

> Therapeutic interventions that enhance neural integration and collaborative inter-hemisphere function may be especially helpful in moving unresolved traumatic states toward resolution. (Siegel, n.d., p. 6)

> The challenge is to take advantage of the brain's integrative capacity. This is achieved by systematically stimulating both the verbal and nonverbal capacities in such ways as to engage total brain functioning in the comprehension, problem solving and subsequent learning experience with respect to the therapeutic issues set forth in treatment. (Jones, 1994, p. 6)

PART III

TREATING CHILDREN AND TEENS
WITH REPEATED EXPOSURE:
CASE EXAMPLES

The final three chapters are devoted to the treatment of children and teens who have experienced developmental or relational trauma. Many have not developed a secure attachment with a primary caregiver, have been exposed to ambient abuse and neglect, to violence in the home, or to multiple separations and losses. These chapters illustrate the application of the NDAT model of treatment with a toddler, a school-age child, and an adolescent, respectively. The case materials demonstrate the application of neurobiology in the treatment process, and how utilizing the right brain in therapy offers maximum therapeutic potential (Jones, 1994).

With the NDAT model, therapy begins by facilitating the return to earlier developmental experiences that promote physical development, attachment behavior, right-brain nonverbal collaborative communication, and affective engagement to redevelop a core concept of mind/body/self. The therapist and child engage in the types of early developmental experiences and interactions that failed to happen earlier in the child's life. Through a process of beginning with right-brain-to-right-brain communication using gesture, sound, facial gaze and reactions, tone of voice, and posture, the therapist is able to create a state of attunement with the client's internal states. When the therapist is in a state of attunement with the client, mutually shared states of co-regulation are achieved that increase affective tolerance and the ability of the child to withstand the rupture and repair sequence (Schore, 2005) that occurs in relationships.

By replicating many of the early developmental experiences that were missed as a result of the lack of an attachment opportunity or as a result of abuse and neglect, it appears possible to rebuild neural pathways for emotions, behavior, and cognition and to restructure internal working models—Bowlby's term for the dynamic and functional aspects of representation (Bretherton, Ridgeway, & Cassidy, 1990). These initial working models of self and caregiver develop from either positive or negative attachment experiences. The initial working models of the self and the caregiver develop whether the attachment experiences are positive or negative. They are a component of the development of the self and the ability to predict how others will behave and to formulate adaptive responses to others in relationships. In my clinical experience, this is followed by an ability to engage the prefrontal structures of the brain that enable judgment, the ability to consider consequences of one's behavior, and the ability to develop wisdom, compassion, and empathy for others.

The case material is presented with special attention to the beginning of therapy and the development of a therapeutic relationship. The last chapter includes specific treatment strategies for adolescents, as they are often particularly challenging to both the novice and the seasoned clinician. Each case includes relevant highlights from sessions over the course of treatment to illustrate the application of neurobiology in the clinical setting.

CHAPTER 7

Treating Toddlers and Preschoolers: Mental Representation in Action

With young children, I have found that assessment and treatment often take place simultaneously. When given the opportunity and tools to tell their stories, they do. Although young children may not have adequate language development, they are able to recall and sequence some aspects of events (Hewitt, 1999; Nelson & Ross, 1980). As language develops from one-word expression at age 1 to full sentences by age 3, children begin to use objects as symbols. They will not tell you about an experience but will re-create that experience using their bodies (Hewitt, 1999). Young children speak the language of the right brain with body, symbol, and play. They do not talk, they act. Their stories do not contain narratives, and the lack of language skill and cognition causes them to share only fragments of their experience in random order. They tend to tell only what is most important to them (Hewitt, 1999) and are not able to provide much detail about an experience or to have an accurate concept of time, the past, or the future. The young child uses play as mastery of traumatic experiences as he replays the event or aspects of the event over and over.

The normal task at this early stage of development is generally to learn to control one's body, temperament, and behavior. The new autonomy achieved in separation and acquiring object constancy propels the child to explore and discover a larger world and to complete the initial developmental separation from the caregiver. Children with a secure attachment and nurturing and consistent caregiving develop the right brain and core self (Schore, 2012). This is a relatively safe experience. For those with relational trauma, these tasks are difficult. They did not experience the secure attachment essential to completing the developmental task of autonomy. They lack development in sensory and motor systems, and lack the repetitive positive experiences that build the structures necessary to organize physically, emotionally, and cognitively. The persistent stress response creates neurochemical changes that alter the development and functioning of the brain (DeBellis, Baum et al., 1999; DeBellis, Keshavan et al.,

1999). There is no internalized template for how the world works and how people behave and respond.

TREATMENT: THE SELF PHASE OF THERAPY

The beginning of therapy is critical to the progression and outcome. When young children arrive for therapy, they are often fearful and shy. When the child and caregiver first enter the therapy setting, I am there to greet them with a warm smile. I say hello to both the mother and child by name. If the child does not respond, I simply smile and say, "That is fine, you don't have to talk." I focus my attention on the parent to give the child time to get a sense of who I am and how I behave. The child will take cues from the parent's level of comfort or discomfort. I invite the child and parent into the studio and offer them a chance to look around and investigate the room, and indicate they may ask any questions about the studio, art supplies, and toys. I do not make any comments or direct the child in any way. After the brief visit, I offer the child control over whether he wants his mother or caregiver to remain in the room or to stay in the waiting room. I repeat to the child that he can leave the studio to visit his mother at any time.

It would seem unnatural for a child in a fear state to immediately separate from his source of comfort. Allowing the child a sense of control over the separation creates a mental representation of control and safety. The mother is close by and the child can easily access that source of comfort. I have found it advantageous for a parent or caregiver to witness my interaction style with her child. Putting the parent at ease helps the child feel at ease with the therapy setting and the therapist.

Young children with developmental or relational trauma often are referred for behavior problems. A common referral is the "out of control" preschooler. Such children are disruptive in the group setting, have lengthy episodes that are described as tantrums, and do not respond well to the usual interventions used in the classroom setting to help them become calm and to cope.

I begin the assessment phase of treatment with a combination of art therapy and play therapy. The studio contains a toddler-size table covered with taped-down white butcher paper, a metal container with washable markers, and a small transparent box of various stickers. A play therapy area is arranged with several animal puppets, male and female multicultural dolls, doll diapers, a doll bed with doll blankets, a dollhouse with furniture and multicultural family figures, and an ambulance, toy cars, a school bus, a few other vehicles, and a pounding toy.

I also have a doctor kit, one of the most utilized toys in the playroom. It has plastic medical devices from a commercial toy medical kit, along with some real medical devices and equipment. I have a stethoscope, infant blood pressure cuff, and syringes without needles. The doctor kit includes several rolls of tape, many adhesive bandages, and gauze pads. Before a young child enters the playroom, I place at least one adhesive bandage on each of the dolls. It is remarkable the number of children who immediately describe what has happened to them by offering a description of what has happened to the dolls. A word of caution: I do not allow children to use items from the doctor kit on me. All the medical play is done with the dolls. Many young children are quite sadistic in their medical play as they enact what has been done to them. One of my ways of reassuring aggressive children of their safety is to remind them I will not ever hurt them and will not let them hurt me. This would not be the case if the child were to intentionally or unintentionally hurt me by, for example, jabbing the syringe into or ripping tape from my arm.

The child is invited to explore the toys. I observe and note the developmental level of the play and the themes of the child's play and art: safety and nurturance, aggression and violence, sexualized, creative, family focused, anxious and controlling, or regressed. I use very little language and do not ask the child questions. If invited, I participate in his art or play by following the child's lead. I do not make comments that may suggest a preferred method or direction for the play.

Another task of assessment is to determine the child's level of sensory and motor functioning. This is done over several sessions with a few activities at the beginning of each session. For example, using the large piece of butcher paper, I invite the child to pick two markers of different colors, one for each hand. I select two different color markers, one for each hand. The instruction is "Begin scribbling when I say, 'Go' and follow directions." I begin scribbling and then ask the child to go fast, then slow, then up and down, back and forth, then switch to making dots, small circles, small lines, and large, fast circles that get smaller and slower and smaller and slower, and put a dot in the center of the smallest circle and stop. I turn the paper over and invite the child to draw anything she would like to. While she draws, I observe, or if she indicates I must draw, I draw a similar image in the same style on my side of the paper.

From these brief activities, I am generally able to assess the child's gross motor and fine motor functioning, motor praxis or motor planning, and ability to regulate the speed of her motor activity. I am also able to assess the child's level of normal graphic development from the image she has drawn. Just as in all aspects of development, developmental norms are established in the sequential, hierarchical development of graphic ability. Although I do not rely on indicators in the drawings for assessment purposes, I am able to recognize nonsubjective indicators of possible neurological impairments in the child's drawings that may indicate neurological deficits or delays.

> CASE NOTE: C. is a 3½-year-old child, severely abused and neglected by substance abusing parents who lived on the streets or in shelters. The child was brought to the attention of the authorities when she was found sitting in a park alone and crying. The mother was the victim of a non-lethal knife wound to the neck that was discovered when law enforcement officials visited the identified home of the found child. Neighbors in the housing complex had recognized C. and told the authorities where to

locate the parents. C. was hospitalized for three days for evaluation and treatment of her apparent malnutrition and child abuse. C's medical exam disclosed bruising over the left side of her chest and over the left clavicle. There were circular burns on both hands, over the prominence beneath each thumb and pinkie finger, and lacerations on her posterior right thigh, right calf, and left calf. C. was discharged from the hospital to a medical foster home where she received both a high-calorie diet and ongoing wound care for her injuries. C. was brought to therapy by her foster mother, a woman skilled at fostering medically and psychologically fragile children.

I met with the foster mother before seeing the child. She described C. as a difficult child. C. was not completely mute, but she did not speak outside the foster home and at times did not speak in the foster home for extended periods. She had a difficult time napping or going to bed at night and exhibited sleep disturbance most nights. She was slow and clumsy with most age-appropriate daily living tasks. C. was fearful of using the toilet and had weekly encopretic episodes. The biological parents were poor historians about the child's developmental milestones, and there were no medical or preschool records. An attempt was made to have C. attend a preschool two mornings a week for contact with other children. She did not do well because she did not speak. She was indifferent or mean to her peers. She was defiant and disruptive or shut down and withdrawn.

When the child and foster mother drove up to the studio for the first session, I opened the door, waved hello, and then stepped away from the doorway. C. arrived and hid behind her foster mother. I greeted the foster mother and offered, "I notice C. does not want me to see her right now and that is okay." C. peeked around with very wide eyes and then quickly hid behind foster mother. To the foster mother, I said, "I just got a peek at C. and I liked seeing her." I added, "You and C. may want to see the toys and art supplies. Whenever you would like you may come in and look around and if you don't want to, that is okay, too." I stepped away and walked toward the studio. The foster mother quietly said, "I think it might be fun to see her toys, C. Let's go take a look."

The foster mother and child followed me into the studio, where C. stood close to her foster mother. After placing her purse and sweater on the table, the foster mother sat on a small chair at the child-size table and I sat opposite them on a short stool. I did not encourage C. to play. Instead I said, "Thank you for coming to see the toys; let me show you what is here," as I showed her the toys, and in particular, a doll with a bandage. I pointed to the drawing paper, markers, and stickers on the table and said, "Those are things for you to use if you want to, and if you don't, that is ok." C. walked a short distance from the foster mother to the toys, stood near the doctor kit and pointed to it. I asked, "Do you want to see more of what is in the doctor kit?" She nodded affirmatively. I opened the kit and showed her the stethoscope, blood pressure cuff, ample bandages and tape, and the other small items in the doctor kit. She then pointed to a newborn-sized doll. I picked up the doll and held it for her to see. She pointed to the bandages in the doctor kit and then pointed to the head of the doll. I pointed to myself then the bandage then the doll's head, and she nodded affirmatively. I silently put the bandage on the doll's head and then showed it to her. I asked if the baby was okay now.

C. ignored me and walked over to her foster mother. The foster mother began to play with the stickers and C. joined her on one side of the small table. I remained on the small stool a bit farther away. C. and her foster mother placed stickers on one sheet of paper making a joint image. I did not interfere with comments or questions. I let the child and the foster mother have their shared experience. As it was obvious C. was losing interest in the stickers, I slowly moved to the small chair opposite them at the table and invited C. and the foster mother to scribble with me on the paper taped to the table. C. was hesitant, so I encouraged the foster mother to begin and said, "C., you can scribble if you want to, and if you don't want to, that is okay." After we began, C. reached for a green marker and began scribbling next to the foster mother's scribbles. I encouraged everyone to move around the paper but C. kept her marks close to those drawn by the foster mother. After a moment, she began to scribble further away from the foster mother as all three of us scribbled on the paper together.

I pointed to the foster mother's blue lines and said, as I traced them with my finger, "I see your blue lines go up and down and over here and then here." I then pointed to C.'s green lines and said, as I traced the line with my finger, "I see C.'s green lines go here, up here, over here, and back and forth here." I offered a new sheet of paper and asked the foster mother to try to follow C's green line on the paper with her blue marker as C. scribbled on the paper. I said to C., "You scribble with green and she will try to follow you with her blue marker." C. began to scribble quickly all over the paper. The foster mother tried but could not keep up. C. laughed and the foster mother laughed with her. I then asked them to switch roles and for C. to follow the foster mother's blue lines with her green marker. The foster mother kindly moved her marker slowly and C. attempted to keep up. Her lack of motor control impeded her ability, and after a few moments, I supplied a new sheet of paper and asked them to switch roles again. The foster mother followed C.'s lines and C. and her foster mother laughed together as they played. When the paper was full, I offered another and suggested they scribble all over the paper together. They filled both sides of the paper with lines as they laughed together. When we were done, I said that I had to let them know that our time together this day was nearly over. C. started to climb on the table. I slowly walked a few steps to the table and said, as I held out my hand to her, "We don't climb on the table because it is not safe and we are always safe here." C. complied by getting off the table but did not take my hand. C. leaned on her foster mother who was sitting on one side of the small table, and I sat down opposite them.

As the session ended, I invited C. and her foster mother to remember all we had done. I began by reminding them that they had come in the door, spent a few moments in the waiting room, and then come into the studio to see the toys. I asked C. if she could show something we had done, and she pointed to the scribbled paper on the table. I agreed we scribbled together. I asked the foster mother if she would like to mention something we had done and she commented on the sticker images she created with C. I thanked them both for coming to the studio, and asked C. if she would come back again another time with her foster mother. She nodded affirmatively. I walked them both to the door and said goodbye. As they drove away, I waved goodbye.

With physical homeostasis or comfort as the goal for the first phase of therapy, maximizing the child's sense of physical safety is the focus of my attention during the first session. Given C.'s history and symptom presentation, I would not expect her to be comfortable with a stranger, to separate from her foster mother who is a source of safety, to participate in art or play, or to speak. To help promote experiences that replicate those missed during the attachment with a caregiver, my first interactions with C. were with her sensory and physical safety in mind. I made every effort to enable her to feel safe and unconditionally accepted. I went back to the earliest levels of development where things were done *for* her, where nothing was expected of her, and where she could function from the most passive stance of observation to participating as desired and able, without any overt or covert pressure or expectations. I did not encourage her to play or speak.

C.'s behavior with her body would be the best indicator of her level of comfort. When they arrived, she stood close to her foster mother, indicating a need for protection. To enable her to feel a sense of protection and safety, I did not try to look at her, even playfully. I did not ask her to move or speak. I merely acknowledged her and then allowed what she was showing me with her body: She wanted to hide. Once she was able to feel in control by hiding, she was able to take the next step forward. I made it easy for her to participate observationally. She was able to indicate yes or no with her body by nodding. For example, I did not ask her, "What would you like to play with?" This would require her to answer, and she did not speak. Doing so would imply an expectation of participation. I had to join with her where she was physically, emotionally, and cognitively and allow her to let me know when she was ready for a broader repertoire of experience and interaction.

And she did by pointing to the doll and bandages. We were communicating nonverbally, with gesture. As C. began to communicate nonverbally, I pointed a few times to let her see that I accepted that style of communication. I did not stay with gestures long, as she was able to understand words and responded with nods most of the time. When she showed interest in the dolls, I did not attempt to engage her in play or conversation. While being attuned to her preferred passive, mute stance, I took an active role to allow her to remain passive and observe the dolls rather than attempt to engage her in play. Mutual co-regulation requires you to stay in the moment with the child. Once I created the state of physical comfort with the doll play, she became a bit more active by pointing to the doll's head and the bandage.

My actions and language are never a step ahead of the child's behavior. For example, when she pointed to the head and bandages, I did not hand them to her. Her pointing indicated her intention in the moment. I always deferred to her state of physical homeostasis rather than attempt to engage her in play. Just as a mother does not place expectations or demands on her infant's course of action, I did not place expectations on C. at this time in therapy. Any pressure, no matter how subtle, for her to talk or take a preferred course of action would be picked up by her right amygdala that was tracking below the surface (Schore, 2012). She was acutely sensitive to signals of danger or threat, so my movements were slow and my voice was calm. I focused on co-regulation of her physical state to create a mental representation that the child was in a safe environment and that she would experience no stress associated with the therapy session. The only time I changed C.'s course of action was when she climbed on the table. This was an opportunity to demonstrate my attention to safety rather than her behavior, essential at this time in therapy.

From the sticker and scribbling activity, I could observe weakness in her gross and fine motor skills, poor motor planning, and poor eye-hand coordination. She was slow in her movements and tired easily, which is typical of medically fragile children. My plan was to include a brief sensory system-building activity at the beginning of each session.

> CASE NOTE: C. returned for the second session with her foster mother. She did not hide, nor did she say hello when greeted. She pulled her foster mother by the hand into the studio. The foster mother placed her sweater and purse on the larger table and sat on the chair at the low table. C. stood close to her. I asked C. if she preferred to play or to use the art supplies. C. immediately went to the dolls and picked up the doll with the bandage on its head. She pointed to the bandage and looked at me. I told her I saw the bandage, and she could do whatever she wanted with it. She slowly pulled on the taped end and one side of the bandage came off. She looked startled and her eyes grew wide. I quickly reassured her it was okay to take off the bandage. She then slowly removed the bandage and ran to show the foster mother the doll's head without the bandage. The foster mother commented, "I guess that baby is all better now." C. returned to the dolls and handed me a bandage and the doll. I asked C. if she wanted me to put the bandage on the doll and she nodded affirmatively. I carefully showed C. how to open the bandage wrapper, separate the little tabs on the bandage

cover, remove the adhesive covers, and place the bandage on the doll's head. I then offered her a bandage and she was able, with minimal help, to remove the wrapper and put the bandage on the doll's arm. She then put four more bandages on the doll's arms, legs, neck, and foot. I commented, "The dolly is hurt and you are helping her get better." C. then covered the dolls with blankets and ran to the foster mother. The foster mother commented, "You fixed those babies up and now they are taking a nap, just like you take a nap." Upon hearing this comment, C.'s posture and muscle tone changed dramatically for a few moments. She stood straight and rigid with her fists clenched. Reading the child's nonverbal, body-based communication, the foster mother said, "Not now, you don't have to take a nap now." C. sat in the small chair and began to rock rhythmically back and forth for a few moments, apparently dissociating as she rocked, seemingly unaware of her surroundings and staring intently.

After a few moments, she handed the foster mother a marker and the foster mother drew a heart on a sheet of paper. The child attempted to draw a heart on a separate sheet of paper but could not. The foster mother invited C. to color the heart she had drawn and mostly filled in with color. C. threw the marker on the floor. I asked C., "Do you want to make your own heart to color instead of helping your foster mother color hers?" She nodded affirmatively. I retrieved a sheet of paper and drew a heart with a faint pencil line while she watched. I turned the paper to her and told her she could draw her own heart with a marker by using my line to help her see the heart shape. She carefully attempted to draw on the line but was not successful and threw the marker further across the room. I said, "Well, I have a better idea to help you make your own heart." On a sheet of paper, I quickly sketched the heart again with a pencil and said, "How about if you hold the marker and I will help you hold it so you can follow the line easier." C. was hesitant, but nodded affirmatively. Before taking her hand in mine, I said, "I will put my hand on top of your hand for a minute while I help you trace the heart, then I will take my hand off your hand." I used my hand to cover my own hand to demonstrate putting my hand on hers and I traced the line we would be drawing around the heart with my finger. I told C. she could say stop anytime and I would stop touching her hand for a minute or a long time. She easily let me put my hand on hers to guide the marker on the outline of the heart. She colored the inside for a few moments with a marker before becoming impatient with the slow progress. I quickly produced an oil pastel with the paper removed and showed her how to color a large space quickly. She did so, and proudly showed the heart to her foster mother.

C. then returned to doll play and removed the blanket, gave each doll a drink from the baby bottle, and put them all in the doll bed. I reminded C. that she had only a few minutes left and asked if we could remember all the things we had done. She ignored me. I reminded her of all the things we had done, including, "I noticed when the dolls were taking a nap and your foster mom said they were taking a nap like you do, that your body showed us you did not want to take a nap." C. did not comment; however, the foster mother said that C. does not like naps or sleeping. I commented, "C. does not like naps or sleeping and she never will have to take a nap or sleep here." C. sighed loudly. She looked at me with eye contact and I looked at her with my left eye to her left eye. We briefly sustained a mutual gaze as the session ended.

C. was demonstrating increased comfort when she attended the second session of therapy. Once again, I did not attempt to alter her course of action or engage her in play. I responded to her nonverbal communications and linking body sensations to affect. I was also responding just as a mother would, by meeting her every need. Bandaging the doll for her and teaching her how to bandage the doll allowed her increased comfort interacting in the environment. This is important to the goal of establishing physical homeostasis. When her foster mother mentioned the babies napping, C. demonstrated a visceral response with her change in muscle tone, posture, and clenched fists. Impressively, the foster mother was able to reassure the child, and C. responded well to her verbal reassurance as her body relaxed. When I brought up the subject at the end of the session, there was a moment of affective engagement demonstrated in the eye contact and mutual gaze.

Although minimal, C. had demonstrated an increased comfort in expressing affect. The previous week she was amenable to coloring on the same paper as the foster mother. This week she resisted doing so when suggested by her foster mother. She expressed her desire for her own heart drawing through frustration and anger that was expressed motorically when she threw the marker. I was able to read that nonverbal signal and my response came to me in the form of an image of a heart that she could copy. After her first and only attempt, I did not encourage her to try to draw the heart again herself. She had already shown me she could not. Instead, I helped her succeed, which left her with the mental representation that she was capable and that I was able and willing to help her when she became frustrated and angry. This is all unconscious. Right-hemisphere-to-right-hemisphere communication takes place by engaging with her in the experience, not talking about an abstract concept. She also had a mental representation that her unspoken needs could be met. I did not want to foster her independence. Rather, I wanted to meet her nonverbal physical and emotional needs. After doing so, I noted she was able to offer nurturance to the dolls in her feeding play. She continued to be mute. I made verbal reference to her state of fear associated with napping and reassured her of her safety, which to her was not having to nap.

Midweek I called the foster mother and asked her to please find a reason to leave the room during the next session to see if C. could tolerate being in the studio without the foster mother present. If the response was neutral, I asked the

foster mother to gradually leave during upcoming sessions for increasingly longer periods of time to use the restroom or take a telephone call, and eventually to
bring things to do that required her to sit at the kitchen table. From the studio, C.
would be able to see her foster mother at the table below the paper partially covering the studio door windows. If C. were to protest her foster mother leaving, we
would postpone this strategy.

> **CASE NOTE:** C. returned for the third session and sat by the dolls. The
> foster mother sat at the small table but did not put her purse down or take
> off her coat. C. played with the dolls for a few minutes, played with the
> doctor kit for a few minutes, and did some scribbling on paper for a few
> minutes. C. began running around the room. The foster mother announced
> she had to leave to use the restroom. C. did not stop running. She started
> hitting the table with her hand loudly and rhythmically as she ran around
> the table, seemingly dissociating. I asked the foster mother, "Are you going
> right to the bathroom and then coming right back to this room?" The fos-
> ter mother said she would be right back. After the foster mother left, C.
> gradually stopped running and hitting the table and went and stood by the
> door of the studio. I said, "Are you are waiting for your foster mother to
> come back because you like to have her in this room with you?" C. nodded
> affirmatively. I said, "We will not trick you. If your foster mother is ever
> going to leave while you are here, we will tell you. She is not leaving you
> today and there is no plan to leave you. She can be right here all the time,
> or she can wait in the waiting area if she has stuff to do." C. looked at me
> and I looked at her with my left eye to her left eye and said, "I will never
> trick you or hurt you here." C. came over and sat next to me by the dolls
> until her foster mother returned. We spent the remainder of the session
> engaged in bandaging and diapering the dolls, feeding them, and scrib-
> bling with the foster mother. We ended the session the same way, with a
> reminder of the session ending soon and a recap of what had been done
> together during the session.

The child's right amygdala was tracking below the surface and her hypermo-
toric activity was most likely in response to noticing, consciously or unconsciously, that the foster mother did not behave as usual by taking off her coat and
putting her purse on the large table. Responding to an instinctive need to co-
regulate the anxiety that C. was expressing in rhythmic and sensory ways of self-
soothing, I actively sought reassurance from the foster mother that she would
return.

C. was demonstrating greater comfort in the therapy environment. She was
less restrained physically, emotionally, and socially. She was also demonstrating
aggression with the doll play. She was able to tolerate the foster mother's depar-
ture and was able to utilize the reassurance of the foster mother's plan to return.

I was planting the idea that her foster mother might at some point be out of the room. C. showed her feelings of comfort and connection when she came and sat by me.

Although it is impossible to direct a young child to engage in problem aspects of her life, C.'s physical comfort and ability to rely on me for comfort indicated I could begin to focus on the content of her play and respond accordingly.

TREATMENT: THE PROBLEM PHASE

CASE NOTE: Upon arrival at the next session, C.'s foster mother announced she had some letters to write and would be sitting in the kitchen. C. was curious about the new items in the studio and did not react. I had covered a large table with butcher paper and had three primary colors of paint in small shallow bowls, along with sponge shapes ready for her to use to stamp images on the paper. She grabbed the sponge of a cat and wanted to begin. I reminded her of safety and gave her an apron to cover her clothes, then helped her sit in the chair comfortably. She spent considerable time stamping many papers with the shapes, enjoying the cause-and-effect aspect of the activity. No attention was paid to content or making an integrated image with the shapes. My comments were, "I see you are making a blue one. I see your arm is stamping that shape hard. I see your arm is making many stars very fast." All comments pertained to motor movement and what she was doing in the space. When she finished stamping with paint, I helped her wash and dry her hands.

C. then explored the doll furniture absentmindedly until she spotted a small toilet. She grabbed it and put it in the doctor kit and shut the lid. I commented, "You don't want to see the toilet." She covered the doctor kit with the blanket and began rhythmically rocking back and forth, apparently dissociating. She seemed unaware of her surroundings and stared intently. After several moments, I quietly said, "You don't want to see the toilet and you put the toilet away so it will be gone." C. picked up a doll and slammed it into the chair. She began hitting the doll with her hand and then picked up the stethoscope from the doctor kit to hit the doll. After a long pause, she lay on the floor for a few moments and I remained silent and still. C. then got up, took the doll out of the chair, and left it lying on the floor. She went to the table and began to scribble with a pencil, apparently distracting herself from her internal affective sensations. I gently patted the doll and said, "Poor baby, poor baby has been left and is sad and scared." C. came over near me and looked at the doll intently. Then she went and got the little toilet out of the box and put the doll on the toilet and waited. I gently patted the doll's shoulder and said, "Poor dolly is scared and sad about the toilet. She is trying it now with our help. She is learning that she does not have to be scared and sad." I repeated this again and waited. After a moment, C. got up, put the toilet in the box with the furniture, put the lid on the box, and gave the dolls a drink of juice. I sat quietly, as did C.

Eventually, she got up, came over beside me, sat, and put her hand on my arm. I patted her hand, looked at her with my left eye to her left eye and said, "I am sorry if you were ever sad and hurt and left alone. I am glad you are okay and are with people who know how to take care of a girl. I am sorry your mom and dad did not know how to take care of a girl. That is why you cannot be with them. You did not do anything bad, and it is not your fault, even if you don't believe it right now." C. looked at me with eye contact, very attentive, but did not respond. After a pause, I reminded her of the session ending soon. She grabbed a book and began looking at the pictures rapidly. I quietly asked her if we could look at the book together and patted the floor next to me. C. brought the book over and sat next to me and we looked at the book for about 30 seconds before she put the book down, stood up, and went to leave with her foster mother.

C.'s reenactment of her surmised experience with the toilet allowed the two of us to have an enactment. Her response to seeing the toy toilet was evident in her body and behavior. Typical of a child this age, putting the toilet in the box and shutting the lid is yet another attempt to escape her affect. With the concrete thinking of early childhood, putting anything out of sight is a way to get rid of it. I did not ask questions or attempt to "find out" her associations to the toilet. Instead, I stayed with her in the moment by responding to her body-based expression. An example of not doing this would have been to ask her what she did not like about the toilet, or to tell me about what happened to her with the toilet. This type of questioning is a shift to cognition but I want to stay with her body-based sensory memory and nonverbal communication. At no time in the session did I ask her any questions. We were sharing a mutually safe and nonthreatening intersubjective space, in a shared affective experience. Using the baby as a symbol of self, she was able to demonstrate her body-based kinesthetic memories as evidenced in her reenactment of an event. She did not have the vocabulary or verbal skills to communicate this linguistically. The placement of her hand on my arm embodied the expression of her affect in that moment.

CASE NOTE: C. returned for another session after missing one session because of a holiday. She was intrigued when she noticed different toys on the table. I gave her about fifteen 1-inch-square wooden blocks and asked her to stack them. She stacked about three before they fell over. She immediately tried again, stacked five blocks, and smiled. I smiled, looking at her left eye with my left eye. She restacked the blocks again and added a sixth to the stack. I looked surprised and praised her for her skill. Then I asked her to learn a new clapping game, Patty-cake. She liked the idea but did not have the skill to clap the other person's opposite hand. I changed the game immediately to a game of clapping each other's hands without the crossover, which she was able to do after a several attempts. I asked what she preferred to do next, and she got up and moved to the drawing table. We engaged in bilateral scribbling and took turns leading each other with our markers around the paper. I reminded her that we would take turns following each other just like she and her foster mother had done the first day they were in the studio. We smiled at each other maintaining left-eye-to-left-eye contact. She laughed while scribbling, whether the leader or the follower.

C. then pointed to the paint on the shelf. I asked, "Are you showing me you want to paint?" She nodded affirmatively. I got an apron, paper, water, a wet cloth, brushes, and paints. I asked her to pick a color and she picked red. I showed her how to pour paint in the palette and told her she could use any paint she wanted. She began with a large brush and made a large picture with many colors and lines but no specific image, as is expected developmentally. When given a new paper, C. made three blue strokes across the paper and looked at me. I used my finger to point to the blue paint strokes as I said, "I see you have used the blue paint and made large blue lines here, here, and here."

She then made two large shapes of blue paint on the paper and began hitting them with the paintbrush. I watched as she turned the paintbrush upside down and began to stab the blue shapes with the pointed end of the brush many times. Her breathing was heavy, her teeth were clenched and bared. She stared intently as she stabbed the blue shapes. She then turned the brush around and hit the shapes with the brush. Not knowing what was occurring symbolically, I said, "You are hitting the big blue one with the brush." She kept hitting the blue shapes harder and then suddenly stopped, put the paintbrush on the table, and crumpled up the paper. She got up, put it in the trash and returned to the painting table. She uttered her first word, "No." I quietly said, "No." C. said, "No." She turned to doll play and fed, diapered, and bandaged the dolls until the end of the session.

The therapy does not occur through delving into the meaning or content of the art or play; rather, it is found by joining with the child in the creation of corrective experiences that physically alter the body and mind in a sequential manner consistent with development and information processing. In this instance, the right hemisphere is activated with the fluid paint media and gross motor movement to elicit affect, or primary process material. C. represented her perceived perpetrator with blue paint and physically altered her perception of the experience by engaging in an affective enactment of stabbing the image. The depth of this experience was reflected in her body expression: intense breathing, focus, and bared teeth. The activation of the lower structures moves the processing to the limbic structures, followed by the higher structures and cognition. Her cognition was concrete, reflected when she put the image in the trash to elimi-

nate the perpetrator or threat. There had been some integration of the experience. She used language associated with the event, her first word in therapy,
"No."

In my telephone call with the foster mother following this session, she
reported that C. was doing better at school with her ability to focus and her ability to participate and was using words with her teacher. C. was also having some
nights without sleep disturbance. She was not as fearful of the toilet, and her
encopresis had improved with fewer weekly episodes. Along with therapy, the
foster parents set up a reward system for her use of the toilet.

> CASE NOTE: During another session, C. was playing with the dollhouse
> and doll furniture. She was putting the family members to bed, waking
> them up for school, and giving them breakfast. When she woke up the
> smallest child doll, she announced that the doll had to use the toilet. As
> she placed the doll on the toilet, she tenderly told the doll, "Don't be
> scared. I will hold your hand. You won't go away." In a left-eye-to-left-eye
> exchange, I asked, "Did anyone ever tell you that you would go away in the
> toilet?" C. said, "Yes, they told me I would go away if I didn't go." I said,
> "People told you that you would go away if you didn't go and that is not
> true. That would never happen. I am sorry someone told you that to try to
> make you go." After a long pause, C. asked, "Why?" I replied, "Sometimes
> people tell children things that are not true to make them do things.
> Sometimes people hurt children to make them do things, and that is not
> okay to do to children. The most important thing is that you will never go
> away in the toilet. I am sorry someone told you that to scare you so you
> would go." C. said, "Now they don't say it." I said, "Now you live with
> people who don't tell you that." After a long pause, C. said in a quiet tone,
> "Now I know." I responded in a quiet tone, "Yes, now you know."

This session offers another example of the importance of allowing young children to take the lead in the play or art. Their stories are not buried deeply by time
or defenses. Given the opportunity and the tools, they will use reenactment with
their body to replay and retell aspects of the event. When C. mentioned the doll
would disappear, that caught my attention. Consistent with the findings of Fivush
and Hamond (1990), unlike children under age 4 who report the mundane
aspects of an event, children near age 4 years report the unusual aspect of an
event. I watch for atypical comments. I have heard many children yell at a doll
on the toilet for going pee in their pants or tell a doll on the toilet that she is too
big for diapers or pull-ups. C.'s comment was unusual. Using her language, I
offered, "Now you know." It was not important for me to know exactly what she
knew, but to validate her knowing. She may have been expressing that she knew
she wouldn't disappear, or she may have been expressing that she knew her parents did not tell her the truth. That is not important. What is important is to
engage in a state of affective attunement, not cognitive communication.

CASE NOTE: C. attended another session and was delighted to have the opportunity to fingerpaint. The fingerpaint paper was inside a shallow tray. A small bucket of water, a wet cloth, and a dry cloth were nearby. I asked C. to please keep the paint inside the tray. I sat across from her at the table and asked her what color she wanted to use first. She pointed to the purple paint. I squeezed about 3 tablespoons of purple paint onto the paper and invited her to put a finger in the paint and smear it around. She did so, then put a few more fingers in the paint and stopped and looked at me. I smiled, looked at her left eye with my left eye, and said quietly, "Are you showing me you are not sure you can put all your fingers in the paint?" She nodded affirmatively. I said, "You can do whatever you want as long as the paint is inside the tray. You can ask me anything you want to know, anytime." I smiled at her while looking at her left eye to left eye. C. painted several papers full of yellow, orange, green and purple paint. As she painted, she began to ask for paint colors by name instead of pointing.

There was a shift in her body and behavior when she asked for the red paint. As I put the red paint on the paper, she stared at the paint and did not touch it. I reminded her she could change her mind about the color. She said she did not want red, and asked for blue. I removed the paper with the red paint and set it off to the side, still visible. She fingerpainted on another paper with the blue paint and then asked for the red paint again. I removed the blue painted paper and placed the paper with the red paint on it in front of C. She quickly hit the red paint with both hands and began smearing it all over the paper. She then began to smear the paint on her hands and arms. I stopped her by stating, "Remember, the paint must stay on the paper inside the tray, not on your body." I wiped most of the paint off her arms. C. returned her hands to the red paint on the paper and then immediately put her painted hands on her chest and said, "The red paint is on my mommy's neck" and began to cry. I silently let her cry for a few moments, and then with my left eye on her left eye, I said, "The red paint was on mommy's neck and that is over and the doctor is helping mommy get better." C. continued to cry for a moment and then stopped. After a long pause, C. said, "I didn't want the blood on mommy's neck." I responded, "You didn't want the blood on your mommy's neck, and I am sorry the blood was on mommy's neck and I am glad she is better now."

After a long pause, C. asked, "Why did that happen?" I responded, "Sometimes people do things that are not safe. It is not okay to do unsafe things and hurt people. That is why daddy must stay in jail until he learns not to do unsafe things. But the most important thing is that you did not do anything wrong and it is not your fault." C. replied, "Boy, you sure do know a lot of stuff." I replied, "Yes, C., I do know a lot of stuff. And you know a lot of stuff, too. You are a very smart girl and a very good girl." C. sighed loudly and smiled. I then said to C., "I am glad you told me about mommy's neck, and it is okay to talk about it any time. It is also okay to cry, because that is how our bodies work. When we feel sad or scared feelings, they want to come out, and they do that by crying. Your mommy is getting better and your daddy is not going to be at home for a while. You will be with your new foster mother for a while. Remember, your mommy is safe with your grandma and your daddy is safe in jail. He is not being hurt and has a bed and food and he is safe." C. sighed loudly. After a pause, I asked C., "Were you worried about that?" She nodded affirmatively.

The kinesthetic, tactile, and visual aspect of the fingerpaint accessed the right-brain visual memories C. had of witnessing the blood on her mother's neck. I would not ask the child if she witnessed the stabbing. I stayed with affective communication. The red color of the paint was a visual traumatic reminder (Pynoos, Steinberg, & Goenjian, 1996). By allowing C. control over the pacing of the experience, she was able to demonstrate what occurred with her body. She was not able to tell about the event. Because she was reenacting the event, I had to contain the imagery so she could manage it. I did not want her to become terrified, so I immediately reframed her visual image to one of the event being over and her mother without the blood. However, when she was grieving, I did not interfere. Grief is a necessary part of healing. I was conveying to C. that it was a normal and healthy response. This was an example of mutual co-regulation in that her experience did not become overwhelming, but at the same time, her affect was not restricted. I did not think about my actions. My actions were formulated by C.'s affect that I felt myself.

Cleaning up the symbolic blood on her arms when she painted on them was a response to the ANS activation displayed in her wide eyes, shallow breathing, and perspiration on her face. The act of stopping her was not planned or from cognition. My feeling was that she had been overstimulated by the fluidity of the media and that I needed to contain the media to bring her back to physical homeostasis. The mutual co-regulation that occurred was the result of being attuned to her body-based affective state. I knew what was required because of the images and sensations that came to my right hemisphere from C.'s right hemisphere.

When C. regained her sense of physical homeostasis, she immediately moved closer to the actual traumatic experience. She smeared the paint on her arms and announced that the paint was on mommy's neck. I normalized her response by validating her perception and emotional experience during the event, and I reassured her that her mother was okay. She continued to move closer to describing the actual experience, using the word *blood* instead of the word *paint* to describe her mother's bloody neck.

After telling C. the event was not her fault, her comment about my "knowing a lot of stuff" may be considered humorous, but it was very important not to smile or laugh in response to such a comment made during such a sensitive discussion. Her concrete cognition could have interpreted my smile or laugh as indicating that what I was saying was a joke or being silly. It is ego-dystonic to use humor in this situation. The child was very serious, and the therapist's responses should be as well.

I offered information about her parents to alleviate fantasies she might have about their whereabouts and what was happening with them. This was an important session because of content but also because C. began talking during this session and talked each session thereafter.

TREATMENT: TRANSFORMATION PHASE

CASE NOTE: C. arrived for another session and went straight to the dolls. She wanted to bathe, powder, diaper, and feed them. She was very tender, being careful not to get soap in their eyes, and spent considerable time sitting next to them. After a time I said, "I see you are sitting by the babies while they sleep." C. responded, "They are not sleeping. They better go to sleep." I replied, "Oh, I see. You are sitting by the babies until they can go to sleep." C. did not respond, but continued to sit for a long time. I said, "I wonder why those babies take so long to get to sleep?" C. averted her eyes and appeared to dissociate as she stared intently in space. I asked C. quietly if she was just thinking about something. She whispered, "No." I whispered back, "Okay." After a long pause, C. went to the table and began playing with stickers. She went back to the dolls and put a bandage on the neck of one doll. She brought it over to show me and I commented, "I see you put a bandage on the neck." C. then put the doll in the doll bed and placed an additional doll and a bear puppet on two different blankets. She began to hit the bear puppet repeatedly. I commented, "What did Mr. Bear do?" C. said, "He can't sleep. He gets a whooping." I said, "Mr. Bear gets a whooping because he cannot sleep." C. said, "Yep." She continued to hit the bear puppet. Then she threw the bear puppet under the table. I reached under the table and patted the bear puppet, and said, "Mr. Bear is sad and hurt. He cannot help it that he cannot sleep." C. watched, then put the bear back in the chair and hit it and threw it under the table. I again reached under the table, patted the bear and said again, "Mr. Bear is sad and hurt. He cannot help it that he cannot sleep." C. then put the bear in the chair and hit the bear with the stethoscope from the doctor kit, dropped the bear on the floor, and kicked the bear under the table. I reached over, patted the bear and repeated, "Mr. Bear gets a whooping because he cannot sleep. He is sad and hurt because he cannot help it that he cannot sleep."

After a long pause, C. pulled the bear puppet out from under the table, got down on her hands and knees, placed her upper body under the table, and waited. I patted her and said, "C. is sad and hurt. C. cannot help it that she cannot sleep. She is not bad and she will not be hit anymore because she cannot sleep." C. stayed in this position for several moments while I repeated those words twice. Then C. moved from under the table and sat next to me silently for a few moments. I looked at C. with my left eye to her left eye and said, "I am sorry you were sad and hurt and I am glad you are safe now with people who will not hurt you. If anyone ever hurts you, you tell your foster mother, your teacher, or your doctor or the policeman. It is not okay to hurt others." After a pause, C. stood up, went and got the dolls and the bear, and fed them all with the baby bottle before putting them to bed with a kiss. She announced, "If people hurt me, I will tell my mommy or my teacher."

Therapy with young children is a moment-to-moment, intimate corrective experience that takes place in an intersubjective space where we both are active participants. I assert that recreating attachment behaviors is necessary in therapy with young children because they need to go back and re-create new internal working models within a relational context. Therapy is not something I am offering the child—it occurs with the child. The therapy takes place in the repetitive replaying fragments of the story for affect tolerance and mastery. The kinesthetic aspect of the play activates the right hemisphere. Given the tools to express it, the imagery of the right hemisphere emerges and the symbolic play is an expression of that imagery. The brain moves the processing to the limbic structures with expression of affect, as was seen when C. hit the doll and threw it under the table. Once the affect is validated, welcomed, and felt as shared experience, information processing moves to the higher structures and cognition. This was evidenced in C.'s ability to witness the doll receive nurturance and figure out a way to get that for herself. Her ability to offer nurturance to the dolls and the bear was evidence of the transformative effect of the play therapy.

> CASE NOTE: C. arrived for another session with a new ethnically matched doll. She gave the doll the same name as herself. She was thrilled to show me the eyes, nose, ears, hair, and toes and how the dress could be removed. C. assured me that the doll did not need a bandage because she was not hurt. The foster mother asked C. if she wanted to tell me the reason she received the new doll. C. said, "I got it because I don't have accidents anymore." The foster mother added, "C. earned the doll by not having accidents in her panties anymore. She learned to use the toilet." I commented to C. with my left eye on her left eye, "C., I am so proud of you for earning the doll. You are such a smart girl and such a good girl." C. smiled proudly and began acting silly.
>
> I led her to the studio and when inside I said, "When I tell you how smart and good you are, does it make you feel silly?" C. did not respond. I reassured her that it was not bad to feel silly. I added, with my left eye to her left eye, "Even if you don't believe it right now, you were never bad. You were a baby and then a little girl who didn't know how to do things and had to learn to do things." I pointed to her doll and said, "Does that baby know how to use the toilet?" C. laughed and said, "No." I said, "That is

right, babies and little girls have to learn to do things. Girls are not supposed to be hit and told they are bad. They are supposed to be helped to
learn, just like your foster mother helps you learn." C. said proudly, "I
learn." I said, "Yes, you learn because you are smart." C. added, "I learn
because I am smart and I talk." I replied, "You are smart and you talk." C.
smiled and we engaged in a moment of mutual gaze.

Herein lies more evidence of the transformative and evolutionary nature of
therapy from the lower structures to the higher. After ten months of nearly weekly
therapy, there had been change, as demonstrated in C.'s free use of language, her
ability to sleep, the abatement of her encopresis, and her ability to accept and
give nurturance. The transformations in her reduction of symptoms, her
improved behavior, and developing concept of self are evident.

TREATMENT: INTEGRATION PHASE

Alternative placement for C. was being considered. The father remained in jail
and the mother refused the drug rehab offered to her during her hospitalization,
and she rejected help with housing. She offered for her daughter to be adopted
"somewhere" and blamed the authorities for putting her husband in jail and
causing her problems. It was apparent to the social service staff that reunification
with C. was not an option.

C.'s foster mother called during the week to let me know C.'s maternal aunt
who lived in another state was willing to consider adopting C. rather than adoption by nonfamily members. The aunt is a preschool assistant, married, with two
sons ages 8 and 11. The aunt planned to visit twice to get to know C. before taking C. to live in her home as part of the family. This brought about an abrupt
termination of the therapy and required using the last two sessions as produc-
tively as possible to prepare the child for the transition from her foster mother
and home to a new home with a stranger. The foster mother and aunt asked for
tips for handling the short weekend visits. They were considering a joint trip to a
theme park for one of the days.

I arranged for a conference call rather than have the foster mother convey
information to C.'s aunt for me. During the call, I began by stating that they were
both showing a great deal of care and concern for C. and the possible move, and
I thanked them for asking for tips. I suggested that the theme park visit might be
very stimulating and that perhaps C. would benefit more from spending time
with her aunt reading books, playing, and getting to know each other in a calmer
setting. The aunt was relieved, as she had been rethinking that decision. I supported her intuition. There was also the strong possibility of neurochemical dysregulation brought on by the stress of a visit with a stranger and the talk of a
potential move. I added that C.'s body might not be able to process incoming
sensory information well or rapidly. Therefore, the overstimulating environment
of the theme park might not be a pleasurable experience for C.

To the aunt I suggested that she let C. know she was her mommy's sister but is not exactly like her mommy. I shared with the aunt the exact words I used with C. about her parents: that they do unsafe things and are not able to take care of a girl. I explained to the aunt the necessity of keeping the language similar and easy to understand. I also recommended the aunt say to the child that she has food, a bed, and toys, that she knows how to keep kids safe, and that she does not hit or hurt them even if they have accidents or cannot sleep. I suggested it would be helpful if the aunt could bring a photo of the house, pets, her room, the kitchen, the bathroom, and so on to offer the child visuals of where she was going and would be living. I suggested making color photocopies of a few photos that C. could keep as transitional objects. The aunt was very receptive and planned to spend the time with C. and let C. take the lead during their visit.

I also recommended that C. might need to continue therapy to address the issues regarding the move, the loss of her mother and father, and possible PTSD that might be triggered over the next few months. I prepared the aunt for a regression in sleep and bathroom behavior and told her that C. might refuse to talk for a time.

> CASE NOTE: C. arrived for the next-to-the-last session with her doll and immediately announced, "I am going to live with my auntie." I smiled and said, "I am so happy that you are going to live with your family and be happy and safe." C. said, "My auntie and my mommy are going to be my mommy now." I said, "That is right, your mommy will always be your mommy and now you have a new mommy too." C. then put all the babies in the sink and gave them all a bath because they were going on a trip. She was able to wash, rinse, dry, diaper, clothe, and feed the babies. When she was finished, I said, "You know exactly how to take care of babies going on a trip. Those babies are just like you. They are cared for, loved, fed, can go to the bathroom, can sleep, and they can do anything now, just like you." C. said, "I have a new family too." I said, "You have a new family too."
>
> After a long pause, I said, "It will be different there, C., but in a good way. You will be safe with your auntie and her family. They know how to be good to you and help you learn instead of hurt you and trick you. Remember, if anyone ever hurts you, you can tell your teacher or your mommy." C. said, "I know. Let's get the babies and say goodnight because tomorrow we are going on a trip." We spent a few minutes talking together about what would be the same and what would be different in her new home. I also reminded her that she would have lots of feelings about her new home and family and would still have feelings about her mom and dad and it was okay to talk to her new family about them.
>
> I also brought up the foster mother. I told C. she would be able to talk on the phone with her but would not see her. C. became agitated and began to run around the room, seemingly dissociating from painful emotions that were arising. I said, "I understand it is hard to think about not

seeing your foster mother. I have an idea." C. gradually stopped running and listened as I told her I had some picture frames. I asked C., "Do you want to decorate a frame and we can put a picture of your foster mother in the frame and you can take it with you to your new home?" C. was delighted and said that her foster mother had given her some pictures to keep and she wanted a frame that was pink. I offered her a raw wooden frame in the shape of a heart and she painted it pink and put stickers of animals on it.

C.'s focus on the care of the dolls may seem to be nurturing play, but it appears to be mastery play as well. The mastery aspect of the play was preparing the dolls for the trip. C. was demonstrating what babies need; attention, nurturance, and care. She was no longer hitting the dolls. The experiences of the past had been integrated. She was moving on behaviorally, emotionally, and cognitively.

CASE NOTE: C. arrived for the last session with her foster mother. They were both looking forward to the aunt's arrival in two days. We had a party with juice, popcorn, and fruit to celebrate C.'s new mommy and new home. The foster mother lovingly told C. that she was happy that C. had a new home. C. looked at her and said, "What will you do without me?" The foster mother truthfully said, "I will do the same things I do every day, but it will not be the same without you. I will miss you, and then someday I may help another girl who needs to find a new family, just like I helped you." C. ate in silence and after a time I said to her, "C., I want to tell you that I am so happy I had time with you and that you shared your very important stories with me. I am so happy you are going to live with your new mommy and be safe and have a fun life." C. said, "I am taking my doll with me and her name is Linda." I replied, "Well, your doll has the same name as me." C. said, "Yes." I remarked that I remembered that the doll used to be named C., and if the doll's name was changed again someday, that was fine. C. said, "Okay."

As the session ended, I told C. I had one more thing to say before we said goodbye. I looked at C with my left eye to her left eye and said, "C., I want you to always remember that you are a smart girl and a good girl. You can grow up and be anyone you want to be, and I am really, really happy to know you and to have had time with you in the playroom." I gave C. a small handmade card telling her what a smart and good girl she was and then I read her a storybook about going to a new home. She wanted to read the book again, so we did. She announced, "I am going to my new home." C. left happily with her foster mother.

I often marvel at the rapid pace of treatment with young children. They are so very expressive in their art and play and respond very positively to a structured, contained, safe environment stocked with tools for expression. Young children require a nonverbal method of expression to access their body-based visual memories and engage in interactive, corrective affective experiences as a mechanism of change in therapy.

C. was fortunate to have such a skilled foster mother who augmented the therapy with her calm, steady, and nurturing personality as well as a structured and predictable environment. C. was helped immensely by this devoted and compassionate person. The repetitive nature of the mastery play was evident in the sessions in between the ones presented in the case material. C. would play many of her stories in fragments or out of context. As she played, the narrative aspect of the play became more evident, indicating movement from the lower to the higher structures as she developed more complexity of thought and was able to verbally convey the narratives about her experiences.

CHAPTER 8

Treating School-Age Children: Out of Control or Out of Body?

The school-age years are a time of change. Away from home and caregivers for much of the day, children interact independently with many other children and adults. They are developing language and motor skills rapidly. They are learning to modify and control their emotions and behavior. Development shifts from body-based learning to academics. Many school-age children feel a great deal of academic and peer pressure. Some are exposed to violence daily—in their home, at school, on television, in videogames and other forms of entertainment, on the streets of their neighborhood and in their community. Unfortunately, many children live in poverty or in environments where substance abuse, child abuse, and neglect are common.

School age is a time when children face other changes and challenges as well: the birth of siblings, going to camp, injuries or illnesses requiring hospitalization, or being diagnosed with a chronic illness. Parents divorce, grandparents pass away, pets die. Some lose parents or older siblings to street violence. These experiences can be incredibly stressful on a child with a *healthy* developmental trajectory, but when these challenges face a child whose system is not adequately developed or supported, they can prove to be more than the school-age child is able to integrate and cope with in a functional way.

The early nonverbal right-hemisphere-to-right-hemisphere communications between infant and caregiver create repetitive attachment interactions that result in states of nonconscious emotional attunement, co-regulation, and experiences of rupture and repair in the relationship (Schore, 2005). These experiences are critical to emotional development and affect regulation. It is widely accepted that the negative effects of child abuse, neglect, and failure to form attachment with a primary caregiver during the first year of life have adverse effects on development and functioning: "From infancy through all later stages of life, the right hemisphere is dominant for the non-conscious reception, expression and communication of emotion, as well as the cognitive and physiological components of emotional processing" (Schore, 2012, p. 58).

The infant begins emotional regulation in nonverbal right-hemisphere-to-right-hemisphere body-based experiences. An example is an infant who wakes in the crib and begins to cry. The attuned mother will respond with visual, auditory, olfactory, and tactile reassurance. The infant engages in a state of mutual co-regulation with the mother that creates physical homeostasis. As the mother repetitively responds in a predictable way, the infant eventually cries and stops for a few moments, self-regulating while awaiting the mother's arrival at the crib. As the infant develops within this reliable and dependable internal working model, he grows in the ability to regulate his or her affect for a greater length of time. A mother who responds in random or unpredictable ways interferes with the maturation of the right hemisphere and thus creates high levels of stress:

> Deficits in function must be associated with defects in the dynamic structural systems, and a theory of the genesis of psychopathology needs to be tied to current developmental neurobiological models of the experience-dependent anatomical maturation of brain systems, especially those involved in socio-emotional functioning. (Schore, 2003b, p. 32)

School-age children referred for art therapy are experiencing behavior and learning problems. Many of them are on medication for attention or mood disorders. Children described as "out of control" often exhibit behavior that includes explosive episodes and lengthy tantrums. They are anxious, oppositional, and defiant, and engage in negative behaviors such as stealing, substance abuse, and skipping school. Others are described as slow learners who are inattentive and disruptive in the classroom.

Many parents with difficult children have tried several approaches to change their child's negative behaviors. However, if the child is operating only with the lower structures of the brain and responding with reactive cognition, she is not able to access the higher structures for awareness and insight about her behavior. The pressures and demands to do something one cannot do become too overwhelming, resulting in primitive and reactive coping behaviors such as hitting and screaming.

This chapter consists of case material drawn from nearly 3 years of therapy with an aggressive and violent school-age child with a history of prenatal exposure to substance abuse, early neglect, and inconsistent and aberrant care during the first 3 years of life. The case material offers specific examples of the facilitation of right-hemisphere-to-right-hemisphere communications and of how to create real and symbolic attachment behavioral experiences that result in states of attunement, co-regulation, and experiences of rupture and repair (Schore, 2005) while in a therapeutic relationship. The case will also illustrate how replicating attachment experiences is critical to the ongoing development of a core concept of mind/body/self (Schore 1994, 2000, 2003a) and for emotional regulation, control of behavior, and demonstrations of empathy. The beginning of therapy is given specific attention, followed by vignettes to illustrate the course of treatment and the outcome.

TREATMENT: THE SELF PHASE OF THERAPY

School-age children are typically willing to participate in art therapy, as it appears less threatening than "talk therapy." Most children like to draw and are able to experiment with a variety of art media comfortably. Many are able to understand trial and error, and some children this age are able to delay gratification. Because they are interested in the aesthetic quality of their art, they may need technical help with the art media. School-age children can become anxious about their art ability as they compare their skill level with that of others. Therefore, they may require validation and support of their effort and expression. Their stories naturally contain narratives. They show an interest in exploring new concepts. Some develop a limited coping ability and are able to use problem solving as a way of coping with frustration.

Although school-age children may be aware of injustices and are not as egocentric as younger children, abused children seldom have empathy for others. Empathy only develops under favorable conditions early in life and is based on emotional connections (Perry & Szalavitz, 2007). Infants who have been emotionally deprived demonstrate a persistently active stress response, and are predisposed to aggression and violence (Perry & Szalavitz, 2007; Perry et al., 1995). This is because damage to neural pathways inhibits the ability to access the higher structures of the brain to modulate the urges from the limbic system (Lewis, 1998).

CASE NOTE: J. was a 6-year-old boy who lived with his biological mother and 14-year-old sister. The biological father's whereabouts were unknown. J. was referred for therapy because of problems at home and school. The mother was a substance abuser after J. was born and left him with a variety of caregivers for extended periods during the first 3 years of his life. The mother was now free of drug use and devoted to improving life for herself and her children. She was seeing a therapist for her own traumatic history of neglect and was participating voluntarily in parenting classes. She had been a very lax parent for most of J.'s life but was beginning to implement rules and structure in an attempt to help her son control his behavior. J. resisted the new rules. He was reacting with defiant and oppositional behavior that had escalated to the point that she could not handle his dangerous behaviors. His time at school was limited to the first two hours because of his disruptive and aggressive behavior in the classroom. He was mean to other children and to animals. His tantrums continued for long periods when he did not get his way. J. had recently charged his mother with a large knife when she attempted to set limits on his behavior. J.'s sister was having behavior problems at home and school and was also in treatment.

J. and his mother arrived for the first session. I stood at the door as they walked up the ramp to the studio, then stepped back slightly. As they entered I greeted J.'s mother first and then J. He quietly said, "Hello." I offered them a brief tour of the studio, and then J.'s mother told him she would be in the waiting area. I reassured J. he could visit his mother at any time. He mentioned that he liked macaroni and cheese as he ate the snacks I offered him.

J. went into the studio, picked up the clay on the table, began to shape it and then banged it on the table. As he did so, he began to talk. He mentioned that he lived at home with a sister who was mean to him, and that he went to a school that was boring. I listened without asking any questions and he eventually stopped talking and stopped touching the clay.

I let school-age children and adolescents know at the beginning of therapy that I would like them to complete a few drawings, then or later, so I can see how they draw. I reassure them it is not a test and that they do not have to be a good artist to do the few drawings.

When I told J. this, he said, "I will do it but I hate to draw so I don't want to draw again." I said, "I see. You will do a few drawings today, but you don't want to spend your time here after today drawing." J. said, "Yes. I like to do other stuff." I said, "Let's do the drawings and then you can have the rest of the time to do whatever stuff you want."

I presented J. with a spectrum of eight markers and a pencil with an eraser and gave him a sheet of 9- by 12-inch drawing paper. I said, "Please draw a picture of a house, any kind you want." He completed the house drawing (see Figure 8.1) and stopped. Then he said, "Now I will draw one with my left hand" (Figure 8.2). I gave him another sheet of paper and asked him to draw a tree (Figure 8.3), a person (Figure 8.4), and an animal (Figure 8.5), and to do a free drawing. He refused to draw the free drawing by stating, "I hate to draw. I like outdoor play best." By the end of this structured activity, J.'s speech was somewhat regressed.

I offered J. a choice of two types of structured media. He chose modeling clay and spent the rest of the session pounding and rubbing the clay. Near the end of the session, I reminded J. that our time was nearly up. I thanked him for coming to the studio and for doing the drawings since I learned that he hated to draw. I walked with him to the door and said goodbye, smiled, and waved goodbye. I told him I looked forward to seeing him next week. He ignored me.

Although J. was a bit shy initially, he had no difficulty separating from his mother to come into the studio. As he began to manipulate the clay, he began to talk, which is very common. When I asked him to draw, he was compliant despite his expressed displeasure with drawing. He was able to state his preferences for other "stuff." Note that I imitate his language, as would a mother with her infant in mother-infant, nonverbal collaborative communication. I used my left eye to look at J.'s left eye when speaking to him. He responded by looking at me with his left eye to my left eye occasionally during the first session. In my clinical experience, the organism unconsciously responds to the experiences that promote the developmental trajectory.

From J.'s drawings, I was able to see evidence of neurological impairment and delay in his normal graphic development. Most children his age are able to draw a square house with a triangle roof and a door and windows (Kellogg, 1969; Lindstrom, 1964; Lowenfeld, 1957). The gross asymmetry, lack of spatial organization and delay in visual perceptual ability are evident. Also, when children say they hate to draw, I have found it is often because they can see that they cannot reproduce their internalized image. One child stated, "My hand won't do what my brain tells it to do." It was not surprising that J. disliked drawing. He was able to see that his drawings were unlike those of his peers. Drawing was an unsatisfying activity because he struggled repeatedly and remained unsuccessful. This often produces feelings of anxiety and shame and creates a negative self introjection with comments such as "I am stupid" or feelings of anger and rage, as the frustration is truly intolerable. Children with these types of delays often do better with three-dimensional media because of the spatial, tactile, and kinesthetic components of the media in the art making experience.

CASE NOTE: I greeted J. at the door when he arrived for the second session, as I did at all future sessions. I offered him a snack of organic macaroni and cheese. He said, surprised, "You remembered!" I responded, "I did remember. And I am happy to make this for you." J. said, "I would like it every time I come here." I said, "I will remember you want it every time you come here, and unless for some reason I am out of macaroni and cheese, you may have it when you come here." J. ate macaroni and cheese nearly every session for the first 2 years of therapy. Later he ate other snacks but wanted his favorite at least once or twice a month.

In the studio, J. began building a structure from cardboard and wood. He tested limits constantly throughout the session with the art media, with demands of me, and especially at the end of the session when he did not want to stop working on his project. Limits were set. He ran around the room, then from the room and out the door , where he jumped on and off large rocks repeatedly. I went to the door, said goodbye, and waved goodbye, as I did at all future sessions.

Having J.'s preferred macaroni and cheese for a snack at the following session was an example of meeting his basic hunger need by offering him warm food, but more important, paying attention to him. His first comment was, "You remembered." Not only was I meeting his basic needs, I was acknowledging him as having a self that had preferences and that those needs could be met in as immediate a manner as possible. The exchange between us was spontaneous. We were engaged in a replication of the experiences inherent in an early growth-producing, infant-mother dyad relationship.

J. was behaving as a much younger child during our second session. He was fascinated with water play, dumped art supplies from the containers, and was not able to end the session even when given two reminders of the remaining time. J. had been sitting for a time working on his sculpture, so when he stood up and ran around the room, the increase in motor movement was not unusual. However, I did note his hyper-motoric behavior and inability to stop running.

> **CASE NOTE:** At the third session, I greeted J. in the usual manner and we began with two sensory-motor activities. The first was to locate beads and coins in a shoebox filled with dried pinto beans. J. was eager to find the objects but had difficulty. He wanted to dump the beans out to find the coins. I said that was not part of the game. He resorted to spilling beans out of the box. I slowly and calmly placed the spilled beans back into the box. J. soon stopped that behavior, slowed down, and was able to find several coins in the box. For the second activity, I invited J. to play a game called "Marker Wars." I assured him it did not involve drawing. J. was delighted with the idea of the game, but it was soon obvious he was not able to meet my markers anywhere on the page even though I moved slowly. I slowed my movement further and he was able to meet one marker, but it was a rare success. I announced we would stop in a few moments. He said, "I want to keep doing the game." We turned the paper over and he did a bit better but still had great difficulty. At the end of this activity, I invited J. to help me "mess up" the paper by both of us scribbling all over the paper.
>
> J. then said he wanted to play with clay. He began with quiet, careful play. Soon it evolved into interactive play during which he was ordering me to do things or "there would be consequences." His play was verbally aggressive and threatening, yet he smiled, enjoying his dominant role. He said he was the smartest kid in his class and that he could make anyone do what he wanted. He stated he had no problems at school, counter to what I knew to be true. He ended the session by running from the room and out the door. I walked to the door and said goodbye. J. ignored me as he had done in the past.

After three sessions, it was evident that J. had sensory and motor delays, was aggressive and domineering, and had difficulty controlling his body and behavior. My initial treatment plan was to focus on replicating missed early developmental experiences in real and symbolic ways along with a child-centered (Landreth, 1991) approach to art and play therapy to accommodate J.'s need for a wide range of affective, behavioral, and emotional experiences. Using psychoanalytic and attachment-based therapy along with the sensory and motor growth facilitating experiences would allow him to gain physical mastery. I would modify my treatment plan and adapt it to treat specific delays once I was better able to assess J.'s specific deficits and areas of competency.

An example of mutual co-regulation occurred during bean box play. J. became increasingly frustrated. He began to spill beans in an attempt to get his way. Rather than dialogue about his motivation or behavior, my act of calmly picking up one bean at a time and putting it back enabled J. to regulate, slow his body down and then succeed at finding the coins in the beans. The act of "doing" had far more of an effect on J.'s regulatory system than attempting to impart insight through dialogue, thereby sending stimulus to the left hemisphere. Staying in the right hemisphere is essential to develop and strengthen the communications of the right hemisphere.

I offered J. many sensory-motor activities, usually one or two each session for 5 to 10 minutes, which he did willingly and enthusiastically. Many of the made-up games had aggressive themes. J. was an aggressive child and needed a way to sublimate his aggression, or at least express it in a socially acceptable way. When he participated in playing Marker Wars, he was not very successful and had tension in his body and arms. The joint scribbling activity to "mess up" the paper allowed him to use wide-range motion to release the tension he was holding in his body and arms through kinesthetic activity. This helped keep J. in a state of physical homeostasis.

> CASE NOTE: J. arrived for the fourth session. I suggested playing a new game I made up called "Whack the Balloon." J. was very enthusiastic. I sat on one side of a long table with a long balloon and J. sat opposite me with a foot-long hard cardboard tube. To play the game I moved the balloon across the table horizontally while J. attempted to whack the balloon with the cardboard tube as the balloon moved. I began by moving the balloon slowly to see if he could hit it, and he could not. I moved the balloon more slowly and he was still unable to hit it. I barely moved the balloon, and he was able to hit it only occasionally. After a few moments of this, I suggested another game called "Drop the Clothespins in the Jar." I offered J. eight clothespins (made from a single piece of wood with a smooth end) and a wide-mouth quart jar. I invited J. to hold the clothespins rounded side down and waist high and try to drop them in the jar. He was not able to get any of the clothespins in the jar, even when he held them below his waist. I invited him to stop, but he said he wanted to keep trying. He was able to get one clothespin on the first round, two on the second, and two on the third. Again, I suggested he stop, but he wanted to keep trying. He continued until he got two or three clothespins in the jar each time. He was thrilled and said, "I like that game."

J. switched to a glue activity for several minutes. I made few comments, only those with reference to safety and offering help if needed. He then requested clay, and as he played, he regressed and talked of "poop." He began banging a large piece of clay on the table harder and harder. J. started to rock and hum rhythmically while he created a large clay object. He stated in a serious tone that he wanted to kill it. He began stabbing it with the scissors, many times, and identified it as something he was going to cook. After a long pause, I reminded J. that the session was going to be over soon and that he could continue next week with the clay object. He carefully wrapped the object in three layers of paper and put it on a shelf under other papers. I did not comment. Before leaving, J. asked if he could hug me. He did. I thanked him for the hug and he left happily, smiling as he walked out the door.

Although there are interpretations that one could infer from the play, I do not make interpretations at this time in therapy. It was clear to me that the use of my left eye on his left eye and my focus on safety during the glue activity allowed J. to engage freely in his ensuing play with the clay. Importantly, I remained non-verbal and unconditionally accepting of his expressions, including "poop" talk, typical of much younger children. I did not ask questions or redirect his behavior in any way. I witnessed the annihilation he was capable of perpetrating without reprimand, questions, or redirection. Just as a mother accepts her infant's "poop" and primitive rage, I was accepting and tolerating of all his language and affective expression. These attachment behaviors propel the organism to respond, as seen in J.'s desire to hug me before leaving. I do not mean to imply that J. was attached to me. What I am saying is that the organism will respond to attachment behaviors with attachment behaviors. This is an excellent example of right-hemisphere-to-right-hemisphere communication, experience, and response. J. was able to leave without running out the door, more evidence of a better ability to handle transitions and control his behavior.

CASE NOTE: J. arrived for his fifth session and immediately retrieved his clay object from under the papers on the shelf. He announced, "It may take another week before I am done with this play." I assured him he could take as long as he needed. As he played with the clay, J. told me that the earlier story he had told me about not having problems at school was not the real story. I thanked him for telling me and asked if he wanted to say more. He did not.

J. told me then about the cuts, injuries, and illnesses he had had in his childhood. I looked carefully at each real and imagined scar and said in a concerned tone, "I see that big scar," or "I see that scar and I am sorry you were hurt." Then J. became demanding and aggressive with me. He pretended to sew my mouth shut and happily pretended to eat candy while I watched. He repeated this many times. Next he pretended he wanted to make me eat so much candy that I would blow up. Rather than respond verbally, I widened my eyes to convey surprise at such a demand. J. laughed. He repeated the play many times. At the end of this play, J. put his clay object on the shelf but did not wrap or hide it.

The last 10 minutes of the session was spent engaged in sensory and motor activity. I asked if he wanted to play a game of his own choosing and he immediately chose the clothespin-in-the-jar game. He was able to get two pins in on the first try and five on the second try. He tried a third time and got only four pins in. "I am still getting really good at this," he said. "Can we do this first thing next time?" I assured him I would have the game ready.

As we prepared to leave the studio, I turned to the sink for a moment and when I turned around, J. was not in sight. I knew he had not left the room, so I pretended to look for him. I said, "Oh no, I can't see J. but I will keep looking until I find him, even if it takes me an hour or a day." As I continued to look, he popped out grinning from behind a large planter and said, "Here I am. Do it again." I said, "Well, our time is almost up," as I turned to the sink to give him an opportunity to hide. When I turned around, J. was gone. I repeated my searching and related comments and J. popped out smiling from his hiding place and said, "Here I am. Do it again." We did this three times before he calmly left with his mother.

After the fifth session of therapy, J.'s mother telephoned me to report that J.'s behavior had improved in school. He was now able to stay through the lunch break, a three-hour increase in his ability to tolerate school. He was less defiant and argumentative with his mother at home, and less aggressive with his older sister. This is not atypical, as the improvements in his sensory and motor functioning were affecting J.'s ability to organize and process incoming sensory information and to tolerate stimulation. The lower structures of J.'s brain were able to function more efficiently, and he had gained considerable physical control over his body. This was an indication that he was capable of moving to greater depth in the therapy.

During the session, J. had been able to admit to problems in school, although he did not elaborate on the topic. He used a much younger tone of voice and demeanor when he made comments about his scars and injuries. He sounded more like an infant asking his mother to look at his "owies." The experience was an emotional communication and J. felt very young and needy in my presence. I spoke to him quietly, as one would an infant, with attention to each injury, and I expressed relief and joy that his hurts had healed. In response, he became aggressive and sadistic in his play, apparently associating nurturance with aggression. J. may have been reacting to this emotional communication with a need to withdraw or dissociate during the play. Or, his behavior may have been triggered by recalling prior injuries. My response to his sadistic play was to respond with visual affective responses because he was progressing in development. I responded to his demanding and sadistic behavior in a nonthreatening way, but slightly differently than in the past. I was careful not to display negative affect that may have conveyed shame or dissatisfaction. Instead, I nonverbally communicated surprise or wonder at this behavior.

J.'s success with the clothespins was evidence that his eye-hand coordination, gross motor control, visual perceptual development, and motor planning were improving. Also, his increased awareness of himself and his skills was reflected in his positive comment about himself.

J.'s hide-and-seek behavior demonstrated a subtle advancement in development. Instead of running out the door with no apparent connection between self and other, he was reaching toward mastery of separation by being sought after. This was a very different expression of need, typical of much younger children. J. demonstrated mastery play when he repeated the behavior several times. His calm demeanor afterward suggested that this mastery play was soothing and comforting at this time in his emotional development.

TREATMENT: THE PROBLEM PHASE OF THERAPY

Although there are no distinct criteria for moving to the problem phase of therapy, it was evident that J. was getting more control over his behavior at home and school. The biggest indicator of moving forward was his admission that he was having problems in school.

> **CASE NOTE:** J. arrived to find the clothespin game ready for him. He was excited. He made numerous attempts until he was able to get nearly all the pins in the jar, every time. After doing this, J. announced, "I am done with that game." I congratulated him and reminded him that he had worked hard to be able to get all the pins in the jar. He then wanted to find coins in the box with pinto beans and was able to find all the coins in the box.
>
> J. then chose to work on a building project with wood, glue, and clay. I retrieved all the items for him and he began to build. As he worked, he mentioned that he was doing better in school and that he was able to stay for lunch. In a left-eye-to-left eye exchange, I said, "I am so proud of you. You are a smart boy and a good boy." After a long pause, J. looked at me and said, "I like you." I thanked him and told him I liked him, too. J. said, "Actually, I love you." I thanked him and said it was a very special thing to say and that I would remember it always. We both were smiling and happy. We engaged in a few moments of mutual gaze. J. worked on the project until the end of the session, when he tested limits by refusing to stop working on his project. Limits were set. He was briefly aggressive in a playful way and continued to test limits by refusing to stop work on his art project. When I firmly stated, "Stop now, please," J. responded and calmly walked to the door, said goodbye, and left with his mother.

Having his requested clothespin game ready for him is another example of being attentive and meeting the child's expression of need. When he was building a structure or other art project, I was quick to respond if he requested something and got it right away, anticipating his need when possible. Anticipating and meeting his needs with the art media and tools replicated missed earlier experiences of having his needs met on a physical level of information processing. Mental representation is used as a therapeutic tool (Proulx, 2002). An attuned mother will anticipate the needs of her young child and respond in a timely manner.

J.'s announcement that he was doing better in school was followed by his declaration of affection. This was another emotional communication between the two of us and led to a period of mutual gaze. Each of us was experiencing these affective moments in response to the other. This was not planned, nor was I thinking consciously. It was within the state of attunement that our interactions were formulating in response to other. We were experiencing shared feeling states that created a here-and-now experience. Dr. Phillip Bromberg has articulated this process beautifully in his book *Awakening the Dreamer:*

> When the analyst finally gives up his attempt to "understand" his patient and allows himself to know his patient through the ongoing intersubjective field they are sharing at that moment, an act of recognition (not understanding) takes place in which words and thoughts come to symbolize experience instead of substitute for it. (2006, p. 11)

J. was testing and retesting limits, indicating a move toward autonomy, yet he was increasingly responsive to my verbal directions. He was also able to listen and follow directions better at home. He still was oppositional and defiant, but J.'s mother had noticed dramatic improvement in his ability to control his angry outbursts.

As the sensory and motor systems strengthen, the information processing is able to reach the higher structures of the brain that are able to inform the lower structures. J.'s mind was now better able to manage his more primitive angry feelings without resorting to angry outbursts of screaming and hitting.

CASE NOTE: In another session, J. participated in playing with cornstarch and water mixed together. He delighted in the sensory aspect of the material. I then offered him a sink full of soapy water to wash his hands and asked him to find the objects in the soapy water. Some were small coins, and some were floating, such as a 1-inch-square piece of sponge. He also found a metal car, a small paintbrush, a small rubber fish, and a small plastic ruler. For the rest of the session, J. was free to select his own art media. J. decided to build with boxes and wood. Once he began, he became very irritable. He used tape and glue to bind things together. He was very controlling. He ordered everything around, including me. He had great difficulty managing the media. He regressed and used baby talk. As he worked, he said in a loud and demanding voice, "Stay there, you box," and "You are going to go here!" Finally he calmed, chatting as he worked. He talked about school and told me, "Kids tease me and then I hit them and then I get in trouble." I responded, "Kids tease you and make you very mad." J. added, "Very mad. But then my teacher gets me in trouble." I said, "Kids tease you and when you get mad and hit them, you get in trouble." After a long pause, J. said, "Next year will be the worst year of my life." I asked him why and he said slowly in a sad tone, "I will have to be in first grade and I will never make it." I reflected his sad affect. "You are sad because you think you will not make it in first grade." J. said sadly, "Yes. I know it will be harder." I replied, "I know you might not believe it now, but I believe you will be ready. You are learning so many new ways to express your feelings and control your body. You and I will keep working together to help you learn more so you will be ready for first grade." After a long pause, in a left-eye-to-left-eye exchange, J. looked at me and asked, "Do you like me?" I said, "Yes, J. I do like you very much. Were you worried about that?" He said, "No, I was just wondering."

J. finished his sculpture and I asked him about it. He said it was called "It's Done." I asked J. if I could comment on his art. He agreed and I said, "I wonder if this sculpture is like you in any way?" J. said, "I don't know." I asked him if I could comment on a way the sculpture reminded me of him. He agreed and I said, "I noticed when you came in here you were mad and your anger was kind of like those boxes that were all over the place. Then your anger got put under control as you ordered those boxes where to go and put them under control with all that tape. Then, together we talked about your fear of first grade and having a plan to help you." J. said with amazement, "That is so cool." I said, "Yes, it is pretty cool what we can learn about ourselves from our art."

As we neared the end of the session, I said to J. in a left-eye-to-left-eye exchange, "I want to thank you for asking me if I like you. I am glad to be able to tell you that I do like you very much and that I think you are a very smart and creative boy." J. said, "I hope I can make it in first grade. I hope people like me." J. left calmly with his mother. We both said goodbye when he left.

J. had been irritable when he arrived. Had I asked him what was "wrong" or "Why are you behaving this way?" it is unlikely that J. could have responded verbally. As the kinesthetic aspect of the art activated the right hemisphere, his angry affect shifted to controlling and regressed speech, a dissociative strategy that he used in his attempt to ward off his emotions of fear and sadness. J. was able to use the art media to metaphorically bind up the feelings so that he did not have to dissociate and could verbally state his fear about first grade. When he asked me if I liked him, it was his way of addressing his fear of not being liked in first grade. Once he expressed his fear openly, the higher structures activated, as demonstrated in his comment that he hoped he could achieve the ability to function in the classroom and be liked by others.

> CASE NOTE: J. arrived for the session and was disorganized, regressed in speech and behavior, and ran around the room. He ran out the front door and spotted a small lizard. He chased the lizard until he picked it up. As he stood holding the lizard, he said, "I am going to rip the head off this lizard." I calmly said, "The lizard may have a family and he belongs with lizards, so I would like him to be with his family." J. said, "I am going to rip his head off right now." I replied, "That lizard will die and his family will be worried about him and wonder where he is tonight. Please put the lizard down so he can go to his family." J. said, "Why should I?" I replied, "How do you think the other lizards will feel when he doesn't come home?" J replied, "I don't care." I said, "Well, I do. He lives here and I am asking you to please put the lizard down." After several moments of contemplation, J. complied and put the lizard carefully on the ground. As we went to the studio together, I asked J. how it felt to put the lizard back without hurting it. He replied, "I don't care. I only did it because you said it was your lizard." I said, "I would like to thank you very much for doing that for me." J. said, "I could have ripped his head off, you know." I replied, "I know you could have, and you didn't. I am proud of you for not hurting the lizard."

With minimal help, J. was able to focus on his art most of the session. He used baby talk at times. He had difficulty ending the session, stalling and refusing to stop the art making, running and hiding for me to find him. He attempted to steal a chalk pastel. I saw him pull it out of his pocket to sneak a peek at it. We were in the waiting area near the door and I quietly asked him to go put it back. He went back to the studio. I did not follow him and had no way of knowing if he returned the item or not. My trusting him was more important than the whereabouts of the pastel. He left with his mother.

J.'s behavior with the lizard was evidence of his aggressive and violent nature. I had no prior experience or planned protocol for handling the situation. My initial cognitive reaction was to set firm limits and demand he not hurt the lizard. I stopped myself from thinking. I shifted my attention to my body. I was feeling an unconscious emotional response of fear and loss. I expressed these feelings to J. by talking about the lizard. Apparently this was what J.'s actions were evoking, because in response he was able to stop his aggressive behavior, and although he did not care about the lizard, he showed some movement toward higher brain structure activation, as he did not hurt the lizard because he perceived that it belonged to me. Some evidence of caring for another was beginning to emerge.

For the next several sessions, J. was oppositional, demanding, mean, and angry. Any attempt to have him identify his feelings was met with an "I don't care." He was often aggressive with the art media and tools, and he constantly tested limits and safety. He dumped art media on the floor, threw art media, and tried to break art media and tools. I would calmly walk behind him, picking up the spilled items saying, "No, no," repeatedly, much like one would with an infant. He often used baby talk. I continued to just accept and tolerate all his behaviors unless it pertained to safety. When he attempted to climb onto the table, I helped him off and said, "It is not safe to walk on the table and my job is to keep us safe." His reply was, "I don't care." I replied, "That's okay if you don't care, but I do care and I will always keep you safe here." His reply was, "I don't care." As we neared the end of the session, he ran and hid for me to find him. I did, and he then ran from the studio to the car. Despite being ignored, I still waved.

In all aspects of development and change, progress is gradual and not always straightforward. Regression is to be expected. Behaviorally and emotionally, J. was in a much younger self-state. He was processing language at a younger developmental level. J. did not notice I was using much younger language with him when I said, "No-no."

> **CASE NOTE:** During another session, J. chose to begin by playing "Marker Wars" and "Whack the Balloon" with me. Then he shifted and announced that he would be making a gift for his mother and that he had a friend at school. When I asked J. to tell me more about his friend, he said his new friend played with him at school every day and that they liked the same things like building and playing outside. I congratulated J. on having a new friend. He said, "I am looking forward to first grade because I have a friend."
>
> As J. worked on the gift for his mother, he wanted to leave the studio to show it to her—a first. I welcomed this new behavior. J. showed his mother what he was making for her. Later in the session, he wanted to show her his progress, which I encouraged. J. was not finished with the gift as we neared the end of the session. He was very angry that there was no more time. As he was leaving, he again tested limits with his mother and me. J.'s mother reminded him there would be consequences if he did not stop. He complied with her verbal directions, a new behavior for J. As he was leaving, his mother reminded him there would be a two-week break from art. They were traveling to visit family for a summer vacation. I said to J. "I will be right here when you get back and I will be very excited to see you and hear about your vacation." He left happily with his mother after offering me a self-initiated goodbye hug.

J. was demonstrating new behaviors with regard to relationship. He left the session to show his mother the art he was making and later was upset when he could not complete her gift. He also responded to her verbal limits at the end of the session, evidence of his ability to regulate his affect and manage his behavior when angry. After the reminder that he would not be at art therapy for two weeks,

J. offered me a self-initiated hug, something unexpected and unique to our relationship.

> CASE NOTE: At the beginning of another session, I asked J. if he would be willing to participate in an experiment. I said, "I am learning about kids who hate to draw, and I will ask you to make two shapes on two papers and that is all." J. said, smiling, "I can help you with your experiment because I hate to draw." I gave J. a white sheet of paper with a black piece of chalk. I held up an image of a large circle and said, "Will you please make one of these." J.'s line went off the page as he tried three times to draw the circle (see Figure 8.6). He said, "I just can't do it." I assured J. that was fine and reminded him this was not a test; it was an experiment. I then gave J. a black piece of paper and a white piece of chalk. I held up my drawn circle again and said, "Will you please draw one of these." J. drew the circle line and it went off the page. He said, "Wait," and started over. This time he was able to make the complete circle (see Figure 8.7) and exclaimed excitedly, "It is so much easier."
>
> When we finished, J. said he wanted to make a wood and glue structure. He became frustrated. I asked, "How do you think you can solve that artistic problem?" J. thought of a possible solution and it worked. I praised him for his thinking, planning, and ability to solve the problem. He accidentally knocked over a box of wooden sticks, and when I asked him to help pick them up, he did. Several times when he was frustrated, I would remind him of his ability to problem-solve, and he would backtrack to where the problem began and start over. J. had to leave the unfinished project until the following week, but he ran to show his mother his progress before leaving the art. J. left the studio and we both said goodbye.

This drawing activity of changing the figure and ground, or drawing with white on black, is an excellent way to determine whether drawing with white chalk on a black background instead of black on white makes a difference in the child's ability to perceive and draw a shape. This indicated that J.'s difficulty with motor praxis, or motor planning, had a visual component, as demonstrated by his ability to do better when the figure and ground were reversed.

J.'s willingness to help pick up the spilled sticks without protest was a new behavior. Just as a mother raises her expectations of a child's behavior as the child indicates he is capable, I was no longer running around picking up things for J. We now engaged in a very different relationship than those days of early developmental behavior and affect regulation. His ability to problem-solve at my suggestion indicated he was able to utilize help offered in a new way. J. was once again showing his mother what he had made, a wonderful transformation of his attention and approval seeking. He was also able to delay gratification by happily leaving his unfinished art project at the studio until the following session.

J.'s new behaviors indicated he was ready to move to the next phase of therapy. There would be movement forward and back, but he was able to maintain the improvements in behavior, to access and tolerate affect, and to have meaningful relationships.

TRANSFORMATION PHASE OF THERAPY

CASE NOTE: J arrived for the session, and during a self-initiated left-eye-to-left-eye exchange, admitted he had stolen a piece of chalk when he first began therapy. I praised him for his honesty and asked how he felt about stealing the chalk. J. reported that he felt bad and that he was glad he told me. I encouraged J. to think of other ways he could have gotten the chalk without stealing, and he was able to come up with two alternatives. I praised him for thinking of good alternatives and for telling me what he had done. We also talked about the link between stealing and his feeling bad, and he said, "I am never going to steal anymore because I don't like how I feel doing it." I offered, "I'm glad you learned something important about yourself, and I am glad you told me about it."

J. participated in playing "Whack the Balloon" and "Marker Wars" before he began working on a wood building project. As he built and rebuilt his project, J. identified himself as a person who wants perfection. This led to a discussion about a quality in him that made his art and building projects more difficult. I mentioned that those who don't care about the outcome can build things fast with little or no frustration. J. was very attentive to this discussion. He stated that he liked that quality in himself and that he was learning to be less frustrated. He then told me that he had several friends at school now. At the end of the session, J. became anxious about wanting to hurry and do many things before leaving. I encouraged J. to stop and identify what emotion he was feeling. He said, "In a hurry and frustrated." I asked, "How can we problem-solve to address your hurry and frustration?" J. said, "I could just sit here and think about what I am going to do next time instead of trying to do it now." I said, "Great thinking!" I also told J. that since he did not have to hurry to build, he could put all the supplies he needed in a box for his work the following session. J. said, "Yes, I am a perfectionist, so it will take me longer than one time to do this." He left with his mother in a calm state and we said goodbye at the door.

In this case note, we begin to see evidence of the development of a moral imperative. J. was expressing guilt and regret and was taking responsibility for his behavior for having stolen chalk from the studio. This was evidence of accessing the higher prefrontal cortex, which holds the ability to know right from wrong and to develop a moral imperative. He had been able to problem-solve and delay gratification during the past two sessions. And, J. was clearly developing a more refined concept of self when he identified himself as a perfectionist with his art. The creation of the self occurred when J. saw himself reflected in the expression of the right hemisphere and in the "doing." To identify himself as a perfectionist outside of the context of his art would likely have had little or no meaning for him.

CASE NOTE: J. arrived for the session and was agitated, nonverbal. He did not say hello. He went directly to the studio and announced his plans for his art. He began and demanded I assist him or do things for him. When I encouraged J. to ask for help in a different way, he did so but with great irritation. He was rude and dismissive and demanded the missing specific art media he had requested prior to this session. Before I could speak, J. said, "You are a liar." I asked J. to tell me more about what he was referring to. J. said, "You are a liar. You said you would have the black clay here and you don't have it here. That makes you a liar." I felt the urge to defend myself but paused, trying to formulate a response. I felt irritation and wanted to let J. know I was not a liar. I wanted to tell him he was so very wrong. I had tried to find clay! I also felt sadness as I realized J. thought I was a liar. As if he could hear my thoughts, J. said, "I know you think you are not a liar but you are."

I was frustrated at not having a response to end this continued misperception. I was on the verge of commenting on his rude and ill-informed response to the missing media. I slowed my thoughts down and realized that this rupture in the relationship had the potential to be important relationally. I said to J. "I wonder what you and I are feeling now." J. said, "What do you mean?" I said, "I wonder what you are feeling about me. You say you think I am a liar. I am wondering if you want to know my feelings about being called a liar." J. said, "I feel mad because I don't have the clay." I said, "I feel sad because you are disappointed and mad. I feel sad, mad, and frustrated because you think I lied to you." J. looked at me puzzled and after a long pause said, "Well maybe you are not a liar if you have a reason." I explained to J. that the store did not have the clay he wanted. After another long pause, J. said, "I didn't know that. I might not have said you were a liar if I knew that." I said, "You might not have said I was a liar if you knew I tried to get the clay?" J. said, "Yes." I replied, "I am really glad we talked about this misunderstanding." J. considered this for a few minutes. After a long pause J. said, "That is like my best friend and me. We don't fight or argue about stuff. We talk about it and then we are still friends." I agreed it sounded just like us. J. added, "Now I just talk about stuff and I don't hit." I said, "Thank you for telling me that you thought I was lying. I will try to remember to tell you about missing art media at the beginning of the session." J. responded, "I won't call you a liar next time."

Near the end of the session, I again thanked J. for talking about our feelings and our misunderstanding. J. left happily with his mother. We both said goodbye. I had consistently waved goodbye to J. after all sessions. He returned the wave goodbye as he left.

This exchange occurred because of a rupture in our relationship. J. thought I was lying and was angry at a perceived betrayal. He was dissociating away from potential feelings of deprivation, loss, disappointment, and possibly abandonment because I had not met his perceived level of need for the art media. I was dissociating away from my feelings of anger, frustration, sadness, and resentment by formulating a cognitive response to defend myself. As noted by Bromberg, "An enactment is a didactic event in which therapist and patient are linked through a dissociated mode of relating, each in a "not-me" state of his own that is affectively responsive to that of the other" (2011, p. 151).

Rather than dissociate away from the relationship with my defensive and punitive thoughts, I was able to bring myself back to the relationship and recognize the potential for affective communication. I departed from my defensive state and invited J. to engage in a dialogue about our mutual feeling states. Had I asked J. what he was feeling, he would have remained in his self-state of betrayed victim. By pondering both of our feeling states in a curious tone, J. was also able to be curious as reflected in his question, "What do you mean?" At that point he was able to listen and dialogue not about who was right or wrong, but about our relationship.

> CASE NOTE: J. arrived and participated in finding different textured objects in a bag. He dropped clothespins in the jar and got in seven of the eight on the first try. Then he decided on a building project using cardboard. He was often frustrated. I prompted him to problem-solve and he was able to do so easily. When I helped him hold something he was working on and I made a mistake, he said, "Try again." I did so, reminding him that when he first began therapy and I made a mistake, he would threaten to hurt or kill me. He replied, "I did?" I said. "Yes, you did. Now it feels so much better when you remind me to just try again." I praised his maturity and his friendliness. J. left happily with his mother. We both said goodbye.

This was a dramatic change. J. had not become agitated or angry when I made a mistake. He was clearly able to regulate his affect in astonishing ways compared to his early days in therapy when he would threaten violence if I did or said something he did not like. As we neared the end of the transformation phase of therapy, I watched for opportunities to mention his earlier ways of behaving and coping, and how they had changed. J. had shown a degree of surprise at his earlier mean and threatening behaviors.

> CASE NOTE: In another session, J. participated in a game of Whack the Balloon. This time he hit the balloon every time and announced, "I am done with that game." I agreed that he had mastered the task. He then

found coins in the bean box and was very adept at finding them quickly. J. began an art project of his choosing but was soon frustrated. He became angry and oppositional. He was encouraged to use his problem-solving skills and prompted to use words to communicate what he needed, if anything. He did so, but was often angry and rejected the suggestions offered. I encouraged J. to talk about what he was feeling, but he did not respond. J. was aggressive with the art media, knocking things over and spilling boxes of materials. I gently said, "J., if you need help picking those up, just let me know." He looked at me surprised and began to pick up the materials. He quietly said, "Would you pick up some of this stuff?" I said, "Okay" and began helping him. When we were finished I said, "What do you say now?" J. said questioningly, "Thank you?" I replied with a warm smile, "You are welcome."

I then suggested J. try splatter painting. I took large 8-foot long pieces of butcher paper outside and gave J. small buckets of primary color paint and large brushes. My instructions were to dip the brush and think of something that bugged him and splatter the paint. He delighted in this activity.

Back inside he started a building project using balsa wood. At the end of the session, he did not want to stop working and was oppositional, defiant, and angry. I validated his feelings, but my limits were enforced and he complied. He knocked over a box of sticks on the way out the door. I tried using the words "No-no" to see if he would notice. After saying it once, J. looked at me with his hands held palms up in front of him and asked, "What is this no-no stuff?" I said, "Oh, knocking those sticks off before leaving reminded me of a younger kid and I guess I spoke to you like a little kid. Sorry." J. laughed and said, "I can't believe you said no-no to me, a big kid." He left calmly. We both said goodbye.

As J. moved on in development, I adjusted my expectations. I expected him to pick up items spilled from containers. I offered help to let him know it was not a power differential issue or punishment. It was simply expected. I expected a please and thank you, another subtle shift in our relationship. I did not want to evoke feelings of shame.

The words "no-no" elicited a strong response. J. noticed that this was language typically spoken to a younger child. He had not noticed that I had used this language frequently in the beginning of therapy when he was in a different stage of emotional development.

During the week, J.'s mother telephoned to say he was increasingly oppositional lately and she asked for tips for handling his behavior. I recommended she look at him when speaking, ask him to repeat instructions, and offer some reward that involved her involvement and attention, such as playing a game or going for a walk together. J.'s mother also reported she had made a particular movement or posture when reaching over J. that caused him to react with extreme fear, anger, and sadness as he cowered from her. She reported he responded well to her reassurance after the incident but was puzzled because she was certain she had never hurt or intimidated her child. His mother also mentioned that J. was staying at school for the entire day with few behavior problems. He was playing well with others and had several friends.

> CASE NOTE: J. arrived for a session and participated in two brief sensory-building activities. He was very successful at both. Then he decided to work with difficult media that involved fine motor skills. After several failed attempts, I reminded him he could take a break and rest. He stated he preferred to keep working so he could learn. He asked for help occasionally instead of demanding help. We took brief turns working on the project.
>
> As we worked together, I mentioned to J. that his mother had told me about him getting really upset earlier in the week. He admitted he had a difficult time and did not know why. We had the following conversation in a left-eye-to-left-eye exchange. I offered, "Maybe that reminded you of when someone else had made you mad, or afraid, or hurt you and your body is remembering. Your body may remember some things you cannot remember. The memories in your body can make you feel the same feelings again. It is normal and it happens sometimes." J. said, "I know what you mean but I don't want to talk about it right now." I reassured J. that he did not have to talk. I told him that I wanted him to have the information about why that might happen so I could help him with his emotions. J. did not comment but moved in closer and rested his elbow on my arm. He remained very calm and focused, and handled frustration and delayed gratification very well at the end of the session. J. said that he was able to stay at school longer and asked if he could switch to a later time. We both said goodbye.

When bringing up a potentially sensitive topic, I wait until the child is engaged in the art making and is focused and calm. A child in a state of physical homeostasis affords a greater potential for affective communication. In this instance, I opened the subject raised by his mother's comment by talking about how one's body remembers things we may have forgotten. Offering a possible explanation by beginning with a focus on his body and expanding to his affective responses, I linked those body sensations to affect. Once the fear or other emotion is described as "normal" by the therapist, the patient's neural system moves the information processing to cognition. This was reflected when J. was able to cognitively recognize a relationship between his recent terrified reaction to his mother's movement and an earlier terrifying experience. If I had asked J. what might have caused his reaction to his mother, it is unlikely he would have been able to verbalize a response. His defense function would have activated in response to the recalled body-based fear. He would most likely have refused to talk about the subject or dissociated.

CASE NOTE: J. was eager for art. I suggested making and flying a kite. J. was very enthusiastic. As we worked, he talked about a girl at school who was hurt on the playground. I asked if he was worried about her and he looked at me and said, "Who cares?" He repeatedly stated that he did not care; nobody cares. I presented some imaginary scenarios, such as, "Would you care if your sister was hurt, or would you care if a friend was hurt?" J. replied to both, "Who cares?" I said in a matter-of-fact tone without shame or condemnation, "Well, I guess you don't care about anybody who gets hurt." J. said again, "No, I don't care." Near the end of the session, after a long pause, J. said, "I might care about some people." I praised J. for thinking about his feelings and for sharing that with me.

J. completed the construction of his kite. Twenty minutes of the session remained to fly the kite. J. was clumsy and tripped often while running. He had difficulty coordinating his arms and legs and managing the kite. He rebuffed offers of help and suggestions. He was frustrated when the time was up and protested that he needed more time. I assured him that he could fly the kite next week if it was not raining. J. did not have difficulty leaving the kite flying for the next session. We both said goodbye as he left happily with his mother.

The thought behind the kite making was to have J. engage in gross motor movement in addition to running to see if he was able to coordinate his arms and legs while flying the kite. I concluded after observing his difficulty running that J. would benefit from gross motor strengthening and motor planning activities.

During the session when J. mentioned that a girl had been hurt on the school playground and offered his usual lack of any regard for the suffering of others, I posed my questions in such a way that I could see if there were any qualifiers for his lack of regard, such as family members or friends. I used a matter-of-fact tone to avoid suggesting shame and to allow him just to see himself reflected in the comment. Allowing time for him to think about that without adding commentary lowered his defenses and enabled his affect to surface and to say that he might care about some people. I offered praise and support for his thinking and for sharing his feelings, but I did not ask him who he cared about. Again, this moves the information processing away from our affective communication to cognition. The content is not as important as the affective experience. Bromberg notes, "If one sees the mind as a nonlinear, self-organizing system, facilitation of mutative change is inherent to the process, not to the content" (2006, p. 138).

CASE NOTE: J. arrived at the next session eager to fly the kite. His running was clumsy and his arm movements uncoordinated. He was not able to get the kite airborne and refused to listen to suggestions for doing so. After many attempts, he became frustrated and blamed the kite. I checked out the kite and declared it was not the kite. I said, "There is an easier way. If you decide to try something different, let me know and I will share that with you." After a long pause, J. quietly said, "Please tell me how to get the kite to fly." I said, "Sure." I helped J. learn to fly the kite. He was successful. He flew the kite with excitement and pride. As he did so, he looked at me and said, "Thank you for helping me." I responded, "You are welcome." J. tested limits at the end of the session by refusing to stop. I reminded him of the rule several times and he finally complied. He left with his kite, eager to show his friend the kite he had made and his new kite-flying skills. We both said goodbye.

J. was still exhibiting a defensive stance with regard to help flying the kite. He wanted to be in control of the situation. To allow him to continue to be in control, I merely commented that I was able to help him if he wanted. Having the experience of asking for help without shame or humiliation allowed him to enjoy the experience and express his appreciation.

> CASE NOTE: J. arrived for the next session and I invited him to make paper airplanes. He was delighted to learn how to fold planes. He picked one design he liked and made several until he had all the steps memorized. As he was trying to staple the rubber band and could not, he said, "I really need your help, please, to hold this." As I held the rubber band to the nose of the plane, J. stapled it and said, "Thank you." I said, "You are welcome." We took the planes outside and flew them back and forth across the yard, both of us picking them up and sending them back. J. was running, and although clumsy and uncoordinated, he kept running and stopping during the entire session, resting only occasionally. He left happily with his mother. We both said goodbye.

J. was now engaging in usual social commentary by using please and thank you without prompting. The plane flying provided the opportunity to run, stop quickly, bend, reach, and throw. All are excellent for gross motor and motor planning skill development.

TREATMENT: INTEGRATION PHASE OF THERAPY

> CASE NOTE: J. arrived and immediately wanted to make more airplanes and fly them. We did so. J.'s airplane went into a tree. He asked how to get it down. I told him I did not know. J. took one second to select a pinecone and weakly tossed it in the air in the direction of the plane. He threw a rock at the plane. It was safe to do this because he was throwing the pinecones and rocks in the direction of an empty acre of land with no buildings. I said, "What a great idea. Only one of us can throw a rock or pinecone at a time because we have to make sure we are safe and do not get hit." J. said, "Okay, no problem." He kept tossing pinecones and rocks with increasing strength and surer aim. Once he nearly hit the airplane and was very

excited. I encouraged him to rest before trying again, but he continued to try to knock down the plane. At the end of the session, he said, "I hope that plane stays in the tree until I come back next week." J. did not test limits at the end of the session. He left happily with his mother, after both of us said goodbye.

Trying to hit a paper plane in a large pine tree is difficult and requires eye-hand coordination and upper arm strength. His accuracy improved. He was able to get the rocks and pinecones higher and closer to the plane with each throw.

CASE NOTE: J. arrived for the next session and went outside to find the plane in the tree. He began to throw sticks, pinecones, and rocks at the plane and said, "I was throwing rocks into the creek to practice so I can get the plane." His arm seemed stronger and his aim better as he tried numerous times to hit the plane. He asked if I could try to hit the plane. I did so but could not hit the plane. J. kept at it. I was totally surprised when he finally hit the plane and it fell from the tree. J. was beside himself with joy. He said, "I knew I could get it if I didn't quit." I said, "You knew you could do it if you didn't quit and I noticed you didn't quit and you succeeded. Way to go, J.!" He ran to tell his mother what he had done. When he returned, he looked at me with his left eye to my left eye and said seriously, "Can we actually shoot more planes in the trees and get them out with rocks and pinecones? " With my left eye on his left eye, I said, "Sure, as long as you continue to be safe." He invited me to shoot planes in the tree, too, and we both tried to hit them for the rest of the session, taking turns throwing. He complied with the turn taking and was able to get another plane out of the tree. He ran to tell his mother the news. He did not test limits at the end of the session. We both said goodbye.

J. wanted very much to acquire this skill and worked diligently to achieve his goal. He was successful. Running to show his mother was an excellent response. J.'s primary relationship with his mother had improved. His mother was able to give him time and attention when he shared his projects with her. He was able to rely on her positive regard for him and his art.

CASE NOTE: J. was excited because his birthday was near and he was planning to have a birthday party with several friends. He made and flew airplanes most of the session. He mentioned that he and his friends were making and flying airplanes at school, but they could not throw rocks if a plane got stuck in the tree. When I asked if he knew the difference between throwing rocks at therapy and throwing rocks at school, J. said, "It is not safe at school because there are so many kids around." I praised J. for his knowledge and for knowing the importance of keeping people safe. J. looked at me and said, "I am safe." I looked at him with my left eye to his left eye and said, "I know you are. You have shown me that you can be trusted, and that is why I let you fly planes and hit them with rocks. And you obey the rule of taking turns throwing to be safe." J asked, "You trust me?" I said, "Yes, J. You have shown you can be trusted. You told me about taking the chalk and deciding not to steal, and you obey the no-rock-throwing rule at school." J. said, "I can be trusted." I replied, "Yes, that is another one of your qualities, just like you identify yourself as a perfection-ist, you are also honest and can be trusted." J. did not test limits at the end of the session. When he left, he walked slowly, and as I stood at the door waving, he waved back and just before he turned away he said, "Love you." Spontaneously I said, "Love you." We both smiled.

Another affective exchange occurred when J. asked about trust. Responding to his question, I presented a larger context for his developing self. In over 30 years of clinical work, I had never said, "Love you" to a client. This was a completely spon-taneous and unplanned comment. And, surprisingly, I did not regret saying it. I was surprised that I did not overanalyze my judgment or motivation. What I do know is that it was not a cognitive response. The exchange was simply in a moment of time. We did not discuss it. Neither of us responded similarly again.

> CASE NOTE: J. arrived and wanted to fly airplanes. He made several, and we flew them around the yard and into the trees, and even attempted to fly several over the roof of the studio. We were having fun. At one point, I was attempting to fly a plane and the rubber band snapped my thumb. It hurt. J. said, "Fly it. Fly your plane." I said, "I just tried it and I snapped my thumb with the rubber band and it hurts. Now I am afraid to do it again because I might hurt myself again." J. was standing across the yard. He put his plane down, ran over to me, and said, with his left eye to my left eye, "Linda, don't be scared. I think you can do it and if you can't, I am right here to help you if you get hurt. If you get hurt again, you don't have to try again." I thanked J. and said, "That was really very helpful for you to say that, J. I am not afraid now, and I think I can try it again." J. said, "You can. You can do it, just be careful." I tried it and did not snap my finger and J. said with excitement, "You did it! You did it!" I reminded J. of how I had felt hurt and afraid and asked him how it felt to help someone who was afraid. He said, "Good. It feels good."

J.'s affective and heartfelt offer of support and help revealed his emerging empathy and compassion. His excitement at my success was also evidence of a greater awareness of others. His experience of feeling good while helping another was evidence of a shift away from his earlier insistence that he "did not care" about the distress of others.

J. was taking a break for the summer. I offered to J.'s mother that we could terminate therapy for the time being, as J. was not having any regulation or behavior problems at home, at school, or in therapy. He was well liked by adults and children and had good social skills. I reassured J's mother that she was welcome to return at any time if he had a setback or if other issues emerged that required further treatment.

It would be remiss not to mention that J's. mother's treatment was successful and she had been applying the skills she learned in parenting classes. J. and his mother were both enjoying spending time together. J.'s older sister was doing well and had discontinued treatment. She had enrolled in dance classes and found a community of friends focused on health and fitness for dance. She was focused on her own health and academic success.

> CASE NOTE: J. arrived for therapy and I told him that we would have only a few sessions left before his summer vacation. I also told him that I thought, maybe, he did not have to come to therapy anymore. J. said, "Yeah, I am pretty busy and I do like to play outside." I said, "Well, why don't we just leave it that if you wish to come back any time, you will let your mom know and we can talk about it." J. said, "Okay."

We spent the next two sessions reviewing the sensory and motor games he had played. He did not have a portfolio of art. Most of J.'s projects were made of three-dimensional media and he took the projects home when they were completed. We reviewed his early behaviors and the ways he had changed. We recalled the games we had played with the art media and hide-and-seek and flying airplanes. He did not test limits at the end of the sessions. Just before he left, I gave him a small gift with a card reminding him of how much I liked him and how thankful I was to be his therapist and make art with him. J. left happily with his mother. We both said goodbye and both waved as he left.

Following summer vacation, J.'s mother called to report that J. was doing very well in school, was sweet in temperament, was kind to others and animals, and had no behavior problems at school. He was doing very well academically, reading books one after another. J. had excellent manners and good social skills with adults and peers. A woman who had not seen J. in several years remarked, "I didn't think he was the same boy. He was so calm, polite, and kind."

Although not every positive change or alteration in J.'s behavior can be attributed to his therapy, it is evident that his sensory and motor delays were causing him difficulty. By engaging in sensory and motor building activities with art and play media, and replicating early missed attachment behaviors, J. made progress. By using a combination of directive and nondirective art and play experiences, J. was able to engage in the developmental building experiences of earlier critical periods. By creating a sense of physical awareness and homeostasis, J.'s information processing shifted to affective communication. Once his emotional needs were met and supported, the cognitive structures activated in both symbolic and concrete ways. And, as demonstrated, it is possible to activate the prefrontal structures. J. displayed a sense of a moral imperative and empathy for others.

CHAPTER 9

Treating Adolescents: Discovering the Self

In his seminal book *On Adolescence*, Peter Blos (1962) describes the search for identity as the major task of adolescence. This does not imply that the self *only* develops in adolescence. The early development of the mind/body concept of self begins within the attachment relationship of the infant and primary caregiver, as documented in earlier chapters. Blos is referring to the maturation of the ego. The emerging self in adolescence is complex. In 1954 Jacobson wrote:

> By a realistic concept of the self we mean one that mirrors correctly this state and the characteristics, the potentialities and abilities, the assets and the limits of our bodily and mental ego: on the one hand, of our appearance, our anatomy and our physiology; on the other hand, of our conscious and preconscious feelings and thoughts, wishes, impulses and attitudes, of our physical and mental activities (quoted in Blos, 1962, p. 191)

The task of developing a separate self in adolescence is difficult for teens. Adolescence is a major time of change physically, emotionally, and cognitively. It is a time of great emotional instability, occurring when the brain is going through reorganization, a repruning of synapses, that results in psychological changes (Spear, 2003). The right-brain neurochemical system underlying regulation and stress coping is reorganized (Schore, 2003a). There is a period of stabilization followed by a secondary growth spurt of the prefrontal cortex at about age 15. Referring to Paul MacLean's triune brain system, Pearce writes:

> At the same time that the prefrontals have their secondary growth spurt, the ancient cerebellum undergoes corresponding growth. The cerebellum is made of extensions of all three brains in our triune system and is involved in just about everything we do, primarily speech and movement. It is made of trillions of granular cells that are quite different from ordinary neural cells. It is noteworthy that the granular cells of the same order are also a significant part of the prefrontal makeup, and that very

strong neural links exist between the prefrontal cortex and the cerebellum. (2002, p. 42)

The prefrontal cortex is connected to all areas of the brain and is able to monitor the brain's neural structures. This part of the brain is involved in advanced cognition, with the ability to make judgments, to control impulses, to consider consequences, and to have empathy and compassion for others. There is more prefrontal change during adolescence than in any other time of life. The overproduction of gray matter is pruned off rapidly, along with the development of white matter, or myelination. White matter insulates the brain's circuitry, creating a more precisely tuned and efficient brain. Before this time, teens have difficulty with reasoning and cognitive functioning (Sowell et al., 2001).

Also at this time in life, adolescents experience the developmental need to separate from parents, what Blos (1962) describes as relinquishing the old object and finding the new as the youth experiments with authority, values, and limits. This time of separation is also a time of loss, as the teen moves toward autonomy and being away from home.

Teens who have had the opportunity to develop an attachment with a primary caregiver in infancy are better able to make the shift toward independence. Without the attachment experiences involved in the maturation of the right brain, it is unlikely that the teen will have formed an early concept of mind/body/self. This usually results in a cascade of increasingly serious emotional and behavioral problems that are symptomatically manifested in the most common diagnoses for adolescents (Schore, 1994). These symptoms include antisocial personality disorder (Bradley, Jenei, & Westen, 2005; Fonagy & Target, 1997; Shi et al., 2012), borderline personality disorder (Schore, 2012), conduct disorder (DeKlyen & Speltz, 2004; Fonagy & Target, 1997), PTSD (Schore, 2001), depression (Cicchetti & Toth, 1998), and suicidality (Adam, Sheldon-Keller, & West, 1996). Traumatic or insecure attachments produce ongoing states of hyperarousal and dissociation that affect the maturation of the right brain, the locus of control over emotions and behavior.

Treating teens is challenging. They are often highly resistant, oppositional, defiant, and withdrawn or narcissistic and arrogant. Unfortunately for parents and therapists, these behaviors are developmentally appropriate. Verbal therapy with teens is very difficult due to their resistance and their use of denial and splitting as primary defenses. Many teens are highly distrustful of adults, often with good reason. One teen with a history of child abuse told me, "I learned not to trust anybody because everyone I trusted hurt me." Teens require a tremendous amount of patience and time. Treatment proceeds very slowly. It takes many months, sometimes longer, for teens to form a therapeutic alliance strong enough to engage in the deeper aspects of therapy. Because of their high level of distrust and resistance, they are constantly checking limits, testing boundaries, and challenging safety by risk taking.

Riley (1999) asserts that the adolescent must be in control of the therapy in order to participate in therapy. I find this to be absolutely true. The narcissistic stance of adolescence (Blos, 1962) is an advantage to a therapist, as teens enjoy having the focus of attention directed at them. I make every effort to avoid asking questions about content, to make interpretations, or to challenge the adolescent on the meaning they apply to their art. Instead, I comment on what I see in the art: line, form, color, shapes, texture, use of space, and other visible aspects. I may comment on movement in the image. Teens are more comfortable exploring the image with the therapist in a symbolic or metaphorical way.

THE ISSUE OF CONTROL

Allowing the teen to be in control of the therapy does not mean there are no rules or limits on behavior. Safety is a primary consideration, and I set immediate limits on any unsafe behavior with a two-word command said in a firm but calm tone, "Stop now." I do not restate or change my language but continue with those two words until the behavior stops. Once the unsafe or dangerous behavior has ceased, I allow the teen to recover a state of physical and emotional homeostasis and then talk about the issue, not necessarily in the same session. I find many teens vie for control immediately. The following three case vignettes illustrate how I address the issue of control.

> CASE NOTE: A teen came to therapy listening to an iPod. His father told him to remove the iPod before going into the studio. The teen ignored his father and went into the studio wearing the headphones. Once in the studio and sitting next to the teen, I said, "Will you please remove your ear buds so I can tell you about the art?" He pulled out one ear bud and listened as I described an art directive. I added, "I prefer you not listen to music, but if you feel safer or more comfortable with it, you can wear it until you are ready to turn it off." The teen returned to listening to music. After several minutes, out came one ear bud, then a few minutes later, another. After a few more minutes, he turned off the device.

It is necessary for teens to have the experience of being in control, not to talk about control. I offer many simple opportunities for control, such as asking if they prefer large, medium, or small paper, broad or thin markers, masking tape or clear tape, a glue gun or glue stick. These choices give teens more opportunity to exercise control, and by changing their physical sense of control, they are able to have control in the middle and higher structures of the brain that control emotions and behavior. The more fragmented and disorganized the client, the more opportunities I offer for him to be in physical control to achieve physical homeostasis. I may ask if one chair or another is more comfortable, if he prefers an increase or decrease in temperature or lighting, or if he has a preferred seating arrangement. The symbolic and unconscious replication of early missed experiences of having physical needs met is an effective tool to facilitate the maturation of the underdeveloped right hemisphere of the brain.

CASE NOTE: A 14-year-old with a history of violent behavior wanted to use a small power tool. Safety glasses are required, yet he insisted he did not need them. I told the teen he must wear the safety glasses while operating the tool. He continued to argue. After a while, I said, "Well, here we are at an impasse, as I am telling you one thing and you are telling me another." The teen became very angry and said, "I don't ever wear safety glasses. I have never hurt myself, and I know I won't get anything in my eye." I said, "That would help if we were arguing about your safety in the past, but I am concerned about your eyes here today." The teen was angry, and refused to use the tool.

After a long pause, I said, "I am not feeling good about what is going on between us with this situation. Do you have any suggestions of a way out of this impasse?" The teen angrily said, "No." I asked, "Can you suggest some other type of eye protection you prefer?" He said, "No." He grabbed the tool and turned it on. I said, "Without eye protection, you cannot use the tool. It is not safe, and I will not let you be unsafe." The teen said angrily, "Okay, then forget it. I won't use it and I quit today." I said, "I am sorry you are quitting, but I would feel worse if you were hurt." After a long pause, the teen said, "I used to wear a different type of safety glasses that were not like these. Do you have the other kind?" I said, "No. Thank you for staying with this to help us resolve our disagreement. If you can describe or draw the glasses you prefer, I will see if I can locate a pair for next week." He described the glasses and said, "I will just wait until next week and try those." At the next session, when I told the teen I did not have the requested glasses as they were not available locally, he replied, "Oh, that is okay. I will just wear these for now." He put on the original pair of safety glasses and began working with the power tool.

Although I have few rules in the studio, safety is my first and main concern. The enactment with the teen is an example of the importance of allowing the teen to save face. Rather than get into a power struggle, I stay in the affective communication mode by moving back from cognition to limbic structures where he can organize the incoming stimuli and I can respond from incoming stimuli. My response of not feeling good about what was occurring between us was neither planned nor a technique. Engaging the teen in the problem-solving process minimizes the power differential in the therapeutic relationship.

CASE NOTE: A severely abused and neglected teen with a lifetime of placements wanted to take some art materials to his group home at the end of a session. I reiterated the limit on taking materials home, yet he did not accept the limit and continued to argue. Then he offered to buy the media.

I refused his offer and explained that he could use as much of the media needed in his art but could not take the media home. He still refused to comply, stating that there may not be any left by the time he returned. I reassured him I would order more to have on hand for his next session. He became more agitated and was hollering that he wanted the media. I quietly said, "S., I promise you I will have as much of this media as you need, even if you need an entire truckload, but you cannot take the media home." He became quiet, broke into a large grin and said, "You really would do that for me, wouldn't you? I know you would get a truckload if I asked for it. I can tell you would do that for me, and I can trust your word, even if I don't need no truckload." He did not ask for the media again.

In this case, we were having an exchange that allowed the relationship to go into a state of dysregulation and disrepair followed by a state of repair. This kind of interaction deepens the relationship. He may not have been able to take the media home; however, his mental representation was that of metaphorically having all he could ever want.

CASE NOTE: A 15-year-old was engaging in high-risk behavior, riding his skateboard through a stop sign without stopping for cross traffic, a game he and his friends referred to as "skateboard roulette." After hearing this, I asked the teen to cut out symbols for eight people or things that were important to him, and to include a symbol for himself. I offered him an assortment of colored paper, a pencil, and scissors to create the symbols. When he was finished, I asked him to arrange them on a blank 9- by 12-inch piece of paper. I then asked if he would be willing to look at the symbols in a new way, and he agreed. I asked him to remove one symbol from the paper. He picked up the symbol for the video game. I asked what his life would be like if that were missing, and he stated, "Boring." I asked if he could live being bored and he stated that he could. I had him return the symbol and remove a different symbol. He selected his computer. I asked what life would be like if he had no computer, and he replied, "Dull." I asked if he could live with dull and he replied, "Yes." I asked him to replace that symbol and remove another. He chose the one for family. I asked what it would be like if he had no family, and he became quiet. After a pause he quietly said, "I would have no family and no place to live." I asked him if he could live with no family and no place to live and he said, "Maybe, but it would be hard." I asked him to return that symbol and pick another. He picked the one that represented him. I asked, "What would it be like if there were no you?" He said sadly and quietly, "They would be really sad and they would miss me." I let that linger for a moment. Then I looked at him with my left eye to his left eye and said, "I cannot be at the stop sign to stop you and your friends from playing skateboard roulette, but I want you to remember that every time one of you plays, you risk taking yourself out of this picture, and you will never be back." Two sessions later, he announced that he and his friends were no longer playing skateboard roulette.

I have found no way to verbally impart insight to teens as the prefrontal structures of the teen brain are not highly functional at this time in their physical development. However, to engage teens in a nonverbal, visual activity that allows them to see themselves reflected in their art in real time provides access to the right hemisphere, a more direct link to the affect. Once the information is processed affectively, it is moved to cognition, and the higher structures for wisdom, judgment, and consequences are engaged.

I stress confidentiality with adolescent clients and groups and agree with Riley (1999) that once you have breached confidentiality with a teen, it is unlikely you will be able to reestablish a sense of trust. Many teens do not trust adults and are seeking to validate that assumption. It takes considerable time to establish rapport with teens and perhaps up to a year of individual therapy for them to reveal the more personal aspects of themselves and their lives. When I introduce the topic of reporting laws, I offer my perception of the difference between privacy and secrecy. Privacy is something one may choose not to talk about that harms no one. I convey that secrecy implies keeping something hidden. I let them know we can keep everything in therapy private, but I cannot keep private any potential or active harm to self or others. I also let teens know that I will not show their art or discuss anything pertaining to therapy with a parent without letting them know first. This reinforces their sense of control over what they share.

Adolescents continually test limits throughout therapy. They do so to see if you are paying attention, to garner a reaction, or to locate boundaries. Rather than maintain a neutral face, I respond in a manner that lets the teen know I am engaged in the conversation, curious, and interested in what he has to say. A therapist's not knowing is a valuable tool with teens. When they do begin to talk about themselves, their friends, or other issues, I often just use the phrase, "Tell me more." This is not a question, and it gives teens full control over what they express. If applicable, I indicate that I don't know much about a subject related to them and ask them to help me learn something about the topic. This gives them the opportunity to be an authority in the exchange.

CASE NOTE: A 17-year-old suffered a gunshot wound while involved in gang violence. When I went to see the teen in his hospital room, he was very resistant to talking and did not want to do any art. Instead of trying to urge him to do something he did not want to do, I simply asked him if he would help me learn what it was like to be a 17-year-old from his culture. He talked for nearly an hour, telling me about his school, people he admired, his food, and his grandmother; he also spoke of some of the discrimination and hardships he had faced in his life.

I allow teens total freedom of expression in their art as long as they make no weapons, drug paraphernalia, or hate-speech-themed art. Adolescence is the most creative time in life (Blos, 1962), another advantage for the art therapist. Combined with the new ability for abstract thinking, their creativity provides a pathway for self-expression and self-discovery. Teens will engage in art making, a process that allows them to nondefensively see themselves reflected in the work they have created. Because the art serves as a container for the affect, teens are able to better tolerate the unconscious becoming conscious. With a fragile ego at this time in development (Blos, 1962), teens typically do not like to regress, to feel transparent, or to feel exposed. For teens, utilizing art is a safe way to communicate metaphorically and symbolically. Effective adolescent therapy requires a delicate balance between expression and containment of affect.

BEGINNING OF THERAPY: THE SELF PHASE

The art and vignettes in the following case come from approximately 1 year of hour-long weekly art therapy sessions.

> CASE NOTE: S. was a 17-year-old male who resided in a group home. He spent the first 9 years of his life with his parents and siblings. The parents engaged in domestic violence, substance abuse, neglect, and abuse of their four children. The family lived in a car, in shelters, and on the streets. S. was extremely violent. He attacked his peers and the group home staff. Two or three times a week, he was handcuffed by law enforcement officers because of his violent outbursts and his threats to harm others. He was AWOL from the group home two to three times a week. S. refused all therapy and had bragged for three years that no one could make him take medication and no one could make him attend therapy. His plan for the future was to commit a horrible crime that would put him in prison so he would be taken care of for the rest of his life.

S.'s assigned therapist at the mental health agency was seeing S. but having little success. The therapist sought an art therapy referral for S. because "he apparently likes art" and his therapist thought S. might be willing to attend an art therapy session. S.'s assigned therapist stated that S. was very resistant to therapy but had agreed to come to art therapy at least once with the caveat that his therapist must attend and participate along with him.

S.'s therapist attended during the beginning sessions, observing and occasionally commenting. He gradually removed himself by leaving the room occasionally, then bringing work to do, and eventually dropping S. off at the studio door. When his agency was no longer able to finance his services, we talked with S. and gave him the option to continue art therapy without having the therapist accompany him, or to stop. S. chose to continue.

Some important aspects of the collaboration merit comment. First, we both met with S. in the initial sessions to provide the mental representation of a male/ female parental dyad. We modeled respect for each other, equal power, and appropriate roles and boundaries. We both verbally supported S. for his willingness to attend, his participation, and his creative art productions.

A familiar figure in S.'s life at this point, the therapist offered him a level of safety and comfort. The therapist was also skilled at mutual co-regulation and could help S. with regulation and coping. When the therapist had to stop attending S.'s art therapy sessions, we did not replicate the emotional abandonment that he had experienced early in life. We carefully prepared S. by letting him know what would change and what would stay the same: S. would come to art therapy alone with transportation provided by the group home staff, and he would continue to see his therapist at his office for the foreseeable future.

Art therapy accesses the unconscious body-based emotional memories of the right brain. S. did not say much about the content of his art during therapy. However, on the ride back to the group home afterward, he verbalized, indicating that there had been information processing in the limbic structures that gave access to the hippocampus, which plays a role in consciously accessible memory. He had a safe person and a contained environment in which to dialogue about what had arisen during the session. That his thoughts had crossed over to the left hemisphere was reflected in the use of language to describe the memory of his abuse and neglect. This aspect of the collaboration was a benefit in S.'s treatment.

> CASE NOTE: When S. arrived at the studio with his therapist, I waved at the door and then stepped back. When they came to the door, I welcomed them to the art studio, greeted the therapist by name, and then greeted S. by name while looking at him with my left eye to his left eye. I continued to look at S. with my left eye to his left eye during most of our interactions throughout the session and in future sessions. I introduced myself to S. and asked, "How is your day going?" He replied, "Fine." I invited S. to look around the kitchen and studio and said he could ask any questions he wished. I offered him a snack. He ate it and then went into the studio.
>
> I had an 11- by 17-inch piece of drawing paper and collage material on the table ready for him, along with glue, a glue brush, and scissors. I sat to the left of S. at a table, and his therapist sat at the corner of the table to the left of S. I invited S. to make a collage to introduce himself to me by cutting out pictures or words from magazines that represented who he is. He insisted his therapist must also participate by making his own collage, and he did. S. began by grabbing the hunting magazines and said, "I am going to get all the guns and knives because I like to kill people." I replied, "Whatever images you choose for your art are acceptable."
>
> I watched carefully as S. calmly cut images of guns and knives from the magazines. As he worked, he made comments about the images he selected. I showed great interest but did not ask questions as to why he

chose them or the meaning he ascribed to the images. As we talked, I noticed his selection of images shifted to boots, gloves, coats, hats, and other survival items. S. is left handed, and some of the magazines had tight bindings, making it difficult to tear out entire pages of the magazines. Just as I noticed his difficulty, S. said, "These pages are hard to cut out of this magazine." I watched him struggle for another moment and had a very clear and strong image of him cutting out the pages with a utility knife. I also had a strong image of myself getting him the utility knife to cut the pages. My left brain immediately pointed out the danger of giving a violent teen a utility knife. However, my right brain was apparently taking in the larger picture: S. was in a physical and emotional state of regulation and was calm. I surprised myself by going to the locked art closet to get a utility knife. As I was walking to the closet, I was reminding myself of the potential danger of giving sharp objects to violent teens and imagined this warning in every art therapy book. However, the image was so strong that I retrieved the tool and carefully handed it to S., saying, "I don't leave these lying around the studio but it will help you cut out those pages. Please use it safely and cut away from your body." S. carefully took the knife, cut out the pages he wanted, and handed me the knife with the blade facing away from me. I placed the knife back in the locked closet and returned to the table.

S. continued working on his collage. He added additional sheets of paper to the original 11- by 17-inch paper to accommodate all his images. Near the end of the session, I offered that the last few minutes of the session are for people to comment about their art if they wish. I began by asking S.'s therapist if he wanted to make any comments about his collage. Modeling for S., the therapist made a few general comments about why he chose few of his images. I asked S. if he wished to comment about any of the images in his collage, and he declined. I asked S. if I could tell him something I learned about him today. He hesitantly agreed, and I said, "I learned that you have courage. You came here today not knowing what to expect or who I was, and you participated in making a collage. Doing those things takes courage." I thanked them both for participating. Before the end of the session, I invited S. to attend art therapy again, but asked him to commit to three sessions so he could get a sense of what art therapy is and how it works. S. pointed to his therapist and said, "I will come if he can come." We all agreed. I thanked S. for attending and said goodbye at the door. As I waved, they drove away.

A short time later, I received a call from S.'s therapist. He said with excitement, "You won't believe what happened in the car on the way home!" He told me that S. had said, "I can have her be my therapist because she takes me as who I am. She was not afraid of me. She knew I could handle that utility knife. At the group home they won't give me a knife or even a fork."

As is common with traumatized teens, S. was defensive. The images he created at the onset of this initial session reflected aggression. But during the session they changed, shifted to those of protection. He tested and expanded limits by adding paper to the page I had given him.

The scenario with the utility knife was something that surprised me. My mental image was so strong that I did something I had never done before. Reflecting on that moment, that choice, as I have many times since, I have concluded that I was not thinking consciously. I was responding to a very strong image that this was what I must do. I want to convey that what I am describing is very different from having a sense of not knowing why one is behaving in a particular manner. Unconsciously, I was aware that S. was in a state of physical homeostasis. There was an adult male therapist familiar with S. in the room. Had I been alone with S., or had he been agitated or in any way hypervigilant, I am certain I would not have provided the tool. S.'s comments, "I can have her be my therapist because she takes me as who I am. She was not afraid of me" were accurate. I was accepting S. unconditionally in the moment, not judging his potential behavior based on what I knew about him. And, I was not at all afraid of S. during the session.

By engaging in a state of mutual co-regulation, we were able to co-create an intersubjective space in which S. could communicate from his right hemisphere. In this state of mutual co-regulation, I was able to receive incoming sensory information from S.'s right hemisphere in subsymbolic, nonverbal affective cues in the form of images, speech and body gesture, tone, and posture. Within the intersubjective realm, I was able to respond to the incoming sensory cues that were stronger than my many cognitive responses of caution or uncertainty. We were both engaged in a preverbal exchange of affective body-based states, a state of affect that was in synchronicity. Getting the utility knife for S. turned out to be the right thing to do, as evidenced in a change in S.'s behavior. After 3 years of refusing therapy, S. had identified me as his therapist after our first session.

What transpired during my initial meeting with S. is described by Schore:

> The capacity of the empathic clinician's right brain primary process system to make not surface but deep contact of mind and body within the intersubjective field is critical to the depth of the change process activated in the therapeutic growth-facilitating environment. (2007, p. 11)

Asking S. to commit to three sessions established an agreement between us, another aspect of the relationship. It was a symbolic representation not only that I was invested in his therapy and wanted to see him but also that he was expected to have enough experience with me, and with art therapy, to make an informed decision about whether this would be something helpful for him. It placed S. in a position of control, along with a way out.

CASE NOTE: S. arrived for the second session accompanied by his therapist. I greeted them at the door and used my left eye to S.'s left eye during

the greeting and throughout the session. I offered S. a snack, which he ate before entering the studio. Once inside, he announced that he wanted to paint. I offered him a selection of paper sizes, and he chose a large piece of paper about 24 inches square, tempera paint, and large brushes. He began by painting the outline of a large yellow house on the left side of the paper and one tall and two shorter trees on the right side of the paper (see Figure 9.1). When he had completed the painting, I asked S. if he would be willing to look at the image in a different way to see if we could learn something new about him. S. agreed.

I asked him to look at the image and describe what it looked like and told him that I was going to write his descriptions on a piece of paper. S. responded, "Colorful." I said, "Great, you know what I mean, so just let me know what it looks like." S. said, "Large, green, rectangular, organized, imperfect, and messy." I then told S. that I would read off each word and he could tell me whether or not it described him. I began by saying, "Are you large?" S. replied, "Yes." I asked S., "Are you colorful?" He replied, "Yes." I then asked S. if he was green and he replied, "Well mostly. I like to garden. I have a watermelon plant but it's not doing well because it is in a small pot with old dirt and not enough dirt. I keep hoping it will grow a watermelon." I asked S., "Are you rectangular?" He said, "No." I asked him, "Are you organized?" He said, "Yes." I then asked S., "Are you imperfect?" He said, "Yes." Lastly, I asked S., "Are you messy?" He replied, "Yes."

His therapist commented in a playful tone about S.'s messy room. Upon hearing this, S., who was sitting in a chair with wheels, twirled in his chair in a circular motion away from the table and over to the wall. I asked S. if he could come back to the table, and he twirled in the chair in a circular motion back to the table. I quietly asked S. if talking about his messy room was too much for him. S. again twirled his chair away from the table and over to the wall. I wheeled my chair directly over to the wall next to him and said, "I wheeled over here to get you and we do not have to talk about your room anymore." Together S. and I wheeled directly back to the table together. As we neared the end of the session, I thanked S. for coming to art therapy and he left with his therapist.

S.'s announcement that he wanted to paint was welcome. I chose medium-size paper and paintbrushes to elicit a moderate amount of affect. He participated fully in the exploration of the image. It is noteworthy that when the therapist made the comment about S. being messy, S. twirled in the chair and twirled back. Spinning while approaching a caregiver has been identified as a behavior of insecurely attached infants (Main, 1983).

CASE NOTE: When S. arrived for the third session with his therapist, I greeted him in the usual manner. I offered him a snack of watermelon, and he said, "You know me so well." He commented about his struggling plant and offered, "I really like watermelon and I also like pizza." Once in the studio, S.'s therapist excused himself and said he had to take a telephone call. He returned later in the session and observed.

I offered S. a sheet of 18- by 24-inch drawing paper and markers. I asked him if he would be willing to do some scribbling with me. He agreed and I asked him to pick a marker and scribble all over the paper until I told him to stop, which he did. I asked him to flip the paper over and, using the same scribbling motion, to scribble his initials. He did so, scribbling two S's. I asked him to use any color markers he preferred and to enhance his initials. After a few moments, I asked him to switch to the oil pastels and continue to enhance his initials. When he did so, he began to add several small S's to the image (see Figure 9.2). When he indicated he was finished, I leaned in his direction and pointed to the large S's and asked in a playful tone, "Do those S's know those S's?" while pointing to the small S's. I sat back. S. pulled far away from me in the opposite direction and said, "I don't know." I moved my body back near him, and while pointing to the small S's, asked again in a playful tone, "Do those S's know those S's?" while pointing to the large S's. S. pulled away but not as far. He responded in a playful tone, "No, they don't really know those S's very much." We both continued in a playful tone as I leaned my body in S.'s direction and asked, "Which ones are in charge?" S. pointed to the large S's as he leaned his body in the direction of mine and said, "These are the ones in charge." I leaned closer to S. and asked, "What would this big S. say to this little one?" S. leaned farther in my direction and said, "It would say, you are small."

As we continued to dialogue about the symbolic content of the image, I kept my left eye on his left eye and eventually both of us were engaged in a rhythmic rocking back and forth for the duration of the discussion about the image. Near the end of the session, I asked S. if there was anything the image needed. He proceeded to cut the encapsulated initials out of the background (see Figure 9.3). I pointed to the white background left behind and asked, "Does that part of the image have anything to say about being cut out?" S. replied, "They don't even know it exists." I asked for clarification and he said adamantly, "The white does not even know it exists and it has nothing to say about it." S. announced he was done. We ended the session in the usual manner.

I had no real knowledge of the symbolic content of the image. It was not the focus of therapy at this time. Offering S. an art experience that explored the self was the goal. Being attuned to S.'s body-based states, I therefore responded to nonverbal and body-based cues that were being communicated to me in a state of mutually engaged conversation. I did not plan to have a rocking experience during the session and had never done so before in the many times I had used this art directive. Our bodies were rocking rhythmically in synchrony, in contrast to S. spinning away from me or toward me as he had done in the earlier session.

Replicating the attachment behaviors aids in the maturation of the right hemisphere. By engaging in dyadic right-hemisphere-to-right-hemisphere communications, we are rebuilding the scaffolding that will allow access to the higher structures for affect regulation and behavioral control.

When asked what the image needed, S. cut out his drawn and colored initials from the stark white background. Although S. did not comment, his tone of speech conveyed satisfaction. Perhaps he was symbolically cutting himself out of a stark and empty past.

During the week, I did something I had never done before. I took some fresh dirt, a flowerpot, and a small amount of plant fertilizer to the group home staff and asked if they would please give the dirt and pot to S. for his watermelon plant and help him apply fertilizer; I knew he would not be allowed to possess fertilizer at the group home.

Soon after, S.'s therapist called to inform me that he would no longer be able to attend art therapy with S. due to his agency's policy. He was apprehensive about S.'s reaction and thought he might terminate. We planned to inform S. of this at the next session so he could decide whether to continue attending art therapy or not.

CASE NOTE: S. arrived for the fourth session with his therapist, who was now bringing work with him and remaining out of the studio room during the art therapy sessions. I offered S. pizza for a snack. He said enthusiastically in a childlike voice, "You know how to take care of me!" He thanked me for the dirt and flowerpot and said he hoped his plant would grow. After he ate, his therapist told S. that he could not continue to bring him to art therapy. He asked S. to think about whether he wanted to come alone or not at all, reminding him that his transportation to and from therapy would be provided by group home staff. S. replied, "I will come alone."

S. and I went to the studio. He asked if his therapist could come in because it was his last time. I agreed, and the therapist observed most of the session with minimal comment. I asked S. if he would be willing to work with some symbols of his choosing. He agreed. I offered him scissors and construction paper and asked him to create symbols with it. With both of us using primarily left-eye-to-left-eye contact throughout the session, I began by asking S. to create three or four symbols that represented his *wants*, things he would like in life but did not need for survival. I asked him to create three or four symbols that represented his *needs*, things he needed in order to get by in the world.

To represent his wants he created Nintendo, a big house, and a vault with money (see Figure 9.4). He made symbols of a small bridge, clothes, and a large bridge to represent his needs (see Figure 9.5). I asked S. to place the symbols that represented pleasure or fun on a paper. He selected Nintendo, a small bridge, some money, and a big house. I asked S. if he wanted to comment, and he said, "I would have fun with Nintendo, and I would like money and I would like a house." I asked S. to replace those symbols with the symbols that represented things he needed for survival. He chose the clothes, the house, money, and a bridge. I asked S. if he wanted to comment, and he said, "I need clothes and a house but it doesn't have to be that big. I need money, but it doesn't have to be a vault full."

Then I asked S. to replace those symbols and select the ones having to do with relationships. He picked the small and the large bridge and placed them on the paper. I then had S. look at all the symbols except the ones depicting relationships and asked, "Is this enough?" S. replied, "No, it's not enough. One needs friends and family." S. spoke a bit about his parents and siblings. He used the large bridge symbol (see Figure 9.6) to illustrate his friends and family on the right with a large center support labeled "You" with a self symbol emerging from the base. S. said, "See? On the left are friends, but that is not enough support. They just aren't there for you. And on the right are family, but they are not there for me, so maybe something can be made from this for support," as he pointed to the center of the bridge. I said, "I will do my best to support you until you find your support." S. then commented that the support of family and friends is not enough or reliable and went on to talk about what it takes to destroy a person's trust. We discussed several scenarios of trust, and he talked about his parents and things they had done and things he had done. After he finished talking, there was a long pause. I said, "It is very hard to live with incapable parents. You did a very good job surviving, and I am glad you survived." S. listened but did not comment. After another pause, I asked S., "Do you want to tell me more about your family?" S. replied quietly and nondefensively, "Not now, maybe when I know you better." I responded, "I am willing to earn that trust."

As the session ended, I thanked S. for telling me about himself and his family and asked if he might like to build a bridge, since the emphasis of the discussion about wants and needs had been on bridges, and S. had mentioned earlier that he liked to build with wood. He said he would like to build a bridge. We ended the session in the usual manner.

The therapist again called me from the car just after dropping S. at the group home. He said, "You won't believe what happened in the car on the way home." For the first time, S. had talked extensively with his therapist about his parents, his siblings, and the child abuse and neglect he and his siblings had suffered in the past.

This had been a powerful and pivotal session. The kinesthetic activity of drawing and cutting symbols accessed the imagery of the right hemisphere. S. was able to talk about the concrete symbols as I appealed to the right hemisphere by creating novel and nonthreatening opportunities for self-exploration. I was moving away from body-based self-exploration to the larger psychological interior self by investigating wants and needs. The imagery of the right hemisphere was expressed in visual form. The visual symbols were projected upon, dialogued about, and contemplated.

Although I began with the technique of wants and needs, it was a tool to facilitate the activation of the right-hemisphere images and body sensations. Once S. was engaged in his own associations and responses to his art, I let him take the lead. I didn't offer my projections or interpretations. I made every effort not to move ahead of him. An example of moving ahead would have been to change my response from offering him support and helping him find his own support to asking him instead, "How can I be of support to you?" My responses were my own body-based responses to S.'s nonverbal communications of the right hemisphere. He elicited protection and I responded accordingly. I did not feel curious or a need for more information. In a state of attunement, we engaged in affective communication, not cognitive discourse.

S. opened the door to his past by sharing details about his family—how he grew up, and how he struggled. My response to this information was predicated on a felt body sensation; S. was struggling to survive what he had experienced. If I had been operating from within my own cognition, I might have responded, "I understand" when S. said he did not want to talk more about his family until he knew me better. Instead, my response that I was willing to earn his trust gave him control over the content of his therapy.

It is not surprising that S. talked with his therapist after the session. Right-hemisphere activation often results in increased verbal dialogue as the information from the body is sent to the limbic system and then to the right hemisphere. The imagery is activated and crosses over to the left hemisphere as reflected in S.'s ability to express himself verbally.

> **CASE NOTE:** After missing a session because of a leg injury, S. arrived for the fifth session with his group home transportation provider. He ate a snack and we went to the studio. I had his image of the bridges available from his earlier session, and invited S. to consider building a bridge. He was eager to do this. He began a process that took four months to complete. The bridge was 3 feet long and sat on a 4-foot by 3-foot heavy cardboard base. It was constructed of wood glue, clay, boxes, paint, plastic foliage, jewels for lights, fish line for cables, and tissue paper (see Figure 9.7). At one end of the bridge was an empty green space with three trees. There was no exit to this area from the bridge. The middle span had supports made of wood and clay, and the bridge had high sides and lights. The other end of the bridge exited directly to a building with a path, lights, windows, and a large silo-style building with a small building next to the silo structure (see Figure 9.8).

NEUROBIOLOGY IN THE CLINICAL SETTING

Use of the NDAT interventions is a way to engage clients in the different phases of their therapies, but it is not a prescription plan for therapy. Once S. chose to engage in a large art project that would take many sessions, I followed his lead and his plans for the art making and the therapy.

A review of the relevant, salient aspects of this case follows. I then provide highlights of the ensuing sessions that illustrate the course of the therapy and the application of neurobiology and the use of the right hemisphere in therapy.

During the building of the bridge, S. had access to tools, including a hammer, a balsawood saw, and a glue gun. These items were monitored. I explained that as long as he used the tools safely they would be available to him. Throughout his therapy, S. used the tools safely every time. He was very attentive to my safety as well as his own, and he always asked if my hands were clear before using the saw or reminded me to keep my hands clear of the hot glue. When the transportation staff person returned to fetch him, S. invited him into the studio as he finished up. I noticed that while the staff person was in the room, S. would pick up the utility knife and announce he was changing the blade. He would test the sharpness of the blade with his finger. I would say to S., "No, that is not safe, please give me that" or just take the item from his hand. S. would smile at the transportation worker. It was evident he was showing the fellow that he could be trusted with tools in this relationship, that he could be told what to do and have things taken away from him without reacting violently.

Another curious result of working within an attachment paradigm is the unique aspect of countertransference. I found myself visualizing S. as an infant and a very young child. I found myself thinking, "I wonder how baby S. is doing today," something I had never experienced. The time between our sessions seemed like weeks to me rather than days. I found myself eagerly looking forward to our sessions and being with him. If he was unable to attend therapy, I was truly disappointed. This has occurred with other teen clients. It is wise to be mindful of the unique and possibly unexpected countertransference that can occur with this model of treatment.

> CASE NOTE: When S. began working on his bridge, I constantly gave him the supplies he needed, offered support, and let him take the lead with his project. As he worked, I noted that he had excellent gross and fine motor skills, visual perceptual skills, and eye-hand coordination. He could draw well and did not demonstrate any delays that required sensory or motor strengthening activities other than those inherent in the art making itself. S. did not talk much as he worked. When he became frustrated, he would make a loud growling sound. I began to respond to S.'s affective communication by matching his sound once and asking, "Is that a grouchy sound, a frustrated sound, or an 'I need help' sound?" S. would tell me,

then, what the sound was conveying. Later, when he made a sound, I
would say, "Do I have it right? Is that frustration?" or "I think I have it. That
means you are irritated." S. would respond, "Very good," or "Excellent
deciphering."

Mothers do not expect their infant to clarify the meaning of their sounds, but
mothers do learn to decipher their infant's nonverbal affective communications.
By replicating these early, missed experiences, I was laying down the foundations
for future affect regulation. S.'s comments are poignant. He recognized what I
was attempting to do. I did not try to communicate with S. by making the sounds
he was making. I make the sound once to convey acceptance and then attempted
to learn what the sound was communicating in order to decipher S.'s body-based
affective communications. Once I learned these sounds and their meaning, they
were abandoned and S. used words to describe his feelings most of the time.

> CASE NOTE: During one session, S. asked for a rolling pin to roll out
> clay. I did not have one but offered that I had a heavy mailing tube that he
> could use to flatten the clay. As I went to retrieve the mailing tube in the
> closet, a strong image came to me. I returned with the mailing tube held to
> my eye and said to S., "I see you." My left hemisphere reminded me that
> this 17-year-old would think I was out of my mind, at best, and perhaps
> even be insulted. S. literally *hurried* to the box of thin cardboard tubes,
> grabbed one, and said, in the voice of a very young child, "Me too. I see
> you. Do it again," and began to giggle and laugh. I held the tube to my eye
> and repeated, "I see you." Peering through his tube at me, he said, "I see
> you too. Do it again." We did this for a few moments. Then S. threw the
> tube on the table and said in the voice of a 17-year-old, "Well, that was
> fun" and returned to his clay project.

Once again, we were in a state of mutual co-regulation and attunement. I had
never used, nor did I plan to use, the cardboard tube in the manner I did with S.
I was responding to the incoming sensory information. S. was communicating to
me with his right hemisphere to mine: "Just as the left brain communicates its
unconscious states to other left brains via linguistic behaviors, so the right brain
communicates its unconscious states to other right brains that are tuned to
receive its communications" (Schore, 2007, p. 9).

With the art making, S. was engaged in kinesthetic experiences that elicited
affect. We were learning to regulate his affect in these very early, developmental
ways. Cognition followed and eventually accessed the prefrontal structures promoting the ability for emotional regulation and behavioral control.

Near the end of one session that included several very frustrating experiences,
S. said, "I am going to smash everything and kill everybody." I asked if we could
problem-solve through the art, and he allowed me to help with one particularly
frustrating step. S. was able to calm down and end the session.

During that week, I spoke to S.'s earlier therapist and let him know I was planning to address S.'s violent comments in the next session. I was concerned that S. might quit or be angry. The therapist agreed that S. might blow up or leave and kindly asked if I would like him to attend the next session with S. I declined his offer. I was confident S. would be able to tolerate the discussion about his violent comment during the previous session.

> CASE NOTE: S. had a snack before coming to the studio. He appeared comfortable as he began work on his project. I told S. that I had something to talk about with him. With my left eye on his left eye, I reminded S. of his comment at the end of the last session about smashing everything and killing everybody. I asked him if I needed to stop letting him use the saw and utility knife because of the risk of violence. S. reached over, put his hand on my arm and said, with his left eye on my left eye, "I will never be violent with you. I will never come after you. You never have to worry about that. I will never hurt you." I said, "Thank you, S. So we have an agreement?" He replied, "Yes." I then said with my left eye to his left eye, "I know I am really going to make you mad sometimes and you are going to be really angry with me. My challenge for you is not to attack me or leave but to use words to tell me what is going on and to deal with what is going on with me." S. responded with his left eye on my left eye: "I think I can do that with you." I said, "Great." We both returned to the bridge project.

Before another session, a staff member from S.'s group home called to say that S. had been AWOL from the home the previous night until 3:00 a.m. and that he had caused the staff a great deal of concern. There had also been involvement with law enforcement. After learning of this incident, I thought about what to do if and when the subject came up in the therapy session. In my cognition, I was formulating a plan. However, my right brain kept interfering with the image of me scolding S. for being AWOL. My left brain kept reminding me of the danger of sounding like a parent with a teen—and the inappropriate behavior of a therapist scolding a client! I was certain I would not do this during the session.

> CASE NOTE: When S. arrived, he reported he had not gone to school that day because he had a stomachache and had been up late. He said that he had been AWOL until 3:00 in the morning. I told S. that I had heard about the incident. The image of me scolding S. hovered. My left brain was reminding me why I should not do so. As I was having this internal debate, S. said, "It's no big deal." The words flew out of my mouth. "I can't believe you were out there! I was worried sick when I heard about it." S. yelled at me, "I had my belt and a butter knife and I can protect myself." I responded, totally out of character, "Oh, no you can't! If there had been someone with a knife or a gun, you could have been hurt, and I am really worried about you doing that and I don't want you to ever do that again." I

was actually pointing a finger at S. during the tail end of my tirade. S. looked at me and said in the tone of a bored and irritated adolescent, "Okay." At the end of the session, S. did not want to leave and said that he wished he had more time.

My outburst had been spontaneous. I was responding to the incoming sensory signals picked up from S.'s right hemisphere. I was doing fine with my cognitive plan until S. said, "It's no big deal." My visceral reaction moved to my limbic system with frustration, irritation, and sadness that S. thought his life was no big deal! S.'s right hemisphere was eliciting a necessary response to accommodate his internal developmental trajectory. The evidence of the effectiveness of my response was change. S. never went AWOL from the group home again.

> CASE NOTES: During another session, S. was very frustrated with his art-making project. I could feel the anger rising. He regressed, using sounds to communicate. After a few moments, he said curtly, "I am taking my bridge home today." I reminded him of our earlier discussion during which he mentioned he wanted to create a space in his room to accommodate the bridge. S. repeated curtly, "I am taking my bridge home today." I offered that it was his and he could do so if he wished. He did not respond. At the end of the session, as S. was leaving with his bridge, I offered that he was welcome to bring it back anytime. S. said emphatically, "I will not be bringing the bridge back." After he left with his bridge, I sketched the bridge on a large piece of butcher paper, and included as many details as I could remember.
>
> S. arrived for the next session with the bridge. He said, "I brought it back because it needs more work." The rapprochement of leaving and returning was enacted metaphorically with the art. I said, "I am so glad you brought it back because I missed seeing your bridge." I showed S. the drawing I had made and said, "I even sketched a picture of the bridge so I could remember it." S. looked at me with his left eye on my left eye and said in a very surprised and childlike voice, "You drew this! I like that you drew this for me." Then his voice became the 17-year-old as he then delighted in pointing out all the items I had forgotten or drawn incorrectly and pointed out how he could have done a better job drawing the bridge from memory. He had abandoned the younger child state for the more appropriate narcissistic stance of adolescence (Blos, 1962) that was emerging.
>
> During another session, S. was frustrated and snapped a large piece of balsa wood in half with one hand. I looked at him, not one bit afraid, but irritated that he was wasting the wood. I thought I was not showing my irritation. S. said, "That is not violent. That is like crumpling up a piece of paper except I am wasting wood." Our right amygdalas were tracking just below the surface.
>
> On another occasion, anticipating S.'s arrival for a session, I went to his portfolio and retrieved the house drawing he had made during the session

illustrating his wants and needs. I set the drawing on the table and recalled thinking at the time that S. might want to build a house in art therapy one day. S. arrived for the session carrying a drawing of the house I had selected and said, "I can't believe you have that house picture out and here I come with a better drawing of that house!" I was amazed. I did not know if something had been communicated at the last session, outside of our conscious memory, but neither S. nor I could consciously figure out how this had occurred.

S. worked on the bridge occasionally but was also building a variety of other balsawood structures. During another session, I mentioned to S. that people had jobs making models. I said that people earned money making such models for architects and described the general process. S. listened but did not respond. A few sessions later, I mentioned to S. that I knew an architect and could ask him if being a model builder required one to be an architect or if one had to be a good artist that could build models. S. said, "Yes, can you find that out for me?" In another session, I told S. I had learned that one only needed to be a skilled model builder to work for an architect.

S. now plans to continue to build models and perhaps get a job as an assistant to a model builder or to become a model builder. No longer does he plan to spend his life in prison. He is now saving photos of his models on a disk to keep track of his successful projects and record the improvements in his skill.

During another session, S. was working on a building project. As he worked, I mentioned that the hard thing for him would be precision. He appeared to prefer to build free form. Model building would require details from drawn plans. S. was curious and interested in learning more about plans drawn for buildings. I retrieved the architectural drawings for my studio and we looked at them together. He easily grasped the concept of building to scale and the importance of working with dimensions. He asked for a ruler so he could measure his building projects. He measured everything, in the process creating a whole new level of frustration for himself. However, S. was very pleased with the improved outcome of his structures.

S. turned 18 and was required by law to leave the referring agency. I had very few sessions for closure. We discussed the fact that he did not have much time to finish his current building project, and we discussed the abruptness of not having many sessions left to conclude his therapy.

CASE NOTE: During the next session, I felt a desire to push S. a bit to see how much of the seeming emotional regulation and behavioral control had been internalized and integrated, especially with the stress of leaving therapy so quickly. In addition, he was facing a new placement. He had two options: either go to a place he did not want to, or go to a place he wanted to attend but had not accepted him previously because of going AWOL and his violent behaviors.

I was sitting opposite S. at the table with his current building project between us. As he worked on his building, I began making suggestions of how he should proceed with the project. When he started to do something, I stopped him and told him there was a better way. S. responded politely by stating, "No, I want it this way." I continued to make suggestions and S. continued, politely, to refuse to use my suggestions. After a few minutes, I began moving things on his project. At one point, I pushed too far and S. yelled in a very loud voice, "No! Will you stop it?" I said, apologetically, "Oh, I am sorry. This is your project and of course, you want it your way. I was excited and was taking over your project and you are right, these are your decisions." Then I looked at S. with my left eye to his left eye and said quietly, "But you did it. You didn't attack me and you didn't leave. You talked to me." With his left eye on my left eye S. quietly said, "Yes, I told you to stop it and you knew I meant to stop it." I replied, "Yes. I heard you loud and clear! You were telling me to stop it before and I wasn't listening. Thank you." S. said, "You are welcome." S. resumed his building project. He was jovial and used humor often during the remainder of the session. I felt a sense of elation.

I was thrilled that S. had developed a self that was capable of tolerating the rupture and repair in our relationship that was necessary for S. to develop affect tolerance. His ability to respond politely to my suggestions illustrated his improved ability for emotional control. When stressed, S. did not revert to the more primitive and reactive lower structures of his brain that are expressed physically. He used language to communicate during a highly charged affective moment, a significant change in his behavior. Instead of leaving, he was able to engage in a mutual repair of the rupture that had occurred. The importance of this interactive repair work is documented by Siegel and Bromberg:

> Missed opportunities for attunement and mis-attunements, whether these occur in psychotherapy, parenting, or other emotional relationships, are unavoidable. Unless repair of these disruptions in attunement is undertaken, toxic senses of shame and humiliation can become serious blocks to interpersonal communication. . . . Repair requires the recognition that a rupture has occurred in the attunement process. A realignment of states between the two individuals is involved. The repair process is an interactive one, requiring the openness of both people in their attempts to reconnect after a rupture. (Siegel, 1999, p. 291)

> The analytic goal is that the experience of the struggle in the here and now will feel increasingly safe to the patient over time, and that safer feeling will, we hope, lead to a gradually more enduring capacity for holding as a symbolized state of internal conflict that which was formally a collision of realities between dissociated self-states. (Bromberg, 2006, p. 34)

Acknowledgment of S.'s power in our relationship was another developmental step. When S. yelled at me, it was an appropriate level of indignation. Rather than engage in a cognitive discussion of how he felt, I stayed engaged in the affective exchange that allowed S. to experience the repair instead of "talk about" the repair. Reciprocity occurred in the next session.

> CASE NOTE: S. arrived for our next-to-last session with a magazine featuring redwood trees and said, "I thought you might like to see the pictures in this magazine." S. did not know of my affinity for redwood trees, nor did he know that I had seen and marveled at the same photos. This was another aspect of two-person biology; it works both ways.
>
> I listened as S. showed me the large redwood tree photo he thought I would enjoy, but the two other images that he focused on were even more stunning. One photo was of the wise and rare spotted owl. S. was about to turn 18 and was being pushed out of the "system" of structure, school, and home onto his own if he did not get into the residential school of his choice, the one that had refused to consider him in the past. The spotted owl, protected for many years, is now being pushed out of its territory by the barred owl.
>
> The other photo was that of the ecosystem that grew in the soil created on a limb or branch fork of the ancient redwood tree. Coincidentally, some of the fine print on the page referred to "partnership . . . in a symbiotic relationship with the support." S. spoke at length of the new growth and the world that was developing out of the older branch (see Figure 9.9).
>
> The resemblance to S.'s early bridge drawing identifying his needs was evident. Arising from the support of his art therapist, S. has sprouted new aspects of himself. His new capacity to regulate his affect and control his behavior reflects his growth. He no longer goes AWOL from the group home and has had no violent outbursts at the home in many months.
>
> S. spent his last session finishing a building project. We reviewed all we had done. I told him of his strengths and the progress he had made. I assured him that my door was always open to him to return if the opportunity came about. He left smiling and said, "Yeah, I like it here, I may come back to visit."

S.'s development of a self, the major task of adolescence, was well under way. He was accepted at the school of his choice because of his improvements in development and in particular, the abatement of violent episodes. At the time of this writing, S. has not been violent toward others for the past 3 years.

I would like to leave you with a thought that has guided my work for many years: "The sage only helps all creatures to find their own nature, but he does not venture to lead them by the nose. He simply reminds people of who they have always been" (Johanson & Kurtz, 1991, p. 134).

Posttraumatic Stress Symptoms in Children After Mild to Moderate Pediatric Trauma: An Examination of Symptom Prevalence, Correlates, Parent-Child Symptom Reporting, and the Efficacy of an Art Therapy Treatment Intervention for Acute Trauma

I. INTRODUCTION

The high incidence of observed PTSD symptoms in a population of acutely injured pediatric trauma patients prompted an investigation to determine the level of PTSD symptoms in the population and to assess the efficacy of an art therapy treatment intervention designed to reduce PTSD symptoms in the acute care setting.

The quantitative experiment utilized a randomized cohort design. Data was collected at an urban Level-I trauma center. Ninety (90) subjects were identified using the hospital daily trauma registry, and met the following criteria: (1) ages 7–17; 2) hospitalized overnight for physical trauma, excluding head trauma, burns, and child abuse.

Children were assessed for presenting PTSD symptoms, and randomized to a control group or intervention group. Follow-up assessments were completed at one month, six months, and 1.5 years following the initial hospitalization.

Sixty-eight percent of the children had significant PTSD symptoms at baseline, 60 percent at one week, and 50 percent at one month. The art therapy treatment intervention did not significantly decrease PTSD symptoms, except in the avoidance and numbing symptom cluster.

II. RATIONALE

Pediatric trauma is the foremost cause of death in children greater than 1 year of age. Each year, over 2 million children require hospitalization after sustaining traumatic injuries. Injured children would appear to be among those at greatest risk for developing PTSD, yet there is surprisingly little empirical research on the development or treatment of psychological sequelae following injury.

The Specific Aims of the Study

Specific Aim 1:

Hypothesis: The incidence rate of significant PTSD symptoms in this population of pediatric trauma patients after the initial traumatic event will be greater than the previously reported rate of 25–33 percent.

Aim: To determine the incidence rate of PTSD in pediatric trauma patients following an acute injury.

Specific Aim 2:

Hypothesis: Children exhibiting significant PTSD symptoms who receive a specific art therapy treatment intervention will show a greater decrease in symptoms when compared at one month, six months, and 1.5 years post-injury with children who do not receive the intervention.

Aim: To determine the effectiveness of a brief psychological intervention in reducing the severity and number of PTSD symptoms.

Specific Aim 3:

Hypothesis: Parents will significantly under-report their child's level of psychological stress following an acute injury.

Aim: To determine the accuracy of parents to assess their child's level of psychological stress following an acute injury.

Specific Aim 4:

Hypothesis: Nursing staff will significantly under-report their patient's level of psychological stress following an acute injury.

Aim: To determine the accuracy of nursing staff to assess their child patient's level of psychological stress following an acute injury.

III. METHODS

This 5-year prospective study was implemented at University of California San Francisco School of Medicine at San Francisco General Hospital and Children's Hospital Oakland, in Oakland, California.

The study population consists of children ages 7–17 hospitalized overnight for injuries resulting from pedestrian and vehicle crashes, falls, gunshots, stabbings and assaults, penetrating injuries, and animal injuries. Children who were victims of physical or sexual abuse, burns or those with severe head injury were excluded. Informed consent was obtained from parents of children meeting enrollment criteria following a detailed explanation of the study by the project coordinator.

Patients who met criteria were interviewed by the study coordinators during their inpatient stay to determine the presence of PTSD symptoms using the Posttraumatic Stress Disorder Reaction Index (PTSD-RI, Child or Adolescent version) developed by Robert Pynoos and colleagues at University of California Los Angeles School of Medicine (Frederick et al., 1992). Patients endorsing at least mild trauma symptoms on the PTSD-RI were randomly assigned to either the standard hospital services group or the intervention group. Patients who did not endorse at least mild PTSD symptoms during initial hospitalization were also followed as a control group to track possible later onset of symptoms and for the purposes of comparison analysis.

In addition, parents were asked to rate their own levels of stress using the Parent Version of the PTSD-RI, and the Post Traumatic Stress Diagnostic Scale (Foa, 1995). Parents were asked to assess their family environment (Moos & Moos, 1994). Previous history of traumatic events, family history and makeup, prior psychiatric diagnosis, prior use of psychiatric services, and prior hospitalization or injury were determined by interviewing the child's parent or caregiver during the initial interview. The child's medical record was used to determine injury severity score (ISS), type of injury, and course of hospitalization (surgeries required, number) and complexity of medical interventions (Therapeutic Intervention Scoring System, TISS), length of hospitalization, length of stay in the Intensive Care Unit (ICU).

The child or adolescent's primary nurse was also asked to rate presence of hyper-arousal PTSD symptoms in children using a modified version of the PTSD-RI during the child's inpatient stay. Interviews with both parents and children were repeated at one month, six months, and 18 months following the child's initial hospitalization.

The Chapman Art Therapy Treatment Intervention (CATTI, Chapman et al. 2001) was implemented with those randomized to the intervention group. The intervention is designed for acute, incident-based trauma, and can be completed in approximately one hour.

IV. RESULTS

A total of 90 subjects were recruited for participation at the time of the child's initial hospitalization over a period of one and a half years. Of this number 29 received the art therapy intervention, 31 received standard hospital treatment, and 30 did not demonstrate PTSD symptoms during the baseline interview. The results presented here represent 71 of the 90 enrolled patients. Of these participants, 74 percent were male and 26 percent were female. The average age of participants was 10.56 (median = 10, sd = 2.6). The ethnic background of participants included the following: Caucasian (n = 39), African American (n = 26), Hispanic (n = 11), Asian/Pacific Islander (n = 5), Native American (n = 1), and "other" (n = 1).

A majority of study participants experienced motor vehicle versus pedestrian/bicycle accidents (n = 33), followed by motor vehicle/motor cycle accidents (n = 21), falls (n = 12), miscellaneous penetrating injuries (n = 7), sports injuries (n = 5), and animal-related injuries (n = 5). The most common types of injuries incurred by study participants included injuries to extremities (30 percent), abdominal/organ injuries (16 percent), external lacerations/contusions (16 percent), multiple systemic injuries (16 percent), mild head injuries (11 percent), chest injuries (8 percent), and vertebrae injuries (8 percent).

A total of 43 percent of all subjects enrolled met diagnostic criteria A, B. C, and D for

PTSD at one month, 30 percent at six months, and 28 percent at 1.5 years post-injury. Parents underreported their child's level of stress, and a high level of parental traumatization, as measured by the PDS, was strongly related to the presence of high child's PTSD-RI score at baseline, one week and one month. Nurses significantly and dramatically underestimated the child's level of distress during the child's initial inpatient treatment.

The art therapy treatment group did not show statistically significant overall PTSD-RI reductions when compared with the standard treatment group. While all groups showed reductions in symptom severity ratings over time, no change in *overall* symptom severity scores could be attributed to intervention status. The art therapy group demonstrated a mean decrease of 8.28 from baseline to one month, while the standard services only group demonstrated a mean decrease of 3.13 from baseline to one month.

Specific symptom clusters were examined to detect differences in reductions of specific symptomatology between groups using ANOVA analysis. Results revealed no significant differences in the reduction of reexperiencing or increased arousal symptoms from baseline to one month between the randomized groups. The art therapy group demonstrated a significant reduction in avoidance/numbing symptoms from baseline to one month (p = .01) when compared to the standard services and no PTSD groups. However, this change was not maintained over time. At six months, the standard treatment group showed a decrease in overall symptom severity of 7.31 from one month, while the art therapy group demonstrated no improvement from one month. In fact, the art therapy group showed a slight, although nonsignificant increase in overall symptom severity. Analysis of specific symptom clusters at six months revealed no significant differences between art therapy and standard services group from baseline to six months. Analysis of changes in severity scores between groups at 1.5 years also revealed no significant differences. While the standard services group demonstrated slightly higher decreases in all symptom clusters at six months and 1.5 years, these changes were not statistically significant.

V. Correlational Data

1. *Anxiety* was observed in 94 percent of subjects: 83 percent exhibited decrease postintervention, correlated with *Expression of Affect* (p Value = .002) and *Creation of Coherent Narrative* (p Value = .002).
2. *Expression of Affect* was observed in 89 percent of subjects and correlated with *Avoidance and Numbing* cluster symptoms (p Value = .044) and *Anxiety* (p Value = .002).
3. *Re-experiencing* cluster symptoms were observed in 17 percent of subjects, correlated with *Increased Arousal* (p Value = .000).
4. *Increased Arousal* cluster symptoms were observed in 22 percent of subjects, correlated with Re-experiencing symptoms.
5. *Avoidance and Numbing* cluster symptoms were observed in 33 percent of subjects, correlated negatively with the *Creation of a Narrative* (p Value = .044) and Ability to Draw Event (p Value .044).
6. *Creation of Coherent Narrative* was completed by 89 percent of subjects, correlated negatively with *Avoidance* (p Value = .044) and with *Anxiety* (p Value = .002).
7. *Misperception Corrected* was observed in 67 percent of subjects, correlated with *Autonomic Nervous Response* (p Value = .005) and *Grief Reaction* (p Value = .015).

Another fascinating finding pertains to the selection of media by acutely injured children. The following three charts illustrate the choice of media during the creation of a coherent narrative of an acute traumatic injury.

VI. Discussion

There are few studies of any treatment designed to address PTSD symptoms in children. Considering the emerging data on the prevalence of PTSD and the effects on behavior and development caused by childhood trauma, the lack of research is concerning. This study is an attempt to assess the level of PTSD in a population of hospitalized trauma patients, and to assess the effectiveness of one brief intervention using an art therapy drawing intervention for children experiencing the effects of trauma.

The results of the study suggest that PTSD symptoms are common in children who have experienced traumatic injuries. The incidence of children meeting all symptom criteria for PTSD was higher than other studies of trauma in this age group.

A single session art therapy treatment intervention helped reduce the overall severity of avoidance/numbing symptoms from baseline to one month, but did not affect overall symptom reduction. The findings should be taken as a starting point for future research with this population.

Many children who are hospitalized do not receive inpatient psychiatric services. In this study, only five patients in the randomized group and one in the "no PTSD" group were referred for evaluation to the hospital's psychiatric consultation services.

Limitations of the study warrant attention. In addition to the small sample size, no assessment was available for acute stress disorder, and the assessment tools are limited for childhood PTSD for this population. The self-selecting nature of the sample may also be problematic, as perhaps the most traumatized children refused participation in the study due to avoidance, suggesting a possible incidence of PTSD that may be higher in the population than the results currently demonstrate. Importantly, there were errors in the randomization as children who had lost a family member were initially erroneously included. Also, no effect size was determined.

The intervention was originally designed to be part of an inpatient pediatric art and play therapy program where rapport was established before the intervention was utilized. In this study, children were seen for the intervention with no prior interaction with the therapists.

This project has and continues to contribute to the field of art therapy. In the specialization of PTSD, the CATTI is utilized by numerous trained clinicians in the U.S. and Europe, and has helped thousands of children in the resolution of PTSD symptoms and disorder. The study and the CATTI have been presented at numerous professional symposia, including the American Academy of Child & Adolescent Psychiatry Annual Meeting, The EMDR International Association Annual Conference, and the Annual Conference of the American Art Therapy Association.

One conclusion that can be drawn from this project is that empirical art therapy research can be done. It is concerning that the art therapy profession is lacking in evidence-based treatment interventions. Many art therapists erroneously assume one has to demonstrate *how* or *why* art therapy works, or the subjective interpretation of the images. Clinical outcome research must demonstrate measurable outcomes, such as the reduction of symptoms, or changes in behavior.

From the correlational data, it is apparent that children willingly draw their stories of acute trauma. From the specific data, the following conclusions can be surmised:

1. A large majority of acutely injured children exhibit anxiety that can be alleviated by a specific, brief drawing intervention for acutely injured children. The ability to express affect and create a visual and verbal narrative of an experience facilitates the abatement of anxiety.
2. A large majority of acutely injured children express affect during the drawing intervention, reducing the tendency to avoid feelings reduces anxiety.
3. Reexperiencing phenomena is not common in acutely injured children, and if so, is consistent with increased arousal cluster symptoms.
4. Increased Arousal symptoms are also fairly uncommon in acutely injured children, and may be associated with re-experiencing cluster symptoms. One may wonder whether this group of children may have more complex trauma histories, as both of these clusters of symptoms are more commonly associated with chronic traumatic experiences.
5. Avoidance symptoms were the most prevalent of the three DSM PTSD symptom clusters. The negative correlation associated with the Creation of a Narrative and Ability to Draw the Event makes sense since the child is asked to do so.
6. This data suggests children want and need to tell their stories. Again, it makes sense to have a negative correlation with Avoidance symptoms since it is unlikely children would exhibit those symptoms when asked to complete a narrative of their experience. Similarly, the negative correlation with anxiety demonstrates a reduction upon completion of a coherent narrative.

The data pertaining to media is also fascinating, as the children do select the most structured media for most of the intervention. The predominant use of blue may be associated with the fact that blue is typically one of two favorite colors of children (Shoots, 1996). Or, perhaps blue represents the need for control or avoidance of threat or stress (Buck, 1966). Or, perhaps it indicates depression (Malchiodi, 1998). The fact that a pencil has an eraser may dictate choice, or perhaps the directive is reminiscent of a school task, requiring a pencil.

Whatever the interpretation, from this data, it is important to consider bringing a pencil to any drawing task for trauma or disaster relief (Hontz, 2006).

There is value in this work for the art therapy profession. The drawings executed in the interventions, along with the videotape of each session, offer a new perspective of how children experience, perceive, remember, and express traumatic experiences and traumatic imagery.

The data is of value to the art therapist who seeks to understand the symbolic and metaphorical content inherent in the drawings of acutely traumatically injured children.

Another conclusion from the study is the fact that traumatically injured hospitalized children do have PTSD symptoms, and that parents and nurses cannot be relied on to accurately assess a child's level of stress. Therefore, it demonstrates the need for trained individuals to offer treatment interventions to provide the psychological component of care for this population in order to offer comprehensive pediatric trauma care.

VII. References

Buck, J. (1966). The house, tree, person clinical assessment technique. Revised Manual. Los Angeles, CA: Western Psychological Services.

Chapman, L., Morabito, D., Ladakakos, C., Schreier, H., & Knudson, M. (2001). The effectiveness of art therapy interventions in reducing post-traumatic stress disorder (PTSD) symptoms in pediatric trauma patients. *Art Therapy: Journal of the American Art Therapy Association,*19(2), 100–104.

Foa, E. (1995). *Post Traumatic Stress Diagnostic Scale Manual.* Minneapolis, MN: National Computer Systems, Inc.

Frederick, C., Pynoos, R., & Nader, K. (1992). *Child Post-Traumatic Stress Reaction Index.* Unpublished instrument.

Hontz, J. (2006, March 20). The healing canvas. *Los Angeles Times,* pp. F1, F11.

Malchiodi, C. (1998). *Understanding children's drawings.* New York, NY: Guilford Press.

Moos, R., & Moos, B. (1994). *Family environmental scale manual.* Mountainview, CA: Consulting Psychologist Press.

Shoots, E. (1996). The effects of stereotypes and situational factors on children's favorite and preferred colors. Retrieved at www.missouriwestern.edu/psychology/research/psy302/fall96/erin_shoots.html

The figures below display the results of this study.

COLOR USED TO DRAW SCRIBBLE

N=26

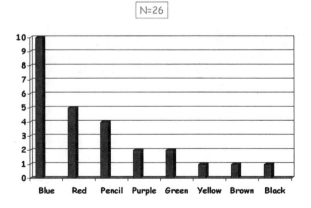

COLOR USED TO DRAW EVENT

N=26

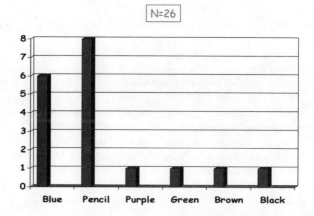

COLOR USED FOR LAST DRAWING

N=28

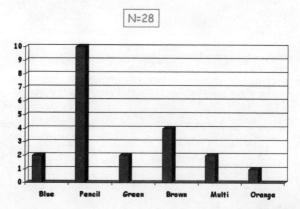

References

Aach-Feldman, S., & Kunkle-Miller, C. (1987). A developmental approach to art therapy. In J. Rubin (Ed.), *Approaches to art therapy* (pp. 251–274). New York, NY: Brunner/ Mazel.

Achenbach, T. M., & Rescorla, L. A. (2000). *ASEBA preschool forms & profiles: An integrated system of multi-informant assessment.* Burlington, VT: Achenbach System of Empirically Based Assessment.

Achtenberg, J., & Lawlis, F. (1980). *Bridges of the bodymind.* Champlain, IL: Institute for Personality and Ability Testing.

Adam, K. S., Sheldon-Keller, A. E., & West, M. (1996). Attachment organization and history of suicidal behavior in clinical adolescents. *Journal of Consulting and Clinical Psychology, 64*(2), 264.

Allen, J., Console, D., & Lewis, L. (1999). Dissociative detachment and memory impairment. Reversible amnesia or encoding failure? *Comprehensive Psychiatry, 40,* 160–171.

Allen, J. P., Hauser, S. T., & Borman-Spurrell, E. (1996). Attachment theory as a framework for understanding sequelae of severe adolescent psychopathology: An 11-year follow-up study. *Journal of Consulting and Clinical Psychology, 64*(2), 254.

American Psychiatric Association. (1994). *Diagnostic and statistical manual of mental disorders* (4th ed.). Washington, DC: American Psychiatric Association.

American Psychiatric Association. (2000). *Diagnostic and statistical manual of mental disorders* (4th ed. text revision). Washington, DC: American Psychiatric Association.

American Psychiatric Association. (2013). *Diagnostic and statistical manual of mental disorders* (5th ed.). Washington, DC: American Psychiatric Association.

Appleton, V. (2001). Avenues of hope: Art therapy and the resolution of trauma. *Art Therapy: Journal of the American Art Therapy Association, 18*(1), 6–13.

Arizmendi, T. (2008). Nonverbal communication in the context of dissociative process. *Psychoanalytic Psychology, 25*(3), 443–457.

Balaban, V. (2006). Psychological assessment of children in disasters and emergencies. *Disasters, 30*(2), 178–198.

Bell, C. (1992). Advocacy, research and service to prevent violence and treat victims. *Hospital and Community Psychiatry, 43*(11), 1134–1136.

Bell, C., & Jenkins, E. (1993). Community violence and children on Chicago's Southside. *Psychiatry, 56,* 46–53.

Berger, R., Pat-Horenczyk, R., & Gelkopf, M. (2007). School-based intervention for prevention and treatment of elementary students' terror-related distress in Israel: A quasi-randomized controlled trial. *Journal of Traumatic Stress, 20*(4), 541–551.

Blos, P. (1962). *On adolescence.* New York, NY: The Free Press.

Bokhorst, C. L., Bakermans-Kranenburg, M. J., Fonagy, P., & Schuengel, C. (2003). The importance of shared environment in mother-infant attachment security: A behavioral genetic study. *Child Development, 74*(6), 1769–1782.

Bokszczanin, A. (2007). PTSD symptoms in children and adolescents 28 months after a flood: Age and gender differences. *Journal of Traumatic Stress, 20*(3), 347–351.

Bowlby, J. (1969). *Attachment and loss, Vol. 1: Attachment.* New York, NY: Basic Books.

Bowlby, J. (1982). Attachment and loss: Retrospect and prospect. *American Journal of Orthopsychiatry, 52*(4), 664–678.

Bradley, R., Jenei, J., & Westen, D. (2005). Etiology of borderline personality disorder: Disentangling the contributions of intercorrelated antecedents. *The Journal of Nervous and Mental Disease, 193*(1), 24–31.

Bremner, J., Randall, P., Vermetten, E., Staib, L., Bronen, R., Mazure, C., & Charney, D. (1997). Magnetic resonance imaging-based measurement of hippocampal volume in posttraumatic stress disorder related to childhood physical and sexual abuse—a pre-liminary report. *Biological Psychiatry, 41*(1), 23–32.

Breslau, N., Kessler, R. C., Chilcoat, H. D., Schultz, L. R., Davis, G. C., & Andreski, P. (1998). Trauma and posttraumatic stress disorder in the community: The 1996 Detroit Area Survey of Trauma. *Archives of General Psychiatry, 55*(7), 626.

Bretherton, I., Ridgeway, D., & Cassidy, J. (1990). Story completion task to assess young children's internal working models of child and parents in the attachment rela-tionship. *Attachment in the preschool years: Theory, research, and intervention,* 300–308.

Briere, J., Johnson, K., Bissada, A., Damon, L., Crouch, J., Gil, E., & Ernst, V. (2001). The Trauma Symptom Checklist for Young Children (TSCYC): Reliability and asso-ciation with abuse exposure in a multi-site study. *Child Abuse & Neglect, 25*(8), 1001–1014.

Bromberg, P. (2006). *Awakening the dreamer: Clinical journeys.* Mahwah, NJ: The Ana-lytic Press.

Bromberg, P. (2011). *The shadow of the tsunami: And the growth of the relational mind.* New York, NY: Routledge.

Bruner, J. S. (1964). The course of cognitive growth. *American Psychologist, 19,* 1–15.

Bruner, J. S. (1973). Organization of early skilled action. *Child Development, 44,* 1–11.

Bucci, W. (2003). Varieties of dissociative experiences: A multiple code account and a discussion of Bromberg's case, "William." *Psychoanalytic Psychology, 20,* 542–557.

Bucci, W. (2007). Dissociation from the perspective of multiple code theory. *Contempo-rary Psychoanalysis, 43*(2), 165–184.

Burns, B. J., Costello, E. J., Angold, A., Tweed, D., Stangl, D., Farmer, E. M., & Erkanli, A. (1995). Children's mental health service use across service sectors. *Health Affairs, 14*(3), 147–159.

Burton, D., Foy, D., Bwanausi, C., Johnson, J., & Moore, L. (1994). The relationship between traumatic exposure, family dysfunction, and post-traumatic stress symptoms in male juvenile offenders. *Journal of Traumatic Stress, 7*(1), 83–93.

Carlson, V., Cicchetti, D., Barnett, D., & Braunwald, K. (1989). Disorganized/disori-ented attachment relationships in maltreated infants. *Developmental Psychology, 25*(4), 525.

Caron, C., & Rutter, M. (2006). Comorbidity in child psychopathology: Concepts, issues and research strategies. *Journal of Child Psychology and Psychiatry, 32*(7), 1063–1080.

Carrion, V. G., Weems, C. F., Eliez, S., Patwardhan, A., Brown, W., Ray, R. D., & Reiss, A. L. (2001). Attenuation of frontal asymmetry in pediatric posttraumatic stress disorder. *Biological Psychiatry, 50*(12), 943–951.

Carrion, V. G., Weems, C. F., Ray, R. D., Glaser, B., Hessl, D., & Reiss, A. L. (2002). Diurnal salivary cortisol in pediatric posttraumatic stress disorder. *Biological Psychiatry, 51*(7), 575–582.

Carrion, V. G., Weems, C. F., & Reiss, A. L. (2007). Stress predicts brain changes in children: A pilot longitudinal study on youth stress, posttraumatic stress disorder, and the hippocampus. *Pediatrics, 119*(3), 509–516.

Casler, L. (1965). The effects of extra tactile stimulation on a group of institutionalized infants. *Genetic Psychology Monographs, 71*(1), 137–175.

Cauffman, E., Feldman, S., Watherman, J., & Steiner, H. (1998). Posttraumatic stress disorder among female juvenile offenders. *Journal of the American Academy of Child & Adolescent Psychiatry, 37*(11), 1209–1216.

Caulfield, R. (2000). Beneficial effects of tactile stimulation on early development. *Early Childhood Education Journal, 27*(4), 255–257.

Centers for Disease Control and Prevention. (2006). Mental health surveillance among children—United States. Retrieved from www.cdc.gov/mmwr/preview/mmwrhtml/su6202a1.htm?s_cid=su6202a1_w

Centers for Disease Control and Prevention. (2011). National and state statistics at a glance: Youth violence. Retrieved from www.cdc.gov/violenceprevention/youthvio lence/stats./index/html

Chapman, L. (2001, April). How do you start your first play therapy session? *California Association for Play Therapy Newsletter, 1*(2), 10–11.

Chapman, L. (2002). A neuro-developmental approach to treating post-traumatic stress disorder and symptoms. *Proceedings of the 33rd Annual Conference of the American Art Therapy Association* (p. 106). Mundelein, IL: American Art Therapy Association.

Chapman, L. (2003). Neuro-developmental art therapy: Treating acute and chronic post-traumatic stress disorder and symptoms. *Proceedings of the 34th Annual Conference of the American Art Therapy Association* (p. 101). Mundelein, IL: American Art Therapy Association.

Chapman, L., Morabito, D., Ladakakos, C., Schreier, H., & Knudson, M. (2001). The effectiveness of art therapy interventions in reducing post-traumatic stress disorder (PTSD) symptoms in pediatric trauma patients. *Art Therapy: Journal of the American Art Therapy Association, 18*(2),100–104.

Chemtob, C. M., Nakashima, J., & Carlson, J. G. (2002). Brief treatment for elementary school children with disaster-related posttraumatic stress disorder: A field study. *Journal of Clinical Psychology, 58*(1), 99–112.

Chiland, C., & Young, J. (Eds.). (1994). *Children and violence.* Northvale, NJ: Jason Aronson.

Children's Defense Fund. (2012). Each day in America: July 2011. www.childrensdefense .org/child-research-data-publications/each-day-in-america.html

Cicchetti, D., & Barnett, D. (1991). Attachment organization in maltreated preschoolers. *Development and Psychopathology, 3*(4), 397–411.

Cicchetti, D., & Rogosch, F. A. (2001). Diverse patterns of neuroendocrine activity in maltreated children. *Development and Psychopathology, 13*(03), 677–693.

Cicchetti, D., & Toth, S. (1998). The development of depression in children and adolescents. *American Psychologist*, 53(2), 221.

Cohen, J., Berliner, L. & Mannarino, A. (2000). Treating traumatized children: A research review and synthesis. *Trauma, Violence & Abuse*, 1(1), 29–46.

Cohn, L. (1993). Art psychotherapy and eye movement desensitization reprocessing (EMDR) technique: An integrated approach. In E. Virshup (Ed.), *California art therapy trends*. Chicago, IL: Magnolia Street Publishers.

Cooper, C., Eslinger, D., Nash, D., Al Zawahri, J., & Stolley, P. (2000). Repeat victims of violence: Report of a large concurrent case-control study. *Archives of Surgery*, 135(7), 837–843.

Cooper, J. C. (1978). *An illustrated encyclopaedia of traditional symbols* (Vol. 66). London, England: Thames and Hudson.

Cozolino, L. (2002). *The neuroscience of psychotherapy; Building and rebuilding the human brain*. New York, NY: Norton.

Damasio, A. R. (2002). How the brain creates the mind. *Scientific American—Special Edition*, 12(1), 4–17.

Daviss, W. B., Mooney, D., Racusin, R., Ford, J. D., Fleischer, A., & McHugo, G. J. (2000). Predicting posttraumatic stress after hospitalization for pediatric injury. *Journal of the American Academy of Child & Adolescent Psychiatry*, 39(5), 576–583.

Deblinger, E., Steer, R. A., & Lippmann, J. (1999). Two-year follow-up study of cognitive behavioral therapy for sexually abused children suffering post-traumatic stress symptoms. *Child Abuse & Neglect*, 23(12), 1371–1378.

De Bellis, M. D., Baum, A. S., Birmaher, B., Keshavan, M. S., Eccard, C. H., Boring, A. M., . . . Ryan, N. D. (1999). Developmental traumatology part I: Biological stress systems. *Biological Psychiatry*, 45(10), 1259–1270.

De Bellis, M. D., Casey, B. J., Dahl, R. E., Birmaher, B., Williamson, D. E., Thomas, K. M., & Ryan, N. D. (2000). A pilot study of amygdala volumes in pediatric generalized anxiety disorder. *Biological Psychiatry*, 48(1), 51–57.

De Bellis, M. D., Chrousos, G. P., Dorn, L. D., Burke, L., Helmers, K., Kling, M. A., & Putnam, F. W. (1994). Hypothalamic-pituitary-adrenal axis dysregulation in sexually abused girls. *Journal of Clinical Endocrinology & Metabolism*, 78(2), 249–255.

De Bellis, M. D., Keshavan, M. S., Clark, D. B., Casey, B. J., Giedd, J. N., Boring, A. M., . . . Ryan, N. D. (1999). Developmental traumatology part II: Brain development. *Biological Psychiatry*, 45(10), 1271–1284.

De Bellis, M. D., Lefter, L., Trickett, P. K., & Putnam, F. W. (1994). Urinary catecholamine excretion in sexually abused girls. *Journal of the American Academy of Child & Adolescent Psychiatry*, 33(3), 320–327.

DeKlyen, M., & Speltz, M. (2004). In J. Hill & B. Maughan (Eds.), *Conduct disorders in childhood and adolescence*. Cambridge, UK: Cambridge University Press.

deVries, A. P. J., Kassam-Adams, N., Cnann, A., Sherman-Slate, E., Gallagher, P., & Winston, F. (1999). Looking beyond the physical injury: Posttraumatic stress disorder in children and parents after a pediatric traffic injury. *Pediatrics Digest*, 104(6), 1293–1299.

Erickson, B., & Egeland, B. (2002). Child neglect. In J. Myers, J. Briere, C. Hendrix, L. Berliner, & T. Reid (Eds.), *The APSAC Handbook on Child Maltreatment* (pp. 4–20). Thousand Oaks, CA: Sage Publications.

Eth, S., & Pynoos, R. (1985). Developmental perspective on psychic trauma in childhood. In R. Figley (Ed.), *Trauma and its wake*. New York, NY: Brunner/Mazel.

Fantz, R. (1961). The origin of form perception. *Scientific American, 204*(5), 66–72.

Feiring, C., Taska, L., & Chen, K. (2002). Trying to understand why horrible things happen: Attribution, shame, and symptom development following sexual abuse. *Child Maltreatment, 7*(1), 25–39.

Felitti, V., & Anda, R. F. (2010). The relationship of adverse childhood experiences to adult medical disease, psychiatric disorders and sexual behavior: Implications for healthcare. In R. A. Lanius, E.Vermetten, & C. Pain (Eds.), *The impact of early life trauma on health and disease: The hidden epidemic* (pp. 77–87). Cambridge, UK: Cambridge University Press.

Figley, C. (1985). *Trauma and its wake* (Vol. 1). New York, NY: Routledge.

Fisher, A. G., & Murray, E. A. (1991). Introduction to sensory integration theory. *Sensory integration: Theory and practice* (pp. 3–26). Philadelphia, PA: FA Davis.

Fivush, R., & Hamond, N. R. (1990). Autobiographical memory across the preschool years: Toward reconceptualizing childhood amnesia. In R. Fivush & J. A. Hudson (Eds.), *Knowing and remembering in young children* (pp. 223–248). New York, NY: Cambridge University Press.

Fonagy, P., & Target, M. (1997). Attachment and reflexive function: Their role in self-organization. *Development and Psychopathology, 9*(04), 679–700.

Ford, J., & Kidd, P. (1998). Early childhood trauma and disorders of extreme stress as predictors of treatment outcomes with chronic post-traumatic stress disorder. *Journal of Traumatic Stress, 11*, 743–761.

Fosha, D. (2003). Dyadic regulation and experiential work with the motion and relatedness in trauma and disorganized attachment. In M. Solomon & D. J. Siegel (Eds.), *Healing trauma: Attachment, mind, body, and brain* (221–281). New York, NY: W. W. Norton.

Frederick, C. J. (1985). Selected foci in the spectrum of posttraumatic stress disorders. In J. Laube & S. Murphy (Eds.), *Perspectives on disaster recovery* (pp. 110–131). Norwalk, CT: Appleton-Century-Crofts.

Garbarino, J. (1993). Children's response to community violence: What do we know? *Infant Mental Health Journal, 14*, 103–115.

Garbarino, J., Dubrow, N., Kostelny, K., & Pardo, C. (1992). *Children in danger: Coping with the consequences of community violence.* San Francisco, CA: Jossey Bass.

Gazzaniga, M. (1998). *The mind's past.* Berkeley, CA: University of California Press.

Gil, E. (1991). *The healing power of play: Working with abused children.* New York, NY: Guilford Press.

Gillis, H. (1993). Individual and small-group psychotherapy for children involved in trauma and disaster. In C. Saylor (Ed.), *Children and disasters.* New York, NY: Plenum Press.

Goenjian, A., Karayan, I., Pynoos, R., Minassian, D., Najarian, L., Steinberg, A., & Fairbanks, L. (1997). Outcome of psychotherapy among early adolescents after trauma. *American Journal of Psychiatry, 154*, 536–542.

Goins, W., Thompson, J., & Simpins, C. (1992). Recurrent intentional injury. *Journal of the National Medical Association, 84*(5), 431–435.

Green, B. L., Korol, M., Grace, M. C., Vary, M. G., Leonard, A. C., Gleser, G. C., & Smitson-Cohen, S. (1991). Children and disaster: Age, gender, and parental effects on PTSD symptoms. *Journal of the American Academy of Child & Adolescent Psychiatry, 30*(6), 945–951.

Green, J., & Goldwyn, R. (2002). Annotation: Attachment disorganization and psychopathology: New findings in attachment research and their potential implications for developmental psychopathology in childhood. *Journal of Child Psychology and Psychiatry, 43*(7), 835–846.

Greenwald, R. (1999). *Eye movement desensitization and reprocessing (EMDR) in child and adolescent psychotherapy.* Northvale, NJ: Jason Aronson.

Grych, J. H., Fincham, F. D., Jouriles, E. N., & McDonald, R. (2000). Interparental conflict and child adjustment: Testing the mediational role of appraisals in the cognitive-contextual framework. *Child Development, 71*(6), 1648–1661.

Gur, R. C. (2002). Declaration of Ruben C. Gur, Ph.D., *Patterson v. Texas* 536 U.S. 984.

Haas-Cohen, N., & Carr, R. (Eds.). (2008). *Art therapy and clinical neuroscience.* Philadelphia, PA: Jessica Kingsley.

Hart, J., Gunnar, M., & Cicchetti, D. (1995). Salivary cortisol in maltreated children: Evidence of relations between neuroendocrine activity and social competence. *Development and Psychopathology, 7*, 11–26.

Hepper, P. G., & Shahidullah, S. (1994). The beginnings of mind—evidence from the behavior of the fetus. *Journal of Reproductive and Infant Psychology, 12*(3), 143–154.

Hewitt, S. (1999). *Assessing allegations of sexual abuse with preschool children: Understanding small voices.* Thousand Oaks, CA: Sage Publications.

Hildyard, K., & Wolfe, D. (2002). Child neglect: Developmental issues and outcomes. *Child Abuse and Neglect, 25*(6–7), 679–695.

Hinz, L. (2009). *Expressive therapies continuum: A framework for using art in therapy.* New York, NY: Routledge.

Horowitz, M. J. (1970). *Image formation and cognition.* New York, NY: Appleton-Century-Crofts.

Howes, D., & Espinosa, M. (1985). The consequences of child abuse for the formation of relationships with peers. *Child Abuse & Neglect, 9*(3), 397–404.

Johanson, G., & Kurtz. R. (1991). *Grace unfolding: Psychotherapy in the spirit of the Tao-te ching.* New York, NY: Crown Publishers.

Jones, J. (1994). The neuropsychology of creative arts therapy. Presentation at 25th Annual Conference of the American Art Therapy Association, San Francisco, CA.

Jung, C. (1916/1958). The structure and dynamics of the psyche. In J. Chodorow (Ed.), *Encountering Jung on active imagination.* Princeton, NJ: Princeton University Press.

Kaplan, F. (2000). *Art, science and art therapy: Repainting the picture.* London, England: Jessica Kingsley.

Kataoka, S. H., Stein, B. D., Jaycox, L. H., Wong, M., Escudero, P., Tu, W., & Fink, A. (2003). A school-based mental health program for traumatized Latino immigrant children. *Journal of the American Academy of Child & Adolescent Psychiatry, 42*(3), 311–318.

Kellogg, R. (1969). *Analyzing children's art.* Palo Alto, CA: National Press Books.

Kennell, J. H., & Klaus, M. H. (1979). Early mother-infant contact: Effects on the mother and the infant. *Bulletin of the Menninger Clinic, 43*(1), 69.

Klaus, M. H., Jerauld, R., Kreger, N. C., McAlpine, W., Steffa, M., & Kennell, J. H. (1972). Maternal attachment. *New England Journal of Medicine, 286*(9), 460–463.

Klaus, M. H., Kennell, J. H., Plumb, N., & Zuehlke, S. (1970). Human maternal behavior at the first contact with her young. *Pediatrics, 46*(2), 187–192.

Klingman, A. (1987). A school-based emergency crisis intervention in a mass school disaster. *Professional Psychology: Research and Practice, 18*(6), 604.

Klorer, P. (2000). *Expressive therapy with troubled children*. Northvale, NJ: Aronson.

Koop, C., & Lundberg, G. (1992). Violence in America: A public health emergency. *Journal of the American Medical Association, 267*(22), 3075–3076.

Kramer, E. (1979). *Childhood and art therapy*. New York, NY: Schocken Books.

Kranowicz, C. (2003). *The out-of-sync child has fun: Activities for kids with sensory integration dysfunction*. New York, NY: Penguin Putnam.

Landreth, G. (1991). *Play therapy: The art of the relationship*. Muncie, IN: Accelerated Development Press.

Lanius, R. A., Williamson, P. C., Densmore, M., Boksman, K., Neufeld, R. W., Gati, J. S., & Menon, R. S. (2004). The nature of traumatic memories: A 4-T fMRI functional connectivity analysis. *American Journal of Psychiatry, 161*(1), 36–44.

Lanius, R. A., Williamson, P. C., Bluhm, R. L., Densmore, M., Boksman, K., Neufeld, R. W., & Menon, R. S. (2005). Functional connectivity of dissociative responses in posttraumatic stress disorder: A functional magnetic resonance imaging investigation. *Biological Psychiatry, 57*(8), 873–884.

Lansky, M. (1991). The transformation of affect in posttraumatic nightmares. *Bulletin of the Menninger Clinic, 55*(4), 470–490.

Lee, J. M. (1970). Emotional reactions to trauma. *Nursing Clinics of North America, 5*(4), 577–587.

Levendosky, A. A., Huth-Bocks, A. C., Semel, M. A., & Shapiro, D. L. (2002). Trauma symptoms in preschool-age children exposed to domestic violence. *Journal of Interpersonal Violence, 17*(2), 150–164.

Levine, P., & Kline, M. (2007). *Trauma through a child's eyes*. Berkeley, CA: North Atlantic Books.

Levy, H. B., Markovic, J., Chaudhry, U., Ahart, S., & Torres, H. (1995). Re-abuse rates in a sample of children followed for 5 years after discharge from a child abuse inpatient assessment program. *Child Abuse & Neglect, 19*(11), 1363–1377.

Lewis, D. (1998). *Guilt by reason of insanity*. New York, NY: Ivy Books.

Lieberman, A. F., Van Horn, P., & Ippen, C. G. (2005). Toward evidence-based treatment: Child-parent psychotherapy with preschoolers exposed to marital violence. *Journal of the American Academy of Child & Adolescent Psychiatry, 44*(12), 1241–1248.

Lindstrom, M. (1964). *Children's art: A study of normal development in children's models of visualization*. Berkeley, CA: University of California Press.

Lowenfeld, V. (1957). *Creative and mental growth* (3rd ed.). New York, NY: Macmillan.

Lusebrink, V. (1990). *Imagery and visual expression in therapy*. New York, NY: Plenum Press.

Lusebrink, V. (2004) Art therapy and the brain: An attempt to understand the underlying processes of art expression in therapy. *Art Therapy: Journal of the American Art Therapy Association, 21*(3), 125–135.

Lyons-Ruth, K. (1996). Attachment relationships among children with aggressive behavior problems: The role of disorganized early attachment patterns. *Journal of Consulting and Clinical Psychology, 64*(1), 64.

Lyons-Ruth, K. (2013). The two person unconscious: Intersubjective dialogue, enactive relational representation, and the emergence of new forms of relational organization. Elaboration of Working paper 3 of the Change Process Study Group of Boston.

Lyons-Ruth, K., & Jacobvitz, D. (1999). *Attachment disorganization: Unresolved loss, relational violence, and lapses in behavioral and attentional strategies*. New York, NY: Guilford.

Lyshak-Stelzer, F., Singer, P., St. John, P., & Chemtob, C. M. (2007). Art therapy for adolescents with posttraumatic stress disorder symptoms: A pilot study. *Art Therapy, 24*(4), 163–169.

Mahler, M. S., Pine, F., & Bergman, A. (1975). *The psychological birth of the infant.* New York, NY: Basic.

Main, M. (1983). Exploration, play, and cognitive functioning related to infant-mother attachment. *Infant Behavior and Development, 6*(2), 167–174.

Main, M., Kaplan, N., & Cassidy, J. (1985). Security in infancy, childhood, and adulthood: A move to the level of representation. *Monographs of the Society for Research in Child Development, 50*(1/2), 66–104.

Malchiodi, C., Kim, D., & Choi, W. (2003). Developmental art therapy. In C. Malchiodi (Ed.), *Handbook of art therapy* (pp. 93–105). New York, NY: Guilford.

Mallett, C. (2003). Socio-historical analysis of juvenile offenders on death row. *Criminal Law Bulletin—Boston, 39*(4), 445–468.

Mancia, M. (2006). Implicit memory and early unrepressed unconscious: Their role in the therapeutic process (how the neurosciences can contribute to psychoanalysis). *The International Journal of Psychoanalysis, 87*(1), 83–103.

Mangeot, S. D., Miller, L. J., McIntosh, D. N., McGrath-Clarke, J., Simon, J., Hagerman, R. J., & Goldson, E. (2007). Sensory modulation dysfunction in children with attention deficit hyperactivity disorder. *Developmental Medicine & Child Neurology, 43*(6), 399–406.

Manning, J. T., Trivers, R. L., Thorhill, R., Singh, D., Denman, J., Eklo, M. H., & Anderton, R. H. (1997). Ear asymmetry and left-side cradling. *Evolution and Human Behavior, 18*(5), 327–340.

McGilchrist, I. (2009). *The master and his emissary: The divided brain and the making of the Western world.* New Haven, CT: Yale University Press.

McLeer, S. V., Deblinger, E., Henry, D., & Orvaschel, H. (1992). Sexually abused children at high risk for post-traumatic stress disorder. *Journal of the American Academy of Child & Adolescent Psychiatry, 31*(5), 875–879.

McNamee, C. M. (2003). Bilateral art: Facilitating systemic integration and balance. *The Arts in Psychotherapy, 30*(5), 283–292.

McNamee, C. M. (2004). Using both sides of the brain: Experiences that integrate art and talk therapy through scribble drawings. *Art Therapy: Journal of the American Art Therapy Association, 21*(3), 136–142.

McNamee, C. M. (2006). Experiences with bilateral art: A retrospective study. *Art Therapy, 23*(1), 7–13.

McNiff, S. (1992). *Art as medicine.* Boston, MA: Shambala Press.

Melillo, R. (2009). *Disconnected kids: The groundbreaking brain balance program for children with autism, ADHD, dyslexia, and other neurological disorders.* New York, NY: Penguin.

Morrison, D. (1985). *Neurobehavioral and perceptual dysfunction in learning disabled children.* Lewiston, NY: Hogrefe.

Mueller, E., & Silverman, N. (1989). Peer relations in maltreated children. In D. Cicchetti & V. Carlson (Eds.), *Child maltreatment: Theory and research on the causes and consequences of child abuse and neglect* (pp. 529–578). Cambridge, UK: Cambridge University Press.

Nader, K., Pynoos, R., Fairbanks, L., Al-Ajeel, M., & Al-Asfour, A. (1993). A preliminary study of PTSD and grief among the children of Kuwait following the Gulf crisis. *British Journal of Clinical Psychology, 32,* 407–416.

Nader, K., Pynoos, R., Fairbanks, L., & Frederick, C. (1990). Children's PTSD reactions one year after a sniper attack at their school. *American Journal of Psychiatry, 147*(11), 1526–1530.

Nelson, K., & Ross, G. (1980). The generalities and specifics of long-term memory in infants and young children. *New Directions for Child and Adolescent Development, 1980*(10), 87–101.

Office of Juvenile Justice and Delinquency Prevention. (2013). *Statistical briefing book.* Retrieved from www.ojjdp.gov/ojstatbb/court/qa06201.asp?qaDate=2010

Ogden, P., & Minton, K. (2000). Sensorimotor psychotherapy: One method for processing traumatic memory. *Traumatology, 6*(3), 149–173.

Ogden, P., Minton, K., & Pain, C. (2006). *Trauma and the body: A sensorimotor approach to psychotherapy.* New York, NY: Norton.

Osofsky, J. D. (Winter, 1999). The impact of violence on children. *Domestic Violence and Children, 9*(3), 33–49.

Pearce, J. C. (1992). *Evolutions end: Claiming the potential of our intelligence.* San Francisco, CA: Harper.

Pearce, J. C. (2002). *The biology of transcendence: A blueprint of the human spirit.* Rochester, VT: Park Street Press.

Perry, B. (1994). Neurobiological sequelae of childhood trauma: PTSD in children. In M. Murburg (Ed.), *Catecholamine function in post-traumatic stress disorder: Emerging concepts* (pp. 233–255). Washington, DC: American Psychiatric Press.

Perry, B. (1997). Incubated in terror: Neurodevelopmental factors in the "cycle of violence." In J. Osofsky (Ed.), *Children in a violent society* (pp. 124–128). New York, NY: Guilford Press.

Perry, B. (2009). Examining child maltreatment through a neurodevelopmental lens: Clinical applications of the neurosequential model of therapeutics. *Journal of Loss and Trauma: International Prospectives on Stress and Coping, 14*(4), 240–255.

Perry, B., & Hambrick, E. (2008). The neurosequential model of therapeutics. *Reclaiming Children and Youth, 17*(3), 38–43.

Perry, B., Pollard, R., Blakely, T., Baker, W., & Vigilante, D. (1995). Childhood trauma, the neurobiology of adaptation, and "use-dependent" development of the brain: How "states" become "traits." *Infant Mental Health Journal, 16,* 271–291.

Perry, B., & Szalavitz, M. (2007). *The boy who was raised as a dog and other stories from a child psychiatrist's notebook: What traumatized children can teach us about loss, love, and healing.* New York, NY: Basic.

Piaget, J. (1964). Development and learning. In R. E. Ripple & V. N. Rockcastle (Eds.), *Piaget rediscovered* (pp. 7–20). New York, NY: W. H. Freeman & Co.

Pine, F. (1985). *Developmental theory and clinical process.* New Haven, CT: Yale University Press.

Proulx, L. (2002). *Strengthening ties: Parent/child dyad art therapy.* London: Kingsley.

Putnam, F. W. (2003). Ten-year research update review: Child sexual abuse. *Journal of the American Academy of Child & Adolescent Psychiatry, 42*(3), 269–278.

Pynoos, R. S. (1996). Exposure to catastrophic violence and disaster in childhood. *Severe stress and mental disturbance in children,* pp. 181–208. Washington, D.C.: American Psychiatric Press, Inc.

Pynoos, R., & Eth, S. (1984). The child as witness to homicide. *Journal of Social Issues, 40*(2), 87–108.

Pynoos, R., & Eth, S. (1986). Witness to violence: The child interview. *Journal of the American Academy of Child Psychiatry, 25*(3), 306–319.

Pynoos, R., Frederick, C., Nader, K., Arroyo, W., Steinberg, A., Eth, S., Nunez, F., & Fairbanks, L. (1987). Life threat and post-traumatic stress in school-age children. *Archives of General Psychiatry, 44,* 1057–1063.

Pynoos, R., Goenjian, A., Tashjian, M., Karakashian, M., Manjikian, R., Manoukian, G., Steinberg, A., & Fairbanks, L. (1993). Post-traumatic stress reactions in children after the 1988 Armenian earthquake. *British Journal of Psychiatry, 163*(2), 239–247.

Pynoos, R., & Nader, K. (1988). Psychological first aid and treatment approach to children exposed to community violence: Research implications. *Journal of Traumatic Stress, 1*(4), 445–473.

Pynoos, R., & Nader, K. (1989). Children's memory and proximity to violence. *Journal of the American Academy of Child and Adolescent Psychiatry, 28*(2), 236–241.

Pynoos, R., & Nader, K. (1990). Children's exposure to violence and traumatic death. *Psychiatric Annals, 20*(6), 334–344.

Pynoos, R., Rodriguez, N., Steinberg, A., Stuber, M., & Frederick, C. (1998). *The UCLA PTSD Reaction Index for DSM-IV (Revision 1).* Los Angeles, CA: UCLA Trauma Psychiatry Program.

Pynoos, R., Steinberg, A., & Goenjian, A. (1996). Traumatic stress in childhood and adolescence: Recent developments and current controversies. In B. van der Kolk, A. McFarlane, & L. Weisaeth (Eds.), *Traumatic stress: The effects of overwhelming experience on mind, body and society* (pp. 303–327). New York, NY: Guilford Press.

Pynoos, R. S., Steinberg, A., & Piacentini, J. C. (1999). A developmental psychopathology model of childhood traumatic stress and intersection with anxiety disorders. *Biological Psychiatry, 46*(11), 1542–1554.

Rausch, S. L., van der Kolk, A. B., Fisler, R. E., Alpert, N. M., Orr, S. P., Savage, C. R., . . . Pitman, R. K. (1996). A symptom provocation study of posttraumatic stress disorder using positron emission tomography and script-driven imagery. *Archives of General Psychiatry, 53*(5), 380–387.

Reich, W., & Welner, Z. (1988). *Revised version of the Diagnostic Interview for Children and Adolescents (DICA-R).* St. Louis, MO: Washington University School of Medicine, Department of Psychiatry.

Reynolds, S., & Lane, S. J. (2009). Sensory overresponsivity and anxiety in children with ADHD. *The American Journal of Occupational Therapy, 63*(4), 433–440.

Riley, S. (1999). *Contemporary art therapy with adolescents.* Philadelphia, PA: Kingsley.

Rogeness, G. A., Javors, M. A., & Pliszka, S. R. (1992). Neurochemistry and child and adolescent psychiatry. *Journal of the American Academy of Child & Adolescent Psychiatry, 31*(5), 765–781.

Rogosch, F., Cicchetti, D., & Aber, L. (1995). The role of child maltreatment in early deviations in cognitive and affective processing abilities and later peer relationship problems. *Development and Psychopathology, 7,* 591–609.

Rossman, M. (2000). *Guided imagery for self-healing.* Tiburon, CA: Kramer.

Runyon, M. K., Deblinger, E., Ryan, E. E., & Thakkar-Kolar, R. (2004). An overview of child physical abuse developing an integrated parent-child cognitive-behavioral treatment approach. *Trauma, Violence, & Abuse, 5*(1), 65–85.

Saigh, P. A., & Bremner, J. (1999). *Posttraumatic stress disorder: A comprehensive text.* Boston, MA: Allyn & Bacon.

Sandler, J., Kennedy, H., & Tyson, R. (1980). *The technique of child psychoanalysis: Discussions with Anna Freud.* Cambridge, MA: Harvard University Press.

Scheeringa, M., Zeanah, C., Drell, M., & Larrieu, J. (1995). Two approaches to the diagnosis of posttraumatic stress disorder in infancy and early childhood. *Journal of the American Academy of Child & Adolescent Psychiatry,* 34(2), 191–200.

Schiffer, F., Teicher, M. H., & Papanicolaou, A. C. (1995). Evoked potential evidence for right brain activity during the recall of traumatic memories. *The Journal of Neuropsychiatry and Clinical Neurosciences,* 7(2), 169–175.

Schore, A. N. (1994). *Affect regulation and the origin of the self: The neurobiology of emotional development.* Hillsdale, NJ: Erlbaum.

Schore, A. N. (1996). The experience-dependent maturation of a regulatory system in the orbital prefrontal cortex and the origin of developmental psychopathology. *Development and Psychopathology,* 8, 59–87.

Schore, A. N. (1999). Attachment, trauma, and the neurobiology of the developing mind. Presentation at the 46th Annual Meeting, American Academy of Child & Adolescent Psychiatry Conference, Chicago, IL.

Schore, A. N. (2000). Attachment and the regulation of the right brain. *Attachment & Human Development,* 2(1), 23–47.

Schore, A. N. (2001). Effects of a secure attachment relationship on right brain development, affect regulation, and infant mental health. *Infant Mental Health Journal,* 22(102), 7–66.

Schore, A. N. (2003a). *Affect regulation and the repair of the self.* New York, NY: Norton.

Schore, A. N. (2003b). *Affect dysregulation and disorders of the self.* New York, NY: Norton.

Schore, A. N. (2005). Back to basics: Attachment, affect regulation, and the developing right brain: Linking developmental neuroscience to pediatrics. *Pediatrics in Review,* 26(6), 204–217.

Schore, A. N. (2007, Summer). Psychoanalytic research progress and process: Developmental affective neuroscience and clinical practice. *Psychologist-Psychoanalyst,* 6–15.

Schore, A. N. (2009a). Relational trauma and the developing right brain: An interface of the psychoanalytic self psychology and neuroscience. *Annals of New York Academy of Science,* 1159, 189–203.

Schore, A. N. (2009b). Attachment trauma and the developing right brain: Origins of pathological dissociation. In P. Dell & J. O'Neil (Eds.), *Dissociation and the dissociative disorders: DSM-V and beyond* (pp. 107–141). New York, NY: Routledge.

Schore, A. N. (2012). *The science of the art of psychotherapy.* New York, NY: Norton.

Schore, J. R., & Schore, A. N. (2008). Modern attachment theory: The central role of affect regulation in development and treatment. *Clinical Social Work Journal,* 36(1), 9–20.

Schreier, H., Ladakakos, C., Morabito, D., Chapman, L., & Knudson, M. (2005). Posttraumatic stress symptoms in children after mild to moderate pediatric trauma: A longitudinal examination of symptom prevalence, correlates, and parent-child symptom reporting. *Journal of Trauma, Injury, Infection and Critical Care,* 58(2), 353–363.

Schutz, L. E. (2005). Broad-perspective perceptual disorder of the right hemisphere. *Neuropsychology Review,* 15(1), 11–27.

Shaw, J. A., Applegate, B., Tanner, S., Perez, D., Rothe, E., Campo-Bowen, A. E., & Lahey, B. L. (1995). Psychological effects of Hurricane Andrew on an elementary school population. *Journal of the American Academy of Child & Adolescent Psychiatry,* 34(9), 1185–1192.

Shelby, J., & Tredinnick, M. (1995). Crisis intervention with survivors of a natural disaster: Lessons from hurricane Andrew. *Journal of Counseling & Development*, 73, 491–497.

Shi, Z., Bureau, J., Easterbrooks, M. A., Zhao, X., & Lyons-Ruth, K. (2012). Childhood maltreatment and prospectively observed quality of early care as predictors of antisocial personality disorder features. *Infant Mental Health Journal*, 33(1), 55–69.

Siegel, D. (n.d.). The developing mind and resolution of trauma: Some ideas about information processing and an interpersonal neurobiology of psychotherapy. Unpublished paper.

Siegel, D. J. (1994). Memory, trauma and child development. Presentation at Child & Adolescent Psychiatry & Allied Professions Conference, San Francisco, CA.

Siegel, D. J. (1999). *The developing mind: Toward a neurobiology of interpersonal development*. New York, NY: Guilford Press.

Siegel, D. J. (2001). Memory: An overview, with emphasis on developmental, interpersonal, and neurobiological aspects. *Journal of the American Academy of Child & Adolescent Psychiatry*, 40(9), 997–1011.

Siegel, D. J. (2002). *The developing mind and the resolution of trauma: Some ideas about information processing and an interpersonal neurobiology of psychotherapy*. Washington, DC: American Psychological Association.

Siegel, D. (2012). *Pocket guide to interpersonal neurobiology: An integrative handbook of the mind*. New York, NY: Norton.

Sims, D. W., Bivins, B. A., Obeid, F. N., Horst, H. M., Sorensen, V. J., & Fath, J. J. (1989). Urban trauma: A chronic recurrent disease. *The Journal of Trauma*, 29(7), 940.

Solomon, J., George, C., & De Jong, A. (1995). Children classified as controlling at age six: Evidence of disorganized representational strategies and aggression at home and at school. *Development and Psychopathology*, 7, 447–463.

Sowell, E., Thompson, P., Holems, D., Jernigan, T., & Toga, A. (2001). Mapping continued brain growth and gray matter density reduction in dorsal frontal cortex: Inverse relationships during post-adolescent brain maturation. *The Journal of Neuroscience*, 21(22), 8819–8829.

Spangler, G., & Grossman, K. (1999). *Individual and physiological correlates of attachment disorganization in infancy*. New York, NY: Guilford.

Spear, L. P. (2003). Neurodevelopment during adolescence. In D. Cachetti and E. Walker (Eds.), *Neurodevelopmental mechanisms in psychopathology* (pp. 62–83). Cambridge, UK: Cambridge University Press.

Springer, C., & Padgett, D. K. (2000). Gender differences in young adolescents' exposure to violence and rates of PTSD symptomatology. *American Journal of Orthopsychiatry*, 70(3), 370–379.

Stein, B. D., Jaycox, L. H., Kataoka, S. H., Wong, M., Tu, W., Elliott, M. N., & Fink, A. (2003). A mental health intervention for schoolchildren exposed to violence. *JAMA: The Journal of the American Medical Association*, 290(5), 603–611.

Steinberg, A. M., Brymer, M. J., Decker, K. B., & Pynoos, R. S. (2004). The University of California at Los Angeles post-traumatic stress disorder reaction index. *Current Psychiatry Reports*, 6(2), 96–100.

Talwar, S. (2007). Accessing traumatic memory through art making: An art therapy trauma protocol (ATTP). *The Arts in Psychotherapy*, 34(1), 22–35.

Tellez, M., Mackersie, R., Marabito, D., Shagoury, D., & Heye, C. (1995). Risks, costs, and the expected complication of re-injury. *The American Journal of Surgery*, 170(6), 660–664.

Terr, L. (1979). Children of Chowchilla: A study of psychic trauma. *Psychoanalytic Study of the Child, 34*, 547–623.

Terr, L. (1981). Forbidden games: Post traumatic child's play. *Journal of the American Academy of Child Psychiatry, 20*, 740–759.

Terr, L. C. (1983). Chowchilla revisited: The effects of psychic trauma four years after a school-bus kidnapping. *American Journal of Psychiatry, 140*(12), 1543–1550.

Terr, L. (1988). What happens to the memories of early childhood trauma? *Journal of the Academy of Child and Adolescent Psychiatry, 27*, 96–104.

Terr, L. (1990). *Too scared to cry.* New York, NY: Harper & Row.

Terr, L. (1991a). Childhood traumas: An outline and overview. *American Journal of Psychiatry, 148*(1), 10–19.

Terr, L. (1991b). Psychiatric consequences of child abuse: Conceptual models. American Academy of Child and Adolescent Psychiatry 38th Annual Meeting, San Francisco, CA.

Terr, L. (1995). *Unchained memories: True stories of traumatic memories lost and found.* New York, NY: Basic Books.

Tomatis, A. (1991). Chant, the healing power of voice and ear. In D. Campbell (Ed.), *Music: Physician for times to come* (pp. 11–28). Wheaton IL: Quest.

Tower, R. (1983). Imagery: Its role in development. In A. A. Skeikh (Ed.), *Imagery: Current theory, research and application.* New York, NY: Wiley.

Tripp, T. (2007). A short-term therapy approach to processing trauma: Art therapy and bilateral stimulation. *Art Therapy, 24*(4), 176–183.

Trowell, J., Kolvin, I., Weeramanthri, T., Sadowski, H., Berelowitz, M., Glasser, D., & Leitch, I. (2002). Psychotherapy for sexually abused girls: Psychopathological outcome findings and patterns of change. *The British Journal of Psychiatry, 180*(3), 234–247.

Uddin, L. Q., Molnar-Szakacs, I., Zaidel, E., & Iacoboni, M. (2006). rTMS to the right inferior parietal lobule disrupts self–other discrimination. *Social Cognitive and Affective Neuroscience, 1*(1), 65–71.

Uhlin, F. (1972). *Art for exceptional children.* Dubuque, IA: Brown.

van der Kolk, B. (1987). *Psychological trauma.* Washington, DC: American Psychiatric Press.

van der Kolk, B. (1994). The body keeps the score: Memory and the evolving psychobiology of post-traumatic stress. *Harvard Review of Psychiatry, 1*(5), 253–265.

van der Kolk, B., Greenberg, M., Orr, S., & Pitman, R. (1989). Endogenous opioids, stress induced analgesia, and posttraumatic stress disorder. *Psychopharmacology Bulletin, 25*(3), 417.

van der Kolk, B., McFarlane, L., & Weisaeth, L. (Eds.). (1996). *Traumatic stress: The effects of overwhelming experience on mind, body and society.* New York, NY: Guilford.

van der Kolk, B., & Van der Hart, O. (1991). The intrusive past: The flexibility of memory and the engraving of trauma. *American Imago, 48*(4), 425–454.

Van IJzendoorn, M., Schuengel, C., & Bakermans-Kraneburg, M. (1999). Disorganized attachment in early childhood: Meta-analysis of precursors, concomitants and sequelae. *Development and Psychopathology, 11*, 225–249.

Veltman, M. W., & Browne, K. D. (2001). Three decades of child maltreatment research implications for the school years. *Trauma, Violence, & Abuse, 2*(3), 215–239.

Wadeson, H. (1980). *Art psychotherapy.* New York, NY: Wiley.

Waters, E., Wippman, J., & Sroufe, L. A. (1979). Attachment, positive affect, and competence in the peer group: Two studies in construct validation. *Child Development,* *50*(3), 821–829.

Weinfield, N. S., Whaley, G. J., & Egeland, B. (2004). Continuity, discontinuity, and coherence in attachment from infancy to late adolescence: Sequelae of organization and disorganization. *Attachment & Human Development, 6*(1), 73–97.

Widom, C. (1989). Does violence beget violence? A critical examination of the literature. *Psychological Bulletin, 106*, 3–28.

Williams, G., & Wood, M. (1977). *Developmental art therapy.* Baltimore, MD: University Park Press.

Wisenberg, M., Scharzwald, J., Waysman, M., Solomon, Z., & Klingman, A. (1993). Coping of school-age children in the sealed room during SCUD missile bombardment and postwar stress reactions. *Journal of Consulting and Clinical Psychology. 61*(3), 462–467.

Wolfe, D. A., Sas, L., & Wekerle, C. (1994). Factors associated with the development of posttraumatic stress disorder among child victims of sexual abuse. *Child Abuse & Neglect, 18*(1), 37–50.

Yule, W. (1993). Technology related disaster. In C. F. Saylor (Ed.), *Children and disasters* (pp. 105–121). New York, NY: Plenum Press.

Ziv, A., Kruglanaski, A. W., & Shulman, D. (1974). Children's psychological reactions to wartime stress. *Journal of Personality and Social Psychology, 30*(1), 24–30.

Index

drawings *(cont.)*
  problems with visual perceptual and motor development seen in, 88–89
  scribble, 25–26
  what happened next, 26–28
"Drop the Clothespins in the Jar" game, 157, 159, 160, 168
drug addiction, 17. *see also* substance abuse
DSM-IV. *see Diagnostic & Statistical Manual, fourth edition (DSM-IV)*
DSM-V, posttraumatic stress disorder in pre-school children included in, 9
dyadic relationships
  infant right-brain development within context of, 80, 81
  therapist-child, mutual co-regulation and, 108–10
dysregulated clients, unique way language used in therapy by, 123

eating disorders, 15
ego, maturation of, 176
EMDR treatment. *see* Eye-Movement Desensitization and Reprocessing (EMDR) treatment
emotional homeostasis, Problem Phase in NDAT model and, 61–62
emotional regulation
  infants and nonverbal right-hemisphere-to-right-hemisphere body-based experiences, 152
  repetitive sensory-motor experiences and, 6
emotional responses, CATTI and, 43–47
empathy, 128
  abused children and frequent lack of, 153
  emerging, in school-age child, 174, 175
  prefrontal cortex and, 177
enactments, defined, 168
encopresis, 132, 142, 147
ETC. *see* expressive therapies continuum (ETC)
event drawings, 26
  intervention with adolescent and, 36
  intervention with school-age child and, 33
exercise balls, 97
exploration of images, in NDAT model, 51–52
explosions, 5, 8
expressive media, Problem Phase in NDAT model and, 63
expressive therapies continuum (ETC), 22
eye-hand coordination, 173
  developing, activities for, 89–90
  developing, in infants and toddlers, 94
Eye-Movement Desensitization and Reprocessing (EMDR) treatment, xxv, 203

family members, metaphoric identification of, 66–68

fantasy, acute trauma in young children and, 11
fathers
  in jail, 124–25, 147
  missing, 153
fear
  in abused children and teens, 15
  acute traumatic episode and, 6
  creating symbol of, 111–12
  of dying, 43–44
  of losing body parts, 44
  painting picture of, 107
  retelling in CATTI and, 34, 35, 37
  trauma-specific, 39
feeling it may happen again, CATTI and suggested responses for, 45
feelings, exploring, Problem Phase in NDAT model and, 64–66
Felitti, V., 18
Ferriero, D., xxii
film violence, xxii
fine motor development
  in children and teens, techniques for, 94–95
  in infants and toddlers, techniques for, 94
  overview of, 94
fine motor functioning, in toddlers, assessing, 131, 135
finger and hand manipulation, developing, in infants and toddlers, 94
fingerpainting
  right-brain visual memories accessed through, 143–44
  Self Phase in NDAT model and, 59
  tactile development in children and teens and, 91
firearms-related deaths, xxi
Fivush, R., 142
flexibility, resistant clients and need for, 103–4
follow-up care plan, CATTI and, 48
foster mother, Self Phase in treatment of toddler and interactions with, 132–39, 140, 142, 147, 149, 150
Friedlander, L., 20
friendships, 164
frontal lobes of brain, 22
functional deficits, defects in dynamic structural systems and, 152

gang violence, xxii, 13–14, 181
gaze aversion, 15, 42
Gazzaniga, M., 106
gender differences, child and adolescent PTSD research on, 4
Gesell Developmental Schedule, 90
granular cells, 176
graphic ability in toddlers, assessing, 131
graphic developmental delays, drawings and evidence of, 155
grasping, 94

Also available from

THE NORTON SERIES ON INTERPERSONAL NEUROBIOLOGY

For complete book details, and to order online, please visit the Series webpage at
www.tiny.cc/1zrsfw